Handbook of
PRACTICAL PHARMACOLOGY

Handbook of
PRACTICAL
PHARMACOLOGY

SHEILA A. RYAN, R.N., M.S.N.

Formerly Dean, Associate Professor, College of Nursing,
Creighton University, Omaha, Nebraska; now Doctoral Student,
College of Nursing, University of Arizona, Tucson, Arizona

BRUCE D. CLAYTON, B.S., Pharm.D.

Associate Professor and Vice Chairman,
Department of Pharmacy Practice, College of Pharmacy,
University of Nebraska Medical Center,
Omaha, Nebraska

SECOND EDITION

The C. V. Mosby Company

ST. LOUIS · TORONTO · LONDON   1980

SECOND EDITION

Copyright ©1980 by The C. V. Mosby Company

All rights reserved. No part of this book may be reproduced in any manner without written permission of the publisher.

Previous edition copyrighted 1977

Printed in the United States of America

The C. V. Mosby Company
11830 Westline Industrial Drive, St. Louis, Missouri 63141

Library of Congress Cataloging in Publication Data

Ryan, Sheila A   1945-
   Handbook of practical pharmacology.

   Bibliography: p.
   Includes index.
   1. Pharmacology—Handbooks, manuals, etc.
2. Chemotherapy—Handbooks, manuals, etc.   I.   Clayton, Bruce D., 1947-   II.   Title.
RM300.R9 1980   615'.1   79-26035
ISBN 0-8016-4240-X

TS/VH/VH   9   8   7   6   5   4   3   2   03/A/367

To
Francine

for her unfailing Support
and Encouragement

BDC

In Memory of a little
sunshine soldier

Ryan Patrick

SAR

Preface to the second edition

The response to our first edition has been most gratifying. The support and suggestions offered by reviewers, colleagues, and students have indicated a need for a second edition of the *Handbook of Practical Pharmacology* with expanded content.

We have maintained the style of the first edition, but have added 90 new drugs, bringing the total number of drugs discussed to over 250. Many of these additions are incorporated into new chapters on thyroactive agents, agents used in the treatment of gout, biologic agents, oral contraceptives, local anesthetics, and skeletal muscle relaxants. Information pertinent to the monitoring and counseling of patients using these agents is presented. A major advancement has been made by adding neonatal and pediatric dosages to many of the monographs, thus making the book useful in the pediatric clinical environment.

We wish to extend a word of thanks to the many students and colleagues who have offered suggestions for improvement of this edition.

Special recognition must go to Francine E. Clayton for her patience, support, and excellent secretarial assistance in the preparation of the second edition. Special thanks is extended to the E. F. Ryan family, the John D. Clayton family, and the Francis H. Purdy family for their support and encouragement.

Sheila A. Ryan
Bruce D. Clayton

Preface to the first edition

No single aspect of patient care demands greater accuracy than drug therapy. The continuing exchange of updated knowledge concerning the more than 7000 principal drugs in today's medical arsenal increases the need for accurate, readily available information. This practical, convenient pocket reference, a thorough compilation of information about the most commonly used single-entity drugs currently on the market, emphasizes the need for knowledge and understanding of precautions and potential drug interactions during administration.

Drugs discussed in the book are categorized in chapters according to their primary pharmacologic activity. Most chapters provide an introduction that briefly discusses pathologic conditions for which the agents are used, how treatment should be approached, and what adjunctive measures should be employed to provide patient comfort and improve therapeutic effectiveness of the agent.

Monographs of drugs are arranged alphabetically by generic name within each chapter. More information about these monographs is contained in the Note to the reader. The individual monograph of each drug lists the generic name and a representative sample of trade names. Under each generic name is the American Hospital Formulary Service number that refers the reader to more detailed information about that drug. The category to which the drug belongs follows the AHFS number.

The first section of each monograph includes primary action and use. Knowledge of the mechanism of action is essential to ensure proper utilization of the drug. The actions discussed include the more important mechanisms sufficient for understanding uses and particular side effects, although the discussions in no way reflect the depth of a primary reference text. The most common and frequent usages for each drug have been included, but no attempt has been made to list historical or investigational uses.

The characteristics section represents a search of the literature for physiologic parameters of the drug. These parameters provide a more complete understanding and thus more effective monitoring of both therapeutic activity and adverse effects. Such characteristics include half-life; extent of protein binding; rates of absorption; onset, peak, and duration of action; sites of metabolism and excretion; and requirements of dosage supplementation in patients undergoing dialysis.

The section on dosage administration in each monograph is more complete than in many other references. It discusses dosage adjustments in relation to sites of administration and indications for use, while placing emphasis on techniques and rates of administration. Flow rate charts are provided for those drugs administered by continuous infusion to provide accuracy in calculations and to allow closer correlation with dosage and patient response.

One of the most valuable and important units of each monograph is that on special remarks and cautions. This section provides more clinically pertinent information about observation and interpretation of drug response. It does not belabor long lists of side effects that are experienced infrequently or that are based only on theoretical considerations. It includes reminders of information that the patient needs for improved understanding and compliance, warnings about interferences with laboratory tests, and use of the drug during pregnancy and lactation.

The concluding section of each monograph provides the health professional with information on significant interactions with other therapeutic agents. Drug interactions are a frequent cause of adverse effects, decreased compliance, and prolonged hospitalizations. Continual awareness of the possibility of interactions and observation for these complications are the responsibility of all health professionals.

No clinically oriented reference would be complete without charts that summarize frequently used data on administration, dosage adjustments, and monitoring. Hence, the appendixes include tables on mathematical conversions, correlation of body surface area with height and weight, pediatric dosage adjustment charts, and tables on excretion of drugs in breast milk and discoloration of excreta secondary to drug metabolism.

Safe monitoring of therapeutic agents carries enormous implications for every health professional. We believe that this book will serve as a review to help ensure the safe administration of medications. Students and practitioners in the health sciences will find this a useful and convenient source of accurate, readily applicable information.

Sheila A. Ryan
Bruce D. Clayton

Acknowledgments

Use of the *American Hospital Formulary Service*

Permission to use the pharmacologic-therapeutic classification system of the *American Hospital Formulary Service* has been granted by the American Society of Hospital Pharmacists. The Society is not responsible for the accuracy of transpositions, or additions, or excerpts from the original context. For complete information concerning all drugs, consult the two-volume *American Hospital Formulary Service*. Permission to use excerpts from the *American Hospital Formulary Service* has been granted by the American Society of Hospital Pharmacists. The Society is not responsible for the accuracy of transpositions or excerpts from the original context. This material is copyrighted by the American Society of Hospital Pharmacists, Inc. All rights reserved.

Use of therapeutic, toxic, and lethal blood level data in the section on characteristics in each monograph

Done, A. K.: The toxic emergency, Emergency Medicine **7:**193-201, May, 1975.

Use of dialysis information in the section on characteristics in each monograph

Bennett, W. M., and others: A guide to drug therapy in renal failure, J.A.M.A. **230:**1544, Dec. 16, 1974. Copyright 1974, American Medical Association.

Use of the illustration in Chapter 4

Adapted from Melmon, K. L., and Morrelli, H. F., editors: Clinical pharmacology: basic principles in therapeutics, New York, 1972, Macmillan Publishing Co., Inc.

We wish to extend a special note of recognition to Dr. Andrew L. Hahn for imparting to our students his thought-provoking judgment, care, and personal concern for patients.

Note to the reader

Trade name

    The trade names represent an arbitrary selection and imply no preference for any brand name or manufacturer.

AHFS

    This number directs the user to the *American Hospital Formulary Service,* a source of more complete information on the drug.

Action and use

    The mechanisms of action provide an overview and are not meant to include minor or proposed mechanisms. The uses are those generally accepted in medical practice today; however, the dosages and uses suggested do not necessarily have specific approval by the Food and Drug Administration. The manufacturer's product information should be consulted for approval.

Characteristics

    A wide degree of clinical variation may alter these parameters. Metabolic and excretory data are based on patients with normal renal and hepatic function. Therapeutic blood level data may vary between laboratories and the specificity of the assay methods used. Toxic and lethal blood level data are often based on a few cases, and toxic effects may be intensified by the ingestion of other drugs.

    The qualitative effect of dialysis on drug removal is indicated by a "No" or a "Yes." A "No" indicates that dosage adjustment is not indicated after either peritoneal dialysis (P) or hemodialysis (H). "Yes" indicates that enough drug is removed in the dialysate to require an extra maintenance dose to ensure adequate therapeutic blood levels. It must be emphasized that even though dosage adjustment may not be required, dialysis may still be beneficial in case of poisoning.

Administration and dosage

    Dosages given are for adults, children, and neonates. The severity of the disease as well as the age and state of health of the patient may alter the dosages. Administration charts are provided for those drugs administered by continuous infusion to provide accuracy in calculations and to allow closer correlation with dosage and patient response. The "Notes" contain particular warnings that relate to administration.

Special remarks and cautions

    Information provided in this section includes:

    The more clinically pertinent side effects. Other sources should be consulted for a complete list of adverse effects.

    Advice that should be given to help promote patient understanding and compliance and to prevent complications in therapy.

    Data provided on laboratory test interferences. The data often refer to tests run by specific methods, many of which are infrequently used. Consult your laboratory for their methods of assay.

    Use of drugs during pregnancy and lactation. Most drugs are not approved for use in pregnancy and many have restrictions concerning pediatric use resulting from a lack of studies in these patient populations. Consult appropriate texts for use if the benefits of therapy outweigh the risks incurred by such therapy.

Drug interactions

Those listed are the more common, potentially significant interactions. If a reaction is suspected, consult texts that provide more complete information.

Contents

Tables

CHAPTER ONE

Antimicrobial agents

Antimicrobial agents
GENERAL INFORMATION

Antimicrobial agents are chemicals that eliminate living organisms pathogenic to the host (that is, the patient). Methods of classifying these agents include (1) mechanism of action (inhibition of protein synthesis, activity on the cell membrane, alteration of nucleic acid metabolism), (2) spectrum of activity (gram-positive organisms, gram-negative organisms, rickettsia, tuberculosis), (3) similarity in chemical structure (penicillins, cephalosporins, aminoglycosides, sulfonamides), and (4) the source (living organisms—bacteria, fungi, or chemical synthesis).

The selection of the antimicrobial agent must be based on sensitivity of the organism, patient variation, and relative toxicity of the agents being considered. If at all possible the infecting organism should be isolated and identified. Culture and sensitivity tests should be completed, and appropriate antibiotic therapy based on the sensitivity results as well as on the clinical judgment of the physician should be initiated.

Host (patient) factors that may alter the response of the infection and therapy include the patient's age, other diseases (diabetes mellitus, malignancy), organ impairment (renal, hepatic, neurologic, immune deficiency), pregnancy, allergy, and concomitant drug therapy.

Special remarks and cautions

Hypersensitivity reactions may develop after exposure to any antimicrobial agent. The severity of allergic reaction ranges from mild rash to fatal anaphylaxis. Allergic reactions may develop within 30 min of administration (anaphylaxis, laryngeal edema, shock, dyspnea, skin reactions) or may occur several days after discontinuance of therapy (skin rashes, drug fever, hemolysis, nephritis, agranulocytosis). All patients must be questioned for previous allergic reactions, and allergy-prone patients must be observed closely.

Antimicrobial agents by any route may predispose a patient to superinfection from nonsusceptible microorganisms. Superinfections occur most frequently with the use of broad-spectrum antibiotics and with agents causing diminished host resistance, such as corticosteroids and antineoplastic agents. Stomatitis, glossitis, itching, and vulvovaginitis are often caused by the candidal species of fungi. Viral infections, such as with the herpes strain, may also occur, especially in the perioral area.

Orally administered antimicrobial agents frequently cause gastrointestinal symptoms of nausea, vomiting, and diarrhea. These adverse effects are often dose related and result from changes in normal flora, irritation, and superinfection.

Patients receiving irrigant solutions over a prolonged period or topical applications to large body surface areas must be observed for toxic effects caused by systemic absorption. Systemic symptomatology may also develop from oral or rectal administration of "nonabsorbable" antibiotics, especially when the intestinal mucosa is inflamed.

The importance of rest as an adjunct to therapy should be emphasized to the patient. Patients should also understand the unique use of the drug for a particular organism and hence should be instructed to neither save nor share their medication. The drug should be continued during the entire prescribed period and not discontinued after symptomatic relief.

Penicillins
GENERAL INFORMATION

The mechanism of action of penicillin on bacteria is interference with cell wall formation. Penicillin is more effective against actively dividing organisms than resting, mature cells.

Penicillin G is the naturally occurring parent of this class of antibiotics. Semisynthetic compounds are made from modification of the parent molecule to alter the spectrum of activity, decrease acid instability, enhance absorption, and diminish enzyme resistance by microorganisms. See Table 1-1 for a comparison of the penicillinase-resistant penicillins.

Special remarks and cautions

Before therapy is initiated, inquiry must be made concerning possible allergy to penicillin. Hypersensitivity reactions ranging from maculopapular rash, urticaria, eosinophilia, and serum sickness to anaphylaxis have occurred in up to 10% of patients receiving penicillin. Patients with a history of hives, asthma, hay fever, and other allergies to drugs must be observed particularly closely.

Dermatologic reactions of varying character and distribution are the most common allergic reactions to penicillin although any manifestation of hypersensitivity, including anaphylaxis, is possible.

The most common side effects of orally administered penicillins are nausea, vomiting, epigastric distress, and diarrhea.

Adverse effects of parenteral therapy include:

1. Neurologic: greater than 60 million units/day of penicillin G or 10 g/day of carbenicillin may produce hallucinations, hyperreflexia, seizures, and delirium. Preexisting neurologic disease or renal dysfunction may predispose a patient to these adverse effects.
2. Electrolyte imbalances: patients receiving large parenteral doses of sodium or potassium penicillin or carbenicillin may display electrolyte disturbances resulting in cardiac arrhythmias, hyperreflexia, convulsions, and coma. Patients with impaired renal function are more prone to these serious side effects.
3. Hematologic: penicillin hypersensitivity may include development of a positive Coombs' test and hemolytic anemia, particularly after high doses (20 million units) and a long duration of therapy. Other hematologic side effects include thrombocytopenia, thrombocytopenic purpura, and agranulocytosis. These are usually readily reversible on discontinuance of therapy.

Drug interactions

Penicillin is a bactericidal antibiotic. It requires actively growing cells to be effective. When it is used concomitantly with bacteriostatic antibiotics its effectiveness may be decreased or destroyed. Examples of bacteriostatic antibiotics are chloramphenicol, erythromycin, and tetracyclines.

Probenecid inhibits the excretion of penicillin by increasing blood levels and prolonging activity. This combination may be used to advantage in the treatment of gonorrhea and other infections where high and prolonged blood levels are indicated.

Excessive antacids may delay or diminish absorption of penicillin.

Hypersensitivity reactions may result from a cross-sensitivity to cephalosporins.

AMOXICILLIN
(Amoxil, Larotid, Polymox)

AHFS 8:12.16
CATEGORY Penicillin antibiotic

Action and use

Amoxicillin is a semisynthetic, broad-spectrum penicillin derivative with an antibacterial activity similar to that of ampicillin.

Characteristics

Amoxicillin is stable in gastric acid and rapidly absorbed on PO administration. Peak serum level: 2 hr. Protein binding: 20% to 25%. Half-life: 60 min. Excretion: 60% unchanged in urine after 8 hr. Dialysis: yes, H; no, P.

Administration and dosage
Adult

PO—250 to 500 mg every 8 hr.
IM—Not available.
IV—Not available.

Pediatric

1. Drops (50 mg/ml):
   a. Under 6 kg (13 lb): 0.5 to 1 ml every 8 hr.
   b. Between 6 and 8 kg (13 to 18 lb): 1 to 2 ml every 8 hr.
2. PO suspension (125 mg/5 ml or 250 mg/5 ml):
   a. Between 8 and 20 kg (18 to 44 lb): 20 to 40 mg/kg/24 hr in divided doses every 8 hr.
   b. Over 20 kg (44 lb): follow adult dosages.

   After reconstitution, amoxicillin drops or suspension may be added to milk, formula, water, or fruit juice to enhance ease of administration.

Special remarks and cautions

See General information on penicillin (p. 3).
Since a parenteral dosage form is not available, amoxicillin is not indicated in the initial treatment of severe, life-threatening infections.

Drug interactions

See General information on penicillin (p. 3).

AMPICILLIN
(Principen, Omnipen, Penbritin, Polycillin)

AHFS 8:12.16
CATEGORY Penicillin antibiotic

Action and use

Ampicillin is a semisynthetic, broad-spectrum penicillin antibiotic effective against gram-positive cocci as well as many groups of gram-negative bacteria. Its primary indication is in the treatment of susceptible gram-negative bacteria including *Escherichia coli, Haemophilus influenzae, Proteus mirabilis,* and species of *Shigella* and *Neisseria.*

Characteristics

Peak plasma level: 5 min (IV), 1 hr (IM), 2 hr (PO). Protein binding: 20% to 25%. Half-life: 90 min. Excretion: 35% of PO dose active in urine, 70% of IM dose active in urine. Dialysis: yes, H; no, P.

Administration and dosage
Adult

PO—250 to 500 mg every 6 hr for respiratory tract, soft tissue, and skin infections. 500 mg every 6 hr for gastrointestinal and urinary tract infections. The presence of food diminishes the absorption of ampicillin.

IM—Same as PO.

IV—Same as PO. Septicemia or bacterial meningitis: 8 to 14 g/day in divided doses every 3 to 4 hr. When given IV, ampicillin must be given at a rate no faster than 100 mg/min to prevent convulsive seizures. Parenteral ampicillin should be administered within 1 hr of reconstitution to prevent significant loss in potency. Dilute the powder with sterile water for injection.

Pediatric
Neonates

IV   1. First 7 days after birth: 25 mg/kg/12 hr.
      2. After 7 days: 33 to 50 mg/kg/8 hr.
      3. After 30 days: 33 to 50 mg/kg/6 hr.

Children under 40 kg (88 lb)

PO—50 to 200 mg/kg/24 hr in divided doses.
IM or IV—As for PO.

Children over 40 kg (88 lb)

PO—1 to 2 g/24 hr in divided doses.
IM or IV—For severe infections 8 to 14 g/24 hr in divided doses.

Special remarks and cautions

See General information on penicillin (p. 3).

When ampicillin is administered to a patient with mononucleosis, there is an 80% to 90% incidence of skin rash.

Drug interactions

See General information on penicillin (p. 3).

Ampicillin may rapidly inactivate gentamicin. They probably should not be mixed together or administered concurrently.

Allopurinol (Zyloprim) and ampicillin used concurrently may manifest a 23% incidence of rash.

CARBENICILLIN, INDANYL SODIUM AND DISODIUM   AHFS 8:12.16

(*Geocillin, Geopen, Pyopen*)   CATEGORY Penicillin antibiotic

Action and use

Carbenicillin is a semisynthetic penicillin derivative. It is the first antibiotic of this class to be effective against *Pseudomonas aeruginosa*. Carbenicillin is indicated in the treatment of severe systemic infections and chronic urinary tract infections caused by susceptible strains of *Proteus, E. coli,* and *Pseudomonas.*

Characteristics

Peak levels: 15 to 30 min (IV), 30 to 120 min (IM). Protein binding: 50% to 60%. Half-life: 60 min. Excretion: 75% to 85% unchanged in urine. Dialysis: yes, H; no, P.

Administration and dosage
Adult

PO—Indanyl sodium salt: 382 to 764 mg 4 times daily for chronic urinary tract infections.

IM—Disodium salt: not more than 2 g of the drug should be administered in each IM injection. For IM use only the powder may be diluted with 0.5% lidocaine solution (without epinephrine) or bacteriostatic water containing 0.9% benzyl alcohol to reduce pain on injection.

IV—Disodium salt: 250 to 500 mg/kg/day to 20 to 30 g/day for *Proteus* or *E. coli,* 30 to 40 g/day for *Pseudomonas.* To keep vein irritation to a minimum, dilute the powder to 1 g/20 ml and administer as slowly as possible. Dilution may be completed with any of the major IV fluids, NS, D-5, D-10, or LR. Rapid IV infusion may produce neurotoxicity manifested by hallucinations, inability to think clearly, and seizures.

Pediatric

Neonates. For severe *Pseudomonas, E. coli, Proteus,* and *H. influenzae* infections, administer IM or by a 15-minute IV infusion.
1. Under 2 kg:
   a. First 7 days after birth: 100 mg/kg/12 hr.
   b. After 7 days: 100 mg/kg/8 hr.
2. Over 2 kg:
   a. First 7 days after birth: 100 mg/kg/12 hr.
   b. After 7 days: 100 mg/kg/6 hr.

Children

IV 1. Severe systemic *Pseudomonas* infections: 400 to 500 mg/kg/24 hr in divided doses.
    2. Severe systemic *E. coli* or *Proteus* infections: 300 to 400 mg/kg/24 hr in divided doses.

Special remarks and cautions

See General information on penicillin (p. 3).

Since resistant organisms may develop, susceptibility testing should be performed prior to and during the course of therapy.

PO administration often produces an unpleasant taste sometimes accompanied by nausea, dry mouth, and furry tongue.

Patients with impaired renal function tend to accumulate carbenicillin. These patients should receive lower doses, and the clinician should monitor coagulation tests and observe for signs of hemorrhage and neurotoxicity. If the patient's creatinine clearance is less than 5 ml/min, therapeutic urine levels will not be achieved.

Carbenicillin disodium has a large sodium content, 5 to 6 mEq/g, and should therefore be used with caution in patients on sodium-restricted diets; their cardiac and electrolyte status should be monitored closely.

Drug interactions

See General information on penicillin (p. 3).

Carbenicillin has been reported to inactivate gentamicin in vitro; therefore give IV at different times or give the gentamicin IM and the carbenicillin IV.

METHICILLIN
(Staphcillin, Celbenin)

AHFS 8:12.16
CATEGORY Penicillin antibiotic

Action and use

Methicillin is a penicillinase-resistant derivative of penicillin. It is used to treat moderate to severe infections caused by penicillinase-producing staphylococci.

Characteristics

Peak serum levels: 30 to 60 min (IM). Protein binding: 35% to 40%. Half-life: 30 min. Excretion: unchanged in urine. Dialysis: no, H, P.

Administration and dosage
Adult

IM—Dissolve 1 g of powder in 1.5 ml sterile water to make a solution of 500 mg/ml. Administer 1 to 2 g every 4 to 6 hr.

IV—Dilute 1 g/50 ml of saline solution and administer at a rate of 10 ml/min. Administer 1 to 2 g every 4 to 6 hr.

Pediatric
Neonates

IV 1. Under 2 kg: 25 mg/kg every 12 hr for the first 2 weeks of age; every 8 hr after 2 weeks of age.
2. Over 2 kg: 25 mg/kg every 8 hr for the first 2 weeks of age; every 6 hr from 2 to 4 weeks of age.

For severe staphylococcal disease or meningitis, 50 mg/kg administered IV on the above schedule is recommended.

Infants and older children. Administer 50 mg/kg every 6 hr.

Special remarks and cautions

See General information on penicillin (p. 3).

Methicillin is an irritant, and pain is a common complaint even on deep IM injection. Rotate sites of injection and observe for signs of inflammation.

Although rare, methicillin may cause interstitial nephritis. The inflammation may result 1 to 4 weeks after therapy is initiated and is fully reversible in the majority of cases after therapy is discontinued. Renal function should be monitored routinely and methicillin should be used with caution in patients with impaired renal function.

Bone marrow suppression is more common with methicillin than with other penicillin derivatives. Agranulocytosis, thrombocytopenia, and anemia have occurred with usual doses of methicillin.

One g of methicillin contains 3 mEq (69 mg) of sodium.

Drug interactions

See General information on penicillin (p. 3).

PENICILLIN G
AHFS 8:12.16

(Pentids, Pfizerpen, Kesso-Pen-G)
CATEGORY Penicillin antibiotic

Action and use

Penicillin G is a bactericidal antibiotic highly effective against many gram-positive streptococci, pneumococci, and nonpenicillinase-producing staphylococci. Other organisms include *Treponema pallidum* (syphilis), *Neisseria gonorrhoeae* (gonorrhea). *N. meningitidis* (meningitis), and *Clostridium*. Most strains of *E. coli, Klebsiella, Proteus, Aerobacter,* and *Pseudomonas* are highly resistant to this form of penicillin.

Characteristics

Peak serum level: 15 to 30 min (IM), 30 to 60 min (PO). Protein binding: 50% to 60%; Half-life: 30 min. Excretion: 60% to 90% of an IM dose unchanged in urine, small amount in feces and milk. Dialysis: no, H, P.

Administration and dosage
Adult

PO—200,000 to 500,000 units every 6 to 8 hr. PO administration of penicillin G should be used only for those microorganisms highly sensitive to it. Penicillin G is partially inactivated by acidic gastric secretions. Adsorption onto food further diminishes absorption. Administer 1 hr before or 2 hr after meals.

IM—300,000 to 4.8 million units depending on the microorganism and severity of infection being treated.

IV—1 million to 80 million units depending on the microorganism and severity of infection being treated.

Pediatric

Premature and full-term neonates. Administer 30,000 to 50,000 units/kg/12 hr IM or IV. For neonates with meningitis administer 75,000 to 125,000 units/kg/12 hr IV.

Children. Administer 25,000 to 50,000 units/kg/24 hr in 4 to 6 divided doses PO, IM, or IV. If PO administer 1/2 hr before meals or 2 hr after meals. For children with life-threatening infections such as meningitis, administer 200,000 to 400,000 units/kg/24 hr.

Special remarks and cautions

See General information on penicillin (p. 3).

One million units of penicillin G potassium contain 1.7 mEq (66 mg) of potassium. One million units of penicillin G sodium contain 1.7 mEq (39 mg) of sodium. Electrolytes must be monitored closely when large doses of sodium or potassium penicillin G are administered IV.

Drug interactions

See General information on penicillin (p. 3).

PENICILLIN V (POTASSIUM PHENOXYMETHYL PENICILLIN)　AHFS 8:12.16
(Compocillin-VK, Pen-Vee-K, V-Cillin K)　CATEGORY Penicillin antibiotic

Action and use

Penicillin V is a natural penicillin derivative similar in spectrum and activity to penicillin G. It is, however, more stable in acid media and better absorbed following PO administration. Average blood levels following PO administration are 2 to 5 times higher than those following equal PO doses of penicillin G potassium. Penicillin V is used to treat mild to moderate streptococcal and pneumococcal infections of the upper respiratory tract, otitis media, scarlet fever, and mild, nonpenicillinase-producing staphylococcal infections of the skin and soft tissues.

Characteristics

Peak serum levels: 30 to 60 min (PO). Protein binding: 55% to 80%; Half-life: 30 min. Excretion: mostly unchanged in urine, small amount in feces and milk. Dialysis: no, H, P.

Administration and dosage
Adult

PO—250 to 500 mg every 6 hr. Food has minimal effects on absorption; however, it is recommended that administration be 1 hr before or 2 hr after meals.

IM—Not available.

IV—Not available.

Pediatric (under 12 years of age)

PO—30 to 50 mg/kg/day in 3 to 4 divided doses.

Special remarks and cautions

See General information on penicillin (p. 3).

TICARCILLIN DISODIUM
(*Ticar*)

AHFS 8:12.16
CATEGORY Penicillin antibiotic

Action and use

Ticarcillin is a semisynthetic penicillin derivative closely related in chemical structure and activity to carbenicillin. Ticarcillin (in combination with other antipseudomonal agents) is used primarily in the treatment of infections caused by *P. aeruginosa*. It may also be used to treat susceptible strains of *Proteus* species and *E. coli*. In the appropriate doses ticarcillin may be useful for the treatment of serious systemic, respiratory tract, urinary tract, or soft tissue or skin infections due to susceptible organisms.

Characteristics

Peak level: 60 min (IM). Duration: 4 to 6 hr (IM). Protein binding: 50% to 65%. Half-life: 70 min. Metabolism: liver. Excretion: 85% to 95% unchanged, 5% to 15% as penicilloic acid, in urine. Dialysis: yes, H, P.

Administration and dosage
Adult

IM—Reconstitute each gram with 2 ml of sterile water for injection. Not more than 2 g of the drug should be administered in each IM injection. For IM use only the powder may be diluted with 1% lidocaine solution (without epinephrine) or bacteriostatic water containing 0.9% benzyl alcohol to reduce pain on injection.

IV   1. Normal renal function: 200 to 350 mg/kg/day in divided doses for systemic, respiratory, and soft tissue infections; 1 g every 6 hr for urinary tract infections.
2. Impaired renal function: loading dose of 3 g followed by subsequent doses (see chart below).

Creatinine clearance rate (CCR)	Dosage
>60 ml/min	3 g every 4 hr
30 to 60 ml/min	2 g every 4 hr
10 to 30 ml/min	2 g every 8 hr
<10 ml/min	2 g every 12 hr (or 1 g IM every 6 hr)

In patients with hepatic dysfunction and a creatinine clearance of less than 10 ml/min administer 2 g/day IV or 1 g every 12 hr IM.

Each gram of ticarcillin should be reconstituted with at least 4 ml of sterile water for injection. The reconstituted solution may be added to usual IV solutions and administered by continuous or intermittent drip. A suggested method is to give one sixth the total daily dose as a 2-hr infusion every 4 hr.

Pediatric
Neonates

1. Under 2 kg: initially 100 mg/kg IM or as a 10 to 20 min IV infusion. Follow every 8 hr with IV infusions of 75 mg/kg during the first week after birth, then increase to 75 mg/kg every 4 to 6 hr.
2. Over 2 kg: initially 100 mg/kg IM or as a 10 to 20 min IV infusion. Follow every 4 to 6 hr with IV infusions of 75 mg/kg during the first 2 weeks after birth, then increase to 100 mg/kg every 4 hr.

Children. For systemic, respiratory, and soft tissue infections, administer IM or IV as for adults. For urinary tract infections in children under 40 kg administer 50 to 100 mg/kg/day IM or IV in divided doses every 6 to 8 hr. For urinary tract infections in children over 40 kg administer as for adults.

Special remarks and cautions

See General information on penicillin (p. 3).

Since resistant organisms may develop, susceptibility testing should be performed prior to and during the course of therapy.

Patients with impaired renal function tend to accumulate ticarcillin. As noted above, these patients should receive lower doses. The clinician should monitor coagulation tests and observe for signs of hemorrhage and neurotoxicity.

Ticarcillin disodium has a high sodium content, (5 to 6.5 mEq/g) and should therefore be used with caution in patients on sodium-restricted diets; their cardiac and electrolyte status should be monitored closely.

Drug interactions

See General information on penicillin (p. 3).

Ticarcillin has been reported to inactivate gentamicin and tobramycin when mixed together; therefore, give IV at different times or give the gentamicin or tobramycin IM and the carbenicillin IV.

Table 1-1. A comparison of penicillinase-resistant penicillins*

AHFS 8:12.16

Penicillin	Peak levels (min)	Duration (hr)	Protein binding (%)	Half-life (min)	Excretion	Dialysis H	Dialysis P	Dosage† Neonate	Dosage† Child	Dosage† Adult
Cloxacillin sodium (Tegopen)	30-60 (PO)	<4	88-96	30	10% active metabolites in urine; small amounts in bile; remainder unchanged in urine	No	No	—	PO: <20 kg: 50 to 100 mg/kg every 6 hr; >20 kg: 250-500 mg every 6 hr	PO: 250-500 mg every 6 hr
Dicloxacillin sodium (Dynapen, Pathocil, Veracillin)	60 (PO) 30-60 (IM)	<4 4-6	96-98	40	Small amounts in bile; the rest unchanged in urine	No	No	—	PO: <40 kg: 12.5-25 mg/kg/day divided into 4 doses; >40 kg: 125-250 mg every 6 hr IM: >40 kg: 25-50 mg/kg/day divided into 4 doses; >40 kg: 250-500 mg every 6 hr	PO: 125-250 mg every 6 hr; ≯1 g every 6 hr IM: 250-500 mg every 6 hr

Drug									
Nafcillin (Unipen)	30-60 (PO, IM)	<4	65-90	60	30% unchanged in urine	No	No	PO: 30-40 mg/kg/day divided into 4 doses. IM: 20 mg/kg/day divided into 2 doses	PO: 50 mg/kg/day divided into 4 doses. IM: 50 mg/kg/day divided into 2 doses. IV: 50 mg/kg/day divided into 6 doses	PO: 250 mg to 1 g every 4-6 hr. IM: 500 mg every 4-6 hr. IV: 500 mg to 1 g every 4 hr
Oxacillin sodium (Prostaphlin)	30 (PO suspension); 60 (PO capsules); 30 (IM)	<4; <4; <4	85-94	30	Metabolite and unchanged drug in urine	No	No	IM and IV: 25 mg/kg/day in 4 divided doses	PO: <20 kg: 50 mg/kg/day divided into 4 doses; >20 kg: 500 mg every 4-6 hr. IM and IV: <20 kg: 50-100 mg/kg/day divided into 4-6 doses; >20 kg: 250-500 mg every 4-6 hr	PO: 500 mg every 4-6 hr. IM and IV: 250 mg to 1 g every 4-6 hr

*For Special remarks and cautions see p. 3; for Drug interactions see p. 3; for discussion of methicillin see p. 7.

†Food interferes with absorption of PO dosage forms. Administer at least 1 hr before or 2 hr after meals.

Cephalosporins
GENERAL INFORMATION

The mechanism of action of cephalosporins is inhibition of mucopeptide synthesis in the bacterial cell wall. The drugs are both bacteriostatic and bactericidal, depending on the concentration of the drug present. The cephalosporins are structurally related to the penicillins, and evidence indicates that the mechanism of action is similar or identical to the penicillins. Cephalosporins are usually resistant to penicillinase; however, strains that may produce destructive enzymes called cephalosporinases are becoming more common.

Cephalosporins are highly effective in the therapy of a variety of mild to severe infections caused by both gram-positive and gram-negative microorganisms. See Table 1-2 for a comparison of cephalosporins.

Special remarks and cautions

Before cephalosporin therapy is initiated, inquiry must be made concerning allergic reactions to cephalosporins and penicillin. Hypersensitivity reactions ranging from maculopapular rash, urticaria, eosinophilia, and serum sickness to anaphylaxis have occurred in about 5% of patients receiving cephalosporins. Patients who are allergy prone, especially to drugs, must be observed particularly closely.

A false-positive reaction for glucose in the urine may occur with Clinitest tablets, but not with Tes-Tape.

Transient elevations of SGOT, SGPT, BUN, serum creatinine, and alkaline phosphatase levels have been observed. Nephrotoxicity, as evidenced by proteinuria, hematuria, casts, decreased creatinine clearance, and decreased urine output, has also occurred.

Neutropenia, leukopenia, thrombocytopenia, and positive direct and indirect Coombs' tests have been reported.

Adverse effects that have occurred with all cephalosporins include oral thrush, gastrointestinal symptoms (especially diarrhea), genital and anal pruritus, genital candidiasis, vaginitis, and vaginal discharge.

Cephalosporins readily cross the placental barrier and are probably secreted in human breast milk. Safe use in pregnancy has not been established.

Drug interactions

Probenecid reduces the renal clearance of the cephalosporins, thereby increasing the plasma concentration. This interaction is potentially more significant with those cephalosporins not metabolized (cephalexin, cefazolin) before excretion.

The possibility of nephrotoxicity may be enhanced by administration of cephalosporins with aminoglycosides (gentamicin, tobramycin, streptomycin, neomycin, kanamycin) and potent diuretics (furosemide, ethacrynic acid).

CEPHALEXIN MONOHYDRATE
(Keflex)

AHFS 8:12.06
CATEGORY Cephalosporin antibiotic

Action and use

Cephalexin is a semisynthetic antibiotic for PO administration. It is used for patients treated initially with a parenteral cephalosporin who require continued antibiotic therapy but whose improved clinical status no longer warrants parenteral administration.

Characteristics

Peak plasma levels: 1 hr. Protein binding: 10% to 15%. Half-life: 1 hr. Metabolism: none. Excretion: more than 90% unchanged within 8 hr in urine. Dialysis: yes, H, P.

Administration and dosage
Adult

PO—250 mg to 1 g every 6 hr.

Pediatric

PO—25 to 50 mg/kg/24 hr in divided doses.

Special remarks and cautions

See General information on cephalosporins (p. 14).

Mild diarrhea is a common side effect of cephalexin. Nausea, vomiting, and abdominal pain also occur.

Drug interactions

See General information on cephalosporins (p. 14).

CEFAZOLIN SODIUM
(Kefzol, Ancef)

AHFS 8:12.06
CATEGORY Cephalosporin antibiotic

Action and use

Cefazolin sodium is a cephalosporin with an action and a spectrum similar to cephalothin, with the following exceptions. It is effective in treating susceptible gram-negative and gram-positive organisms of the respiratory and genitourinary tract and staphylococcal infections of bones and joints. It is not recommended for use in gram-negative skin and soft tissue infections, endocarditis, meningitis, or peritonitis.

Characteristics

Peak plasma levels: 60 min (IM). Protein binding: 75% to 80%; Half-life: 100 min. Excretion: 80% unchanged in urine in 24 hr. Dialysis: no, H, P.

Administration and dosage
Adult

PO—Not available.

IM—250 mg to 1 g every 6 to 8 hr.

IV—250 mg to 1.5 g every 6 to 8 hr. Dilute 500 mg to 1 g of reconstituted cefazolin in a minimum of 10 ml of sterile water for injection. Inject slowly over 5 min through the tubing or directly into the vein. Cefazolin is stable after reconstitution for 24 hr at room temperature and for 96 hr if stored under refrigeration.

NOTE: As a result of minimal metabolism and major excretion via the kidneys, dosage adjustment is required in patients with impaired renal function.

Pediatric

Neonates. Safety for use in premature infants and infants under 1 month of age has not been established. The use of cefazolin is not recommended in these patients.

Children

IM or IV   1. Mild to moderate infections: 25 to 50 mg/kg/24 hr (10 to 20 mg/16 to 24 hr) in divided doses.
2. Life-threatening infections: to 100 mg/kg/24 hr in divided doses.

Special remarks and cautions

See General information on cephalosporins (p. 14).

A specific advantage of cefazolin over other parenteral cephalosporins is the relative pain-free IM injection.

Drug interactions

See General information on cephalosporins (p. 14).

CEPHALOTHIN SODIUM
(Keflin)

AHFS 8:12.06
CATEGORY Cephalosporin antibiotic

Action and use

Cephalothin is indicated in the treatment of respiratory and urinary tract, soft tissue and skin, gastrointestinal tract, bone and joint, and septicemic infections. Susceptible organisms include strains of *Diplococcus pneumoniae, Klebsiella, H. influenzae, E. coli, P. mirabilis, Salmonella, Shigella,* penicillinase- and nonpenicillinase-producing staphylococci, and group A beta-hemolytic streptococci.

Characteristics

Peak plasma level: 30 min (IM). Protein binding: 56% to 60%. Half-life: 40 min. Metabolism: 20% to 30% to a weakly active metabolite. Excretion: 60% to 80% unchanged, 20% to 30% as weakly active metabolite, in urine. Dialysis: yes, H, P.

Administration and dosage
Adult

PO—Not available.

IM—500 mg to 1 g every 4 to 6 hr.

IV—Mild to moderate infections: 500 mg to 1 g every 4 to 6 hr; life-threatening infections: 1 g to 2 g every 4 to 6 hr. Dosage adjustment is required in impaired renal function.

RATE—1 g diluted in 10 ml of diluent and administered over 5 min. Solutions stored at room temperature should be used within 6 hr after reconstitution. The concentrated solution will darken, especially at room temperature.

Pediatric

IM or IV—80 to 160 mg/kg/24 hr (40 to 80 mg/lb) in divided doses.

RATE—As for adult dosages.

Special remarks and cautions

Pain, tenderness, and induration is common following repeated IM injections. Rotate injection sites and observe for inflammation. Thrombophlebitis is a relatively common complication of IV therapy. It is associated with doses of more than 6 g daily for longer than 3 days. Some studies indicate that in-line filters may be successful in reducing venous irritation.

See General information on cephalosporins (p. 14).

Drug interactions

See General information on cephalosporins (p. 14).

Table 1-2. A comparison of the cephalosporins*

Cephalosporin	Peak levels	Duration (hr)	Protein binding (%)	Half-life (min)	Excretion	Dialysis H	Dialysis P	Dosage† Neonate	Dosage† Child	Dosage† Adult
Cephamandole naftate (Mandol)	10 min	—	67-74	42-55	Excreted unchanged in urine	Yes	Yes	Not recommended	IM or IV: 50-100 mg/kg/day in 3 to 6 divided doses	IM or IV: 0.5 to 1 g every 4 to 8 hr; do not exceed 12 g/day
Cefoxitin sodium (Mefoxin)	5 min	—	~70	40-60	Excreted unchanged in urine	Yes	Yes	Not recommended	Not recommended	IM or IV: 1 g every 6 to 8 hr; do not exceed 12 g/day
Cephaloglycin dihydrate (Kafocin)	2 hr (PO)	6-8	0-30	90	90%-98% metabolized in liver to other active forms; 2%-10% excreted unchanged in urine	Yes	Yes	—	PO: 25-50 mg/kg/day in 4 divided doses	PO: 250-500 mg every 6 hr.
Cephaloridine (Loridine)	30-60 min (IM)	6 (IM)	0-30	50-100	75% excreted unchanged in urine	Yes	Yes	—	IM or IV: 30-50 mg/kg/day in 2 to 4 divided doses	IM or IV: 250 mg to 1 g 2 to 4 times daily; do not exceed 4 g/day
Cephapirin sodium (Cefadyl)	30 min (IM)	6 (IM); 3 (IV)	45-50	20-50	70% excreted unchanged in urine	Yes	Yes	—	IM or IV: 40-80 mg/kg/day in 4 divided doses	IM or IV: 500 mg to 1 g every 4 to 6 hr
Cephradine (Anspor, Velosef)	60 min (PO); 1-2 hr (IM)	—	0-20	40-120	Excreted unchanged in urine	Yes	Yes	—	PO: 25-50 mg/kg/day in 4 divided doses IM or IV: 50-100 mg/kg/day in 4 divided doses	PO: 250-500 mg every 6 hr. IM or IV: 500 mg to 1 g every 6 hr Do not exceed 8 g/day

*See also cephalexin (p. 15), cefazolin (p. 16), and cephalothin (p. 17); for Special remarks and cautions see p. 14; for Drug interactions see p. 14.
†Food interferes with PO dosage forms. Administer at least 1 hr before or 2 hr after meals. Dosage adjustment is required in patients with renal failure; see manufacturer's recommendations.

Aminoglycosides
GENERAL INFORMATION

Aminoglycoside antibiotics are an important class of antibacterial agents used in moderate to severe infections. The aminoglycosides act directly on the 30 S ribosomal subunit of bacterial cells, causing mutations of the genetic code required for normal protein synthesis. High concentrations of aminoglycosides are bactericidal, while low concentrations are bacteriostatic. Resting cells are less susceptible to the drug than are multiplying bacteria. Aminoglycosides are primarily effective against gram-negative bacterial infections. As a result of the widespread use of aminoglycosides, resistant strains of microorganisms have rapidly emerged. Combination therapy with other antibiotics with an alternate mechanism of action is often used to inhibit the emergence of resistant strains.

Special remarks and cautions

A relatively common, dose-related side effect of the aminoglycosides is ototoxicity. It may affect the vestibular branch of the eighth cranial nerve, resulting in dizziness, vertigo, tinnitus, and roaring in the ears. Damage to the cochlear branch of the eighth cranial nerve may result in deafness. Instruct the patient to report any of these toxic effects. Withhold the next dose pending consultation with the physician. Audiometric studies are recommended during prolonged or with increased dosage therapy.

Other neurologic dysfunctions include peripheral neuritis causing tingling and numbness usually around the mouth and of the hands and neuromuscular blockade that may result in respiratory depression and/or paralysis.

Renal damage is a potential toxic effect of aminoglycoside therapy. Nephrotoxicity may be manifested by oliguria, granular casts in the urine, proteinuria, and increased BUN and serum creatinine levels. Input and output as well as a progressive decrease in daily urine volume or changes in visual characteristics should be reported.

Skin rashes, eosinophilia, fever, blood dyscrasias, stomatitis, and anaphylaxis are among the hypersensitivity reactions that may follow the administration of aminoglycosides.

Blood dyscrasias are rare, but may include neutropenia, agranulocytosis, aplastic anemia, and thrombocytopenia with purpura.

Other rare adverse effects include loss of hair, increased salivation, hypotension, hypertension, anorexia, weight loss, and joint pain.

Transient hepatosplenomegaly has occurred with elevated serum transaminase levels and hyperbilirubinemia.

Drug interactions

Cephalosporins, especially cephaloridine (Loridine), may enhance the nephrotoxic potential of the aminoglycosides.

Ethacrynic acid (Edecrin) and furosemide (Lasix) may enhance the ototoxicity of aminoglycosides.

Aminoglycoside antibiotics, alone and in combination with skeletal muscle relaxants (succinylcholine, tubocurarine, pancuronium bromide) may produce respiratory paralysis. This interaction has occurred 48 hr postoperatively and is independent of the route of administration. Calcium and reversible cholinesterase inhibitors (neostigmine—Prostigmin, edrophonium—Tensilon) have been effective in reversing the paralysis.

AMIKACIN SULFATE
(Amikin)

AHFS 8:12.28

CATEGORY Aminoglycoside antibiotic

Action and use

Amikacin is an aminoglycoside antibiotic used in the short-term treatment of serious infections caused by susceptible bacteria. Clinical studies indicate that amikacin may be effective against P. aeruginosa, E. coli, and Proteus, Providencia, Klebsiella, Enterobacter, and Serratia species resistant to gentamicin and/or tobramycin. Amikacin is also active against Staphylococcus aureus and S. epidermidis. Because of potential toxicity amikacin should not be used for minor infections or against bacteria susceptible to less toxic drugs. Use should be restricted to 2 weeks.

Characteristics

Peak levels: 60 min (IM). Duration: to 12 hr. Protein binding: less than 11%. Half-life: 2 to 3 hr. Excretion: unchanged in urine. Dialysis: yes, H; poor, P.

Administration and dosage
Adult

IM OR IV
1. Normal renal function: 15 mg/kg/day in 2 to 4 equally divided doses. Do not exceed 1.5 g per day. When administered IV dilute the dose with 100 to 200 ml of standard IV solution and infuse over 30 to 60 min.
2. Impaired renal function
   a. Normal dosage at prolonged intervals:

   $$\text{serum creatinine } (100 \text{ mg/100 ml}) \times 9 = \text{Dose interval (hr)}$$

   Example: If the serum creatinine is 3, administer the single recommended dose (7.5 mg/kg) every 27 hr.
   b. Reduced dosage at fixed time intervals:

   $$\text{loading dose } = 7.5 \text{ mg/kg}$$

   Maintenance dose every 12 hours =

   $$\frac{\text{Observed CCR (ml/min)}}{\text{Normal CCR (ml/min)}} \times \text{Calculated loading dose (mg)}$$

   Example: If a patient weighs 60 kg and has a steady creatinine clearance of 35 ml/min:

   $$\frac{35 \text{ ml/min}}{100 \text{ ml/min}} \times (60 \text{ kg} \times 7.5 \text{ mg/kg}) = 157 \text{ mg/12 hr}$$

Pediatric
Neonates

IM or IV—Loading: 10 mg/kg; maintenance: 7.5 mg/kg every 12 hr. Infuse IV over 1 to 2 hr.

Older infants and children

IM or IV— 15 mg/kg/day in 2 to 4 equally divided doses. Infuse IV over 30 to 60 min.

Special remarks and cautions

See General information on aminoglycosides (p. 19).

Drug interactions

See General information on aminoglycosides (p. 19).

GENTAMICIN SULFATE
(Garamycin)

AHFS 8:12.28
CATEGORY Aminoglycoside antibiotic

Action and use

At present gentamicin is the most widely used aminoglycoside. Its mode of action is similar to that of the other members of this class. As a result of potential toxicity and the development of resistant organisms, gentamicin should only be used in severe infections caused by susceptible gram-negative organisms such as *P. aeruginosa* and *E. coli; Proteus, Klebsiella, Enterobacter,* and *Serratia* species; and most *Salmonella* and *Shigella* species.

Characteristics

Peak plasma level: 1 to 1½ hr (IM). Protein binding: 25% to 30%; Half-life: 2 hr. Excretion: unchanged in urine. Toxic level: 10 to 12 μg/ml. Dialysis: yes, H; no, P.

Administration and dosage
Adult

PO—Not available.

IM—As for IV.

IV   1. Normal renal function:
   - a. Urinary tract infection: 3 mg/kg/24 hr.
   - b. Other infections: 3 to 5 mg/kg/24 hr.
   - c. Life-threatening infections: at least 5 mg/kg/24 hr reduced to 3 mg/kg/24 hr as soon as clinically indicated.

The usual adult dose is 60 mg 3 times daily for those patients weighing less than 60 kg (132 lb) and 80 mg 3 times daily for those patients weighing more than 60 kg (132 lb).

  2. Renal failure (see Table 1-3). Dilute with saline solution or dextrose 5% to a concentration not greater than 1 mg/ml. Administer over 30 to 60 min. Alkalinization of the urine provides greater urinary concentrations for treating urinary tract infections.

Pediatric
Neonates

IV   1. First 7 days after birth (premature or full-term): 2.5 mg/kg/12 hr.
  2. After 7 days: 2.5 mg/kg/8 hr.

Children (normal renal function). Administer 2 to 2.5 mg/kg/8 hr. Dilute with saline solution or dextrose 5% to a concentration not greater than 1 mg/ml. Administer over a 1- to 2-hr period. Do not mix with other drugs.

Special remarks and cautions

See General information on aminoglycosides (p. 19).

As a result of potentially severe neurotoxicity and nephrotoxicity, monitoring of renal and eighth cranial nerve function is recommended.

Drug interactions

See General information on aminoglycosides (p. 19).

As a result of chemical and physical incompatibilities, carbenicillin slowly inactivates gentamicin. Do not mix together prior to infusion.

Gentamicin and heparin are chemically incompatible. Do not mix together prior to infusion.

Table 1-3. Gentamicin dosage in renal failure*

CCR (ml/min)	< 2	4	8	10	20	30	40	50	60	70+
mg/kg/8 hr	0.13	0.2	0.26	0.33	0.6	0.8	1.0	1.3	1.5	1.7
	mg/8 hr	mg/8 hr	mg/8 hr	mg/8 hr	mg/8 hr	mg/8 hr	mg/8 hr	mg/8 hr	mg/8 hr	mg/8 hr
50 kg (110 lb) L.D. = 85 mg	6.5	10	13	16.5	30	40	50	65	75	85
60 kg (132 lb) L.D. = 102 mg	7.8	12	15.6	20	36	48	60	78	90	102
70 kg (154 lb) L.D. = 120 mg	9	14	18	23	42	56	70	91	105	120
80 kg (176 lb) L.D. = 136 mg	10	16	21	26	48	64	80	104	120	136
90 kg (198 lb) L.D. = 153 mg	12	18	24	30	54	72	90	117	135	153
100 kg (220 lb) L.D. = 170 mg	13	20	26	33	60	80	100	130	150	170

*Modified from Chan, R. A., et al.: Ann. Intern. Med. **76**:773-778, 1972.
+For patients with creatinine clearance greater than 70 ml/min, this dosage provides 5 mg/kg/day. In non-life-threatening infections this dosage should be reduced to 3 mg/kg/day or 1 mg/kg/8 hr.

KEY:

CCR—Creatinine clearance rate (ml/min × 1.73 m^2)
L.D.—Loading dose of 1.7 mg/kg followed every 8 hr by the calculated maintenance dose

KANAMYCIN SULFATE
(Kantrex)

AHFS 8:12.28
CATEGORY Aminoglycoside antibiotic

Action and use

Kanamycin is an aminoglycoside used in the short-term treatment of susceptible strains of *E. coli, Proteus, Enterobacter, Klebsiella pneumoniae,* and *S. marcescens.* Kanamycin is not effective against *P. aeruginosa.* PO administration has been useful in suppression of normal bacterial flora in the bowel when treating hepatic coma.

Characteristics

Peak plasma level: 1 hr (IM). Protein binding: 0% to 3%. Half-life: 2.5 hr. Excretion: 40% to 80% unchanged in urine in 24 hr; Dialysis: yes, H, P.

Administration and dosage
Adult

PO—8 to 12 g/day in divided doses.

IM—7.5 mg/kg/12 hr or 15 mg/kg/24 hr in equally divided doses 3 to 4 times daily. Rotate sites of injection.

NOTE: IV administration should be used only if clinical conditions prevent IM administration.

IV—15 mg/kg/24 hr. Add the contents of a 500 mg vial to 200 ml of saline solution or dextrose 5% (providing a solution of 2.5 mg/ml) and administer at 60 to 80 gtt/min. Dosages must not exceed 1.5 g/day regardless of the patient's weight. In renal failure the dosing interval is determined by the following formula:

$$\text{Serum creatinine (mg/100 ml)} \times 9 = \text{Dose interval (hr)}$$

Example: If the serum creatinine is 3, administer the recommended dose (7.5 mg/kg) every 27 hr.

Pediatric

Neonates. Consult the following chart* for neonatal dosages.

Birth weight (g)	≤7 days of age	>7 days of age
≤ 2000 g	7.5 mg/kg every 12 hr	10 mg/kg every 12 hr
> 2000 g	10 mg/kg every 12 hr	10 mg/kg every 8 hr

*Modified from Eichenwald, H., and McCracken, G. H., Jr.: J. Pediatr. **93**:339, 1978.

Children. As for adult dosages.

Special remarks and cautions

See General information on aminoglycosides (p. 19).

Drug interactions

See General information on aminoglycosides (p. 19).

NEOMYCIN SULFATE

AHFS 8:12.28

(*Mycifradin, Neobiotic*)

CATEGORY Aminoglycoside antibiotic

Action and use

Neomycin has the same actions as the other aminoglycosides but is potentially more toxic, especially when administered parenterally. When no other therapy is effective, intramuscular neomycin may be used in the treatment of urinary tract infections caused by susceptible strains of *P. aeruginosa, K. pneumoniae, P. vulgaris, E. coli, Aerobacter aerogenes,* and *Salmonella* and *Shigella* species.

Neomycin is poorly absorbed (only 3%) from the gastrointestinal tract. It is effective in suppressing normal gastrointestinal bacterial flora when treating hepatic coma, diarrhea caused by enteropathogenic *E. coli,* and in preoperative preparation for abdominal surgery.

Characteristics

Half-life: 2 hr. Excretion: 97% unchanged in feces after PO administration, 30% to 50% unchanged in urine after parenteral administration. Dialysis: yes, H; no, P.

Administration and dosage
Adult and pediatric

PO   1. Hepatic coma: 4 to 12 g/day.
    2. Infectious diarrhea: 50 mg/kg/day in divided doses.
    3. Preoperative bowel sterilization: low-residue diet and 40 mg of neomycin sulfate per *pound* (90 mg/kg) in 6 equally divided doses (1 dose every 4 hr) for 2 to 3 days after the use of a cathartic and if there is no bowel obstruction.

IM— 15 mg/kg/day in 4 divided doses. The total daily dose should not exceed 1 g of neomycin sulfate. Therapy should not be continued beyond 10 days. Reconstitute by adding 2 ml of normal saline solution (0.9%) to a 0.5 g vial of neomycin sulfate powder, making a solution of 250 mg/ml.

NOTE: IM use is not recommended in pediatric patients.

Special remarks and cautions

Neomycin is commonly used in many topical and irrigant preparations. Long-term or high-dose irrigant solutions other than in the bladder or frequent topical administration on large body surface areas may result in systemic adverse effects of neomycin.

See General information on aminoglycosides (p. 19).

Drug interactions

Neomycin may inhibit the production and/or absorption of vitamin K from the gut. This may be significant in patients receiving oral anticoagulants (warfarin), resulting in increased bleeding tendency and elevated prothrombin time levels.

See General information on aminoglycosides (p. 19).

TOBRAMYCIN SULFATE

(Nebcin)

AHFS 8:12.28
CATEGORY Aminoglycoside antibiotic

Action and use

Tobramycin is a bactericidal agent with a mechanism of action similar to the other aminoglycosides. The spectrum of tobramycin activity is quite similar to gentamicin; however, tobramycin appears to be 2 to 4 times more active against *P. aeruginosa*, on a weight basis.

Characteristics

Peak plasma levels: 30 to 90 min (IM). Half-life: 1½ to 3 hr. Metabolism: insignificant. Excretion: 60% to 90% unchanged in urine in 24 hr. Dialysis: yes, H; no, P.

Administration and dosage
Adult

IM 1. Normal renal function (see Table 1-4):
    a. Serious infection: 1 mg/kg/8 hr (3 mg/kg/day).
    b. Life-threatening infection: 1.66 mg/kg/8 hr (5 mg/kg/day).
  2. Impaired renal function: see Table 1-4.

IV—As for IM administration, dilute the recommended dosage in 50 to 100 ml of dextrose 5% or saline solution and infuse over 20 to 60 min. Administration in less than 20 min may result in toxic serum levels. Tobramycin should not be physically premixed with other medications.

Pediatric
Neonates (under 1 week)

IM—Up to 2 mg/kg/12 hr (4 mg/kg/day).
IV—As for children and older infants.

Children and older infants (normal renal function)

IM 1. Serious infection: 1 mg/kg/8 hr (3 mg/kg/day).
  2. Life-threatening infection: to 1.66 mg/kg/8 hr (5 mg/kg/day).

IV—Dilute with saline solution or dextrose 5% to a concentration of about 1 mg/ml and administer over 20 to 60 min. Do not mix with other medications.

Special remarks and cautions

See General information on aminoglycosides (p. 19).

Drug interactions

See General information on aminoglycosides (p. 19).

Table 1-4. Tobramycin administration*

CRs (mg/100 ml)	10	7.6	5.3	3.3	2.4	1.9	1.6	1.4	1.3		>70
CCR (ml/min)	0	2	5	10	20	30	40	50	60	70	>70
mg/kg/8 hr	0.06 / 0.10	0.08 / 0.13	0.10 / 0.16	0.18 / 0.3	0.28 / 0.46	0.36 / 0.6	0.45 / 0.74	0.55 / 0.9	0.65 / 1	0.75 / 1.2	1 / 1.66
	mg/8 hr	mg/8 hr	mg/8 hr	mg/8 hr	mg/8 hr	mg/8 hr	mg/8 hr	mg/8 hr	mg/8 hr	mg/8 hr	mg/8 hr
40 kg (88 lb) L.D. = 40 mg	2.4 / 4	3 / 5	4 / 7	7.2 / 12	11 / 18	15 / 24	18 / 30	22 / 36	26 / 43	30 / 50	40 / 66
50 kg (110 lb) L.D. = 50 mg	3 / 5	5 / 7	5 / 8	9 / 15	14 / 23	18 / 30	23 / 37	28 / 45	33 / 54	38 / 62	50 / 83
60 kg (132 lb) L.D. = 60 mg	3.5 / 6	5 / 8	6 / 10	11 / 18	17 / 28	22 / 36	27 / 45	33 / 55	39 / 65	45 / 75	60 / 100
70 kg (154 lb) L.D. = 70 mg	4 / 7	5.4 / 9	7 / 12	13 / 21	20 / 33	25 / 42	32 / 52	38 / 64	46 / 75	53 / 88	70 / 116
80 kg (176 lb) L.D. = 80 mg	5 / 8	6.4 / 10	8 / 13	14 / 24	22 / 37	29 / 48	36 / 60	44 / 73	52 / 87	60 / 100	80 / 133
90 kg (198 lb) L.D. = 90 mg	5.5 / 9	7 / 12	9 / 15	16 / 27	25 / 42	32 / 54	40 / 68	50 / 83	59 / 98	68 / 113	90 / 150
100 kg (220 lb) L.D. = 100 mg	6 / 10	8 / 13	10 / 17	18 / 30	28 / 47	36 / 60	45 / 75	55 / 91	65 / 108	75 / 125	100 / 166

*Modified from Nebcin–Tobramycin sulfate product information, Eli Lilly Co.

KEY:

A — Dosage adjustment for serious infections with renal dysfunction
B — Adjustment of maximum dosage for life-threatening infections with renal dysfunction. REDUCE AS SOON AS POSSIBLE.
CRS — Serum creatinine level (mg/100 ml)
CCR — Creatinine clearance rate (ml/min)
L.D. — Loading dose followed at 8 hr by the appropriate maintenance dose

Sulfonamides
GENERAL INFORMATION

Sulfonamides are bacteriostatic agents that competitively inhibit bacterial synthesis of folic acid from para-aminobenzoic acid (PABA). Only organisms that synthesize folic acid are inhibited by sulfonamides.

Special remarks and cautions

As a result of the increasing frequency of organisms resistant to sulfonamides and the relative unreliability of in vitro sulfonamide sensitivity tests, clinical response must be carefully monitored, especially in the treatment of chronic and recurrent urinary tract infections.

Sulfonamides are a class of drugs with many side effects that may occur in nearly all organs.

1. Gastrointestinal:
   a. Nausea, vomiting, anorexia, and diarrhea are among the more common side effects.
   b. Stomatitis, pancreatitis, hepatitis, and abdominal pains have been reported.
2. Hematologic:
   a. Agranulocytosis may occur 10 to 14 days after therapy is initiated.
   b. Acute hemolytic anemia may occur in the first week of therapy as a result of hypersensitivity or glucose-6-phosphate dehydrogenase deficiency.
   c. Other blood dyscrasias include thrombocytopenia, aplastic anemia, and leukopenia. Signs of blood dyscrasias include sore throat, pallor, fever, purpura, jaundice, and weakness. Routine blood studies should be performed in patients receiving sulfonamides longer than 14 days.
3. Dermatologic:
   a. Patients should be cautioned to avoid unnecessary exposure to sunlight or ultraviolet light since photosensitivity may occur.
   b. Rash, pruritus, and exfoliative dermatitis may also occur. Since many serious adverse effects of sulfonamide therapy may be heralded by a rash, sulfonamide therapy should be discontinued at once if a rash does develop.
4. Renal: crystalluria caused by precipitation of a sulfonamide in the urinary tract may result in urolithiasis, oliguria, hematuria, proteinuria, and obstruction anuria. Input and output should be monitored, and collected urine should be observed for changes in coloration and sediment. Fluid intake should be encouraged to at least 1.5 L/ day.
5. Neurologic: dizziness, headache, mental depression, confusion, acute psychosis, drowsiness, tinnitus, and restlessness occur occasionally.

Sulfonamides may cause hypothyroidism and will suppress ^{131}I uptake for about 7 days after sulfonamide therapy is discontinued.

Drug interactions

Although apparently infrequent, local anesthetics that are derivatives of PABA (benzocaine, procaine, tetracaine) may antagonize the antibacterial activity of sulfonamides. Local infections have occurred in areas of procaine infiltration while patients were receiving sulfonamide therapy.

Sulfonylurea oral hypoglycemics (tolbutamide, acetohexamide, tolazamide, chlorpropamide) may be displaced from protein-binding sites, resulting in hypoglycemia.

Sulfonamides may displace warfarin from protein-binding sites, enhancing anticoagulation and prolonging the prothrombin time.

Sulfonamides may displace methotrexate from protein-binding sites, resulting in enhanced methotrexate toxicity.

SULFASALAZINE
(Azulfidine)

AHFS 8:24
CATEGORY Sulfonamide

Action and use

Sulfasalazine is a sulfonamide derivative poorly absorbed from the gastrointestinal tract. It does not have antibacterial properties although the intestinal flora may split the drug into sulfapyridine and a salicylate. Its exact mechanism of action is unknown. It is indicated in the treatment of ulcerative colitis, especially with prolonged administration when it may be effective in reducing the number of relapses in patients receiving maintenance therapy.

Administration and dosage
Adult

PO—Initially, 4 to 12 g daily in 4 to 8 divided doses. The usual adult maintenance dosage is 500 mg 4 times daily.
IM—Not available.
IV—Not available.

Pediatric (over 2 months of age)

PO—Initial, 40 to 60 mg/kg/24 hr in 3 to 6 doses; maintenance, 30 mg/kg/24 hr divided into 4 doses.

Special remarks and cautions

Common side effects include nausea, vomiting, anorexia, and gastric distress.
Sulfasalazine is partially absorbed from the gastrointestinal tract. Its metabolites may impart an orange-yellow color to an alkaline urine.
Patients who are sensitive to either salicylates or sulfonamides must use caution with this drug.
This drug has been reported to cause pancreatitis, with marked elevations in serum amylase.
See General information on sulfonamides (p. 27).

Drug interactions

See General information on sulfonamides (p. 27).

SULFAMETHOXAZOLE
(Gantanol)

AHFS 8:24
CATEGORY Sulfonamide antibiotic

Action and use

Similar to sulfisoxazole (p. 30).

Characteristics

Peak levels: 3 to 4 hr. Duration: about 12 hr. Protein binding: about 50% to 70%. Half-life: 10 to 11 hr. Metabolism: hepatic acetylation and glucuronidation. Excretion: 10% to 30% unchanged in urine. Dialysis: yes, H.

Administration and dosage
Adult

PO 1. Mild to moderate infections: 2 g initially, followed by 1 g 2 times daily.
    2. Severe infections: 2 g initially, followed by 1 g 3 times daily.
IM—Not available.
IV—Not available.

Pediatric (over 2 months of age)

NOTE: Sulfamethoxazole must not be administered to infants under 2 months of age.
PO—50 to 60 mg/kg (23 to 27 mg/lb) initially, followed by 25 to 30 mg/kg/24 hr in 2 divided doses. Do not exceed 75 mg/kg/24 hr.

Special remarks and cautions

See General information on sulfonamides (p. 27).

Drug interactions

See General information on sulfonamides (p. 27).

SULFISOXAZOLE

(Gantrisin)

AHFS 8:24
CATEGORY Sulfonamide antibiotic

Action and use

Sulfisoxazole is a short-acting sulfonamide that differs from other agents in this class because it is distributed only in extracellular body fluid. It is used in acute urinary tract infections caused by susceptible *E. coli, Klebsiella, S. aureus, P. mirabilis,* and *P. vulgaris.*

Characteristics

Protein binding: 80% to 90%. Half-life: 3 to 4 hr; Metabolism: hepatic acetylation 30%. Excretion: 95% in urine, 30% in acetylated form, in 24 hr. Therapeutic level: 9 to 10 mg/100 ml. Dialysis: yes, H, P.

Administration and dosage
Adult

PO—2 to 4 g initially, followed by 1 to 2 g every 4 to 6 hr.

IM—4 to 5 g every 12 hr. Injectable Gantrisin may be given without dilution.

IV—4 to 5 g every 12 hr. The 40% (2 g) injectable Gantrisin solution must be diluted to a 5% concentration. Dilute one 5-ml ampule with 35 ml of sterile distilled water. This provides a solution containing 50 mg/ml. Diluents other than sterile water may cause precipitation. Administration with other parenteral fluids is not recommended. Maximal urinary concentrations may be attained by alkalinizing the urine with sodium bicarbonate.

Pediatric (over 2 months of age)

NOTE: Sulfisoxazole must not be administered to infants under 2 months of age.

PO—75 mg/kg initially, followed by 150 mg/kg/24 hr in 4 to 6 divided doses. Total daily dose should not exceed 6 g.

IM—50 mg/kg initially, followed by 100 mg/kg/24 hr in 2 to 3 divided doses. Not more than 2 ml of the injection should be given IM in any one site.

IV—As for IM but divided in 4 equal doses.

Special remarks and cautions

See General information on sulfonamides (p. 27).

Sulfisoxazole may cause a hypersensitivity reaction, resulting in hepatitis with jaundice.

Sulfisoxazole may interfere with Urobilistix, resulting in a false-positive urine urobilinogen test.

Drug interactions

Sulfisoxazole may displace thiopental from protein-binding sites, potentiating the effects of thiopental anesthesia.

Sulfisoxazole has been shown to displace phenytoin (Dilantin) from protein-binding sites, resulting in higher active serum levels of the anticonvulsant.

Methotrexate may be displaced from protein-binding sites to the extent of increasing active methotrexate levels as much as 25%, thus enhancing the potential for methotrexate toxicity.

CO-TRIMOXAZOLE
(Bactrim, Septra)

AHFS 8:24
CATEGORY Combination sulfonamide-pyrimidine

Action and use

Co-trimoxazole is one of the few antibacterial combination products available. It contains sulfamethoxazole (p. 29) and trimethoprim in a 5:1 ratio. Trimethoprim and sulfamethoxazole act synergistically by blocking the formation of folic acid and the utilization of folic acid already formed by bacteria. This does not affect human use of folic acid since mammalian cells do not synthesize folic acid and are not as susceptible to trimethoprim, but utilize what is provided by the diet. Co-trimoxazole is used for acute and chronic urinary tract infections caused by susceptible *E. coli, Klebsiella* and *Enterobacter* species, *P. mirabilis, P. vulgaris,* and *P. morgani.* Co-trimoxazole is also approved for use in treating pneumonia caused by *Pneumocystis carinii* and otitis media caused by *H. influenzae* and *S. pneumoniae.* Investigations are currently under way for its use against other pathogenic organisms.

Characteristics

Sulfamethoxazole—see p. 29.
Trimethoprim—peak plasma levels: 1½ to 3 h. Protein binding: 30% to 70%. Half-life: 6 to 17 hr. Metabolism: hepatic. Excretion: 50% to 75%, unchanged in urine, 20% to 30% as metabolites in urine. Dialysis: yes, H.

Administration and dosage

Co-trimoxazole is available in the following dosage forms:
1. Tablets:
   a. 400 mg of sulfamethoxazole and 80 mg of trimethoprim.
   b. 800 mg of sulfamethoxayole and 160 mg of trimethoprim.
2. PO suspension: 200 mg of sulfamethoxazole and 40 mg of trimethoprim in flavored syrup/5 ml.

For urinary tract infections:

Adult

PO—800 mg of sulfamethoxazole and 160 mg of trimethoprim every 12 hr (see Special remarks and cautions).

Pediatric

Infants. Not recommended for use in infants under 2 months of age. See dosages for children.

Children

PO—40 mg/kg/24 hr of sulfamethoxazole and 8 mg/kg/24 hr of trimethoprim given in 2 divided doses (see Special remarks and cautions).

For *P. Carinii* pneumonitis:

Adult and pediatric

PO—100 mg/kg/24 hr of sulfamethoxazole and 20 mg/kg/24 hr of trimethoprim given in equally divided doses every 6 hr.
With renal impairment:
For patients with a creatinine clearance above 30 ml/min, use the above recommendations. For patients with a creatinine clearance between 15 and 30 ml/min give half (½) the

total daily recommended dose once every 24 hr. Do not use in patients with a creatinine clearance below 15 ml/min.

Special remarks and cautions

Patients must maintain adequate fluid intake to prevent crystalluria.

This combination of drugs may produce megaloblastic anemia due to interference with folic acid and vitamin B_{12} metabolism. Patients especially susceptible are those with low folic acid and vitamin B_{12} levels or those receiving pyrimethamine (Daraprim), a folic acid antagonist.

Teratogenic effects such as cleft palate have been reported in laboratory animals. Co-trimoxazole should not be used by pregnant or nursing women.

See General information on sulfonamides (p. 27).

Drug interactions

Leucovorin (folinic acid) may interfere with the antibacterial activity of co-trimoxazole, but may also be used to treat hematologic toxicities induced by co-trimoxazole.

See General information on sulfonamides (p. 27).

Other antibiotics
CHLORAMPHENICOL
(Chloromycetin, Amphicol, Mychel)

AHFS 8:12.08
CATEGORY Antibiotic

Action and use

Chloramphenicol is a bacteriostatic antibiotic that inhibits protein synthesis in susceptible organisms by binding to 50 S subunits of ribosomes, thus interfering with the formation of the peptide bond. Chloramphenicol may be the drug of choice in treatment of *Salmonella typhi* and *H. influenzae* meningitis. It may also be quite effective in rickettsial infections and in gram-negative bacteria causing bacteremia or meningitis. *It must not be used in the treatment of trivial infections or when it is not indicated, as in colds, influenza, throat infections, or as a prophylactic agent to prevent bacterial infection.*

Characteristics

Onset: 30 min. Peak plasma level: 2 hr (PO). Duration: 12 to 18 hr. Protein binding: 60%; Half-life: 3 to 4 hr. Metabolism: hepatic; Excretion: 80% to 90% in urine in 24 hours, 5% to 10% active; Dialysis: No, H, P.

Administration and dosage
Adult

PO 1. Normal renal and hepatic function: 50 mg/kg/day in 4 equally divided doses at 6-hr intervals. Moderately resistant organisms may require 100 mg/kg/day in divided doses. Reduce to 50 mg/kg/day as soon as clinically possible.
2. Impaired renal and/or hepatic function: 25 mg/kg/day in 4 equally divided doses.

IM— Not recommended because of maintenance of inadequate blood levels and poor clinical response.

IV— As recommended for PO administration for normal or impaired renal and hepatic function. Reconstitute by adding 11 ml of sterile water for injection or dextrose 5% to 1 g of chloramphenicol to make a solution containing 100 mg/ml. Administer the calculated dose intravenously over a 1-min period. PO therapy should replace parenteral therapy as soon as possible.

Pediatric

PO 1. Newborn infants and children in whom immature hepatic and/or renal function is suspected: 25 mg/kg/24 hr in 4 equally divided doses.
2. Infant over 2 weeks of age: to 50 mg/kg/24 hr in 4 equally divided doses.

IM— Not recommended.

IV— As for PO dosages. Administer IV over 1 min. Use only chloramphenicol sodium succinate IV in children. Do not use chloramphenicol in 50% *N,N*-dimethylacetamide (Chloromycetin solution). PO therapy should replace parenteral therapy as soon as possible.

Special remarks and cautions

Serious and fatal blood dyscrasias (aplastic anemia, hypoplastic anemia, thrombocytopenia, and agranulocytosis) are known to occur after administration of chloramphenicol. Two types of bone marrow suppression occur, one dose-related and reversible, the other nondose-related and irreversible. Various studies indicated an occurrence of this second type as 1 in 20 to 40 thousand; it may occur weeks to months after the discontinuance of the drug. It is recommended that baseline blood studies should be followed by periodic blood studies every 2 days and that the drug be discontinued as soon as clinically feasible. Early signs of blood dyscrasias include sore throat, malaise, elevated temperature, and petechiae.

Neurologic toxicities include headache, mental depression, confusion, and delirium.

Gastrointestinal side effects include nausea, vomiting, diarrhea, glossitis, stomatitis, and unpleasant taste in mouth.

Allergic manifestations to chloramphenicol include several types of rashes, hemorrhages, urticaria, and anaphylaxis.

Chloramphenicol produces "gray syndrome" in the fetus and neonatal infants. The syndrome results from immature metabolic enzyme systems. Chloramphenicol readily crosses the placental barrier and is secreted in breast milk and so must be used with extreme caution during pregnancy and in nursing women.

Chloramphenicol may cause a false-positive reaction when determining glucose content in the urine by the Clinitest method.

Drug interactions

Chloramphenicol markedly inhibits the metabolism of oral anticoagulants (warfarin). The prothrombin time must be monitored closely and the patient advised to watch for signs of overanticoagulation (easy bruisability, melena, or any episode of bleeding).

Chloramphenicol prolongs the half-life of oral hypoglycemic agents (tolbutamide, chlorpropamide). Reduction of the dosage of the oral hypoglycemic may be required, and the patient advised of signs of hypoglycemia (faintness, pallor, diaphoresis, increased irritability, seizures, or coma).

Chloramphenicol reduces the metabolism of phenytoin (Dilantin), doubling the half-life. Patients may develop manifestations of phenytoin toxicity such as nystagmus, ataxia, malaise, and lethargy. Reduction in the phenytoin dosage may be required.

CLINDAMYCIN
(Cleocin)

AHFS 8:12.28
CATEGORY Antibiotic

Action and use

Clindamycin is a bacteriostatic antibiotic that exerts its action by inhibiting protein formation. This agent's spectrum of activity includes gram-positive aerobic staphylococci, pneumococci, and streptococci and a variety of gram-positive and gram-negative anaerobes.

Characteristics

Peak plasma level: 1 hr (PO). Protein binding: 94%; Half-life; 2 to 2½ hr. Metabolism: hepatic. Excretion: 10% unchanged in urine. Dialysis: no, H, P.

Administration and dosage
Adult

PO—150 to 300 mg every 6 hr in mild to moderate infections; 300 to 450 mg every 6 hr in severe infections. To avoid thickening of the PO suspension, do not refrigerate. The solution is stable for 2 weeks at room temperature.

IM—600 to 2700 mg/24 hr. Do not exceed 600 mg/injection. Pain, induration, and sterile abscesses have been reported. Deep IM injection is recommended to help minimize this reaction.

IV—600 to 2700 mg/24 hr. Dilute to less than 6 mg/ml. Administer at a rate less than 30 mg/min. Administration by IV push is not recommended.

Pediatric (over 1 month of age)

PO 1. Suspension:
    a. Mild infections: 8 to 12 mg/kg/24 hr in divided doses.
    b. Moderate infections: 13 to 16 mg/kg/24 hr in divided doses.
    c. Severe infections: 17 to 25 mg/kg/24 hr in divided doses. In patients weighing 10 kg or less the minimum PO dose recommended is 37.5 mg (½ teaspoon) 3 times daily.
  2. Capsules:
    a. Mild to moderate infections: 8 to 16 mg/kg/24 hr in divided doses.
    b. Severe infections: 16 to 20 mg/kg/24 hr in divided doses.
    Capsules should be taken with a full glass of water to prevent esophageal irritation.

IM 1. Mild to moderate infections: 15 to 25 mg/kg/24 hrs in 3 to 4 divided doses.
  2. Severe infections: 25 to 40 mg/kg/24 hr in 3 or 4 divided doses. It is recommended that children be given no less than 300 mg/day regardless of body weight.

IV—As for IM use. Dilute to less than 6 mg/ml and administer at a rate less than 30 mg/min.

Special remarks and cautions

Severe and persistent diarrhea may develop from the use of this drug. If significant diarrhea results (more than 5 bowel movements per day), the drug should be discontinued. The use of opiates, meperidine, and diphenoxylate with atropine (Lomotil) may prolong and/or worsen the condition. Large doses of kaolin-pectin (Kaopectate) may be effective in diminishing the diarrhea.

Hypersensitivity reactions often manifested by rashes, jaundice, abnormal liver function tests, and bone marrow suppression have been reported in patients being treated with this agent.

Bitter taste caused by possible secretion of clindamycin in saliva has been reported with both oral and parenteral administration.

Drug interactions

Kaolin-pectin may physically absorb clindamycin and impare absorption from the gastrointestinal tract.

Antagonism has been reported between clindamycin and erythromycin when administered concomitantly.

Clindamycin may potentiate neuromuscular blockade in patients recovering from the effects of surgical muscle relaxants (tubocurarine, succinylcholine, gallamine triethiodide [Flaxedil]) and antibiotics (gentamicin, streptomycin, kanamycin, amikacin, and tobramycin).

ERYTHROMYCIN
(Ilosone, Erythrocin, E-Mycin, Ilotycin)

AHFS 8:12.12
CATEGORY Macrolide antibiotic

Action and use

The mechanism of action of erythromycin is inhibition of protein synthesis in susceptible microorganisms. This bacteriostatic agent is indicated as an alternate drug of choice in
the treatment of mild to moderate infections produced by group A beta-hemolytic streptococcus, alpha-hemolytic streptococcus (viridans group), *S. aureus, D. pneumoniae, T. pallidum,* and *Corynelbacterium diphtheriae.* Erythromycin may also be used as an alternate
antibiotic against susceptible organisms in patients allergic to penicillin.

Characteristics

Peak plasma level: 1 to 4 hr (PO). Protein binding: 73%. Half-life: 1⅕ hr. Excretion:
primarily fecal, 2% to 5% unchanged in urine (PO), 12% to 15% unchanged in urine (IV).
Dialysis: no, H, P.

Administration and dosage
Adult

PO—250 mg 4 times a day for 10 to 14 days. Administer at least 1 hr before or 2 hr after
    meals.
IM—100 mg every 4 to 6 hr. As a result of pain on injection, adequate dosages for the
    treatment of serious or severe infections with IM erythromycin are difficult to achieve.
    IM injection of erythromycin may also result in sterile abscess formation and necro-
    sis.
IV—15 to 20 mg/kg/day. If erythromycin is to be given IV, the medication should be given
    by intermittent rapid infusion. One fourth of the total daily dose can be given in 20 to 60
    min by infusion of 250 to 500 mg as an initial solution added to 100 to 250 ml of saline
    solution or dextrose 5%. Thrombophlebitis after IV infusion is a relatively common side
    effect.

Pediatric

PO—30 to 50 mg/kg/24 hr in 4 divided doses. For severe infections this dose may be
    doubled.
IM—Not recommended in infants or children.
IV—15 to 20 mg/kg/24 hr in 3 divided doses.

Special remarks and cautions

The most common side effects of oral erythromycin products are epigastric distress with
possible nausea and vomiting.

The administration of erythromycin estolate (Ilosone) has been associated with an
allergic type of cholestatic hepatitis. Some patients receiving Ilosone for more than 2 weeks
or in repeated courses have developed jaundice accompanied by right upper quadrant pain,
fever, nausea, vomiting, eosinophilia, and leukocytosis.

Since erythromycin is principally excreted via the liver, caution should be exercised in
administering the antibiotic to patients with imparied hepatic function.

Drug interactions

The use of bacteriostatic erythromycin is not recommended in patients receiving bactericidal antibiotics, such as penicillin. If used concomitantly, start the penicillin several hours
before the erythromycin and use adequate doses of each antibiotic.

TETRACYCLINE

AHFS 8:24.24

(Panmycin, Sumycin, Mysteclin, Achromycin V, Tetracyn)

CATEGORY   Tetracycline antibiotic

Action and use

Tetracycline is a bacteriostatic agent that attaches to ribosomes, preventing the binding of transfer-RNA and thus inhibiting protein synthesis in susceptible organisms. Tetracycline is recommended as an alternative for patients hypersensitive to other antibiotics. It is used primarily for the treatment of gram-positive organisms resistant to penicillin, gram-negative bacillary infections, and rickettsial diseases. Because many strains of organisms are becoming resistant to tetracyclines, culture and sensitivity tests are recommended.

Characteristics

Protein binding: 25% to 30%. Half-life: 7 to 11 hr. Metabolism: hepatic. Excretion: 20% to 55% unchanged in urine. Dialysis: no, H, P. See Table 1-5 for a comparison of the tetracyclines.

Administration and dosage
Adult

PO—250 to 500 mg every 6 hr. Administer 1 hr before or 2 hr after the intake of food, milk, or antacids.

IM—250 to 300 mg every 8 to 12 hr. IM injections may cause pain and induration, which may be minimized by deep injections. Patients placed on IM tetracycline should be switched to the PO form as soon as possible.

IV—250 to 500 mg every 6 to 12 hr by infusion over 30 min to 1 hr. Rapid infusions or prolonged therapy may result in a relatively high incidence of thrombophlebitis. Nausea, vomiting, fever, chills, and hypotension may result from rapid infusion and dosages greater than 750 mg.

NOTE: Patients who are pregnant or who have impaired hepatic or renal dysfunction may accumulate toxic serum levels of tetracycline. These patients may also develop further azotemia, hyperphosphatemia, and acidosis caused by enhanced catabolism. Dosages should be reduced to one third to one half the normal dose, or the dosage interval extended 2 to 3 times the normal interval. Administration is not recommended if the creatinine clearance is less than 10 ml/min.

Special remarks and cautions

Anorexia, nausea, vomiting, and diarrhea are common side effects.

Photosensitivity manifested by an exaggerated sunburn reaction has been observed. Patients should be cautioned to avoid unnecessary direct sunlight or ultraviolet light and to watch for early erythema when exposed.

The use of tetracycline during tooth development (the last half of pregnancy, infancy, and childhood to 8 years of age) may cause enamel hypoplasia and permanent staining of the teeth (yellow, gray, or brown). Tetracycline therefore should not be used in this age group unless other drugs are not likely to be effective or are contraindicated.

Tetracyclines are present in the milk of lactating women; therefore infant nourishment by formula is recommended during the mother's tetracycline therapy.

In long-term therapy routine evaluation of the hematopoietic, hepatic, and renal organs should be performed. Leukocytosis, neutropenia, hemolytic anemia, elevated transaminases, bilirubin, alkaline phosphatase, and blood urea nitrogen have been reported. All may be caused by toxicity from tetracycline, so plans for clinical therapy must be reevaluated.

Tetracycline may produce a false-positive urine glucose using Clinitest and a false-negative value when using Clinistix or Tes-tape. These results may actually be caused by ascorbic acid that is used as a stabilizer in parenteral formulations of tetracycline.

Drug interactions

Iron, milk, food, and antacids containing magnesium, calcium, or aluminum inhibit the absorption of tetracycline. PO tetracycline should be administered 1 hr before or 2 hr after these products.

Tetracycline has been shown to decrease plasma prothrombin activity through several postulated mechanisms. Patients receiving tetracycline and anticoagulants (warfarin) should have frequent evaluation of the prothrombin time and may require a reduction in the dosage of the oral anticoagulant.

Nephrotoxicity and fatalities have resulted from concomitant use of methoxyflurane (Penthrane) and tetracycline.

The use of bactericidal antibiotics (cephalosporins, penicillins) with bacteriostatic antibiotics such as tetracycline is not recommended except in special situations.

DOXYCYCLINE
(Vibramycin)

AHFS 8:12.24
CATEGORY Tetracycline antibiotic

Action and use

Doxycycline has a mechanism of action and spectrum of antibacterial activity against both gram-positive and gram-negative organisms similar to tetracycline. A particular advantage of doxycycline is its use in patients with renal insufficiency. Serum levels do not accumulate and there is no significant rise in the BUN level as often occurs with other tetracyclines in patients with renal dysfunction.

Characteristics

Protein binding: 25% to 93%. Half-life: 14 to 22 hr. Metabolism: hepatic. Excretion: 90% fecal, inactive. Dialysis: no, H, P.

Administration and dosage
Adult

PO—First 24 hr: 100 mg every 12 hr; maintenance: 100 to 200 mg/day.
IM—Not available.
IV—First 24 hr: 200 mg; maintenance: 100 to 200 mg/day.
NOTE: PO therapy should be instituted as soon as possible. The duration of infusion may vary with the dose, but is usually 1 to 4 hr. A recommended minimum infusion time for 100 mg of a 0.5 mg/ml solution is 1 hr. Rapid infusions or prolonged therapy may result in a relatively high incidence of thrombophlebitis. Nausea, vomiting, fever, chills, and hypotension may result from rapid infusion.

Special remarks and cautions

See the Special remarks and cautions of tetracycline (p. 38).

If gastric irritation occurs, doxycycline may be given with food or milk. Absorption is not significantly influenced by food or milk as with other tetracyclines.

Drug interactions

See the Drug interactions of tetracycline (above).

Phenytoin (Dilantin) and carbamazepine (Tegretol) may significantly shorten the serum half-life of doxycycline, reducing its therapeutic efficacy.

AHFS 8:12.24

Table 1-5. A comparison of the tetracyclines*

Tetracycline	Peak levels	Duration (hr)	Protein binding (%)	Half-life (hr)	Excretion	Dialysis H	Dialysis P	Dosage† Neonate	Dosage† Child	Dosage† Adult
Chlortetracycline (Aureomycin)	2-4 hr (PO)	—	43-70	9	10%-15% excreted unchanged in urine	No	No	PO: 100 mg/kg/day in 2 divided doses; IV: 10-15 mg/kg/day in 2 divided doses	PO: 25-50 mg/kg/day in 4 divided doses; IV: 10-20 mg/kg/day in 2 divided doses	PO: 250 mg every 6 hr; IV: 250-500 mg every 6-12 hr; Do not exceed 2 g daily
Demeclocycline (Declomycin)	—	24-48	36-91	10-17	10%-25% excreted unchanged in urine	No	No	—	PO: 6-12 mg/kg/day in 2-4 divided doses	PO: 600 mg daily in 2-4 divided doses
Methacycline (Rondomycin)	—	24-48	75-90	11-14	50% excreted unchanged in urine	No	No	—	PO: 6-12 mg/kg/day in 2-4 divided doses	PO: 600 mg daily in 2-4 divided doses
Minocycline (Minocin, Vectrin)	2 hr (PO)	12	70-75	11-18	12% excreted unchanged in urine	?	?	—	PO or IV: 4 mg/kg initially; 2 mg/kg every 12 hr	PO or IV: 200 mg initially; 100 mg every 12 hr
Oxytetracycline (Terramycin)	2-4 hr (PO)	—	20-35	5	10%-35% excreted unchanged in urine	No	No	PO: 100 mg/kg/day in 2 divided doses; IV: 10-15 mg/kg/day in 2 divided doses	PO: 25-50 mg/kg/day in 2-4 divided doses; IM: 15-25 mg/kg/day in 2-4 divided doses; IV: 10-20 mg/kg/day in 2 divided doses	PO: 250 mg every 6 hr; IM: 100-250 mg every 12 hr; IV: 250-500 mg every 6-12 hr; Do not exceed 2 g daily

*For Special remarks and cautions see p. 38; for Drug interactions see p. 38; for discussion on doxycycline see p. 39; for discussion on tetracycline see p. 38.

†Food interferes with absorption of PO dosage forms. Administer at least 1 hr before or 2 hr after meals.

SPECTINOMYCIN HYDROCHLORIDE
(*Trobicin*)

AHFS 8:12.28
CATEGORY Antibiotic

Action and use

Spectinomycin binds to and inhibits the 30 S ribosomal unit required for protein synthesis of the bacterial cell.

The drug is a bacteriostatic agent used specifically for the treatment of acute gonorrheal urethritis and proctitis in the male and acute gonorrheal cervicitis and proctitis in the female when caused by susceptible strains of *N. gonorrhoeae.* A particular advantage is that most strains of the organism respond to one administration of the recommended dosage.

Characteristics

Peak serum level: 1 hr (IM). Protein binding: insignificant. Metabolism: insignificant. Excretion: active form in urine.

Administration and dosage

IM—A 20-gauge needle is recommended. IM injections should be made deep into the upper outer quadrant of the gluteal muscle. Male: 2 g (5 ml); female: 2 to 4 g (5 to 10 ml) divided into 2 sites.

NOTE: Safety for use in infants and children has not been established.

Special remarks and cautions

Spectinomycin provides an alternative to penicillin in the treatment of acute, susceptible gonococcal infections. It is not effective in the treatment of syphilis.

Pain at the site of injection is a common side effect.

Urticaria, nausea, chills, and fever are other possible side effects of single-dose therapy.

Safe use in pregnancy has not been established.

Drug interactions

None have specifically been reported.

Urinary antimicrobial agents
METHENAMINE MANDELATE
(Mandelamine)

AHFS 8:36
CATEGORY Urinary antibacterial agent

Action and use

Methenamine mandelate is essentially inactive until it is concentrated and excreted in an acidic urine. Methenamine, in an acidic environment such as an acid urine, produces ammonia and formaldehyde. Formaldehyde is a nonspecific antibacterial agent effective against both gram-positive and gram-negative organisms. The acid portion of the methenamine salt (mandelic acid) provides antiseptic properties while aiding in urinary acidification.

Methenamine mandelate is used in the antibacterial treatment of pyelonephritis, cystitis, pyelitis, and other chronic urinary tract infections. It should not be used alone in the control of acute infections. If urinary acidification is unattainable because of ammonia-producing bacteria such as *P. aeruginosa* or *A. aerogenes,* methenamine therapy is not recommended.

Administration and dosage
Adult

PO—1 g 4 times daily, after meals and at bedtime.

Pediatric
Under 6 years of age

PO—250 mg/13.5 kg 4 times daily. Do not crush the tablets prior to administration.

Six to 12 years of age

PO—50 mg 4 times daily.

Special remarks and cautions

The optimal effect of methenamine occurs in urine with a pH of 5.5 or less. Test the urine with pH paper to determine whether a urinary acidifier, such as ascorbic acid 500 mg 4 times daily, may be required.

Side effects include nausea, vomiting, skin rash, and pruritus.

Drug interactions

Acetazolamide (Diamox) and sodium bicarbonate tend to render the urine more aklaline, preventing proper conversion of methenamine to free formaldehyde in the urine.

Sulfamethizole (Thiosulfil) may form an unsoluble precipitate in acidic urine. Therefore concomitant use of methenamine salts and sulfamethizole should be avoided.

NALIDIXIC ACID
(NegGram)

AHFS 8:36
CATEGORY Urinary antibacterial agent

Action and use

Although the exact mechanism of action is unknown, nalidixic acid has marked antibacterial activity against gram-negative bacteria. The agent is bactericidal and is effective over a wide urinary pH range.

Nalidixic acid is indicated for the treatment of urinary tract infections caused by susceptible gram-negative microorganisms.

Characteristics

Protein binding: 93% to 97%. Half-life: 8 hr. Metabolism: hepatic, inactive. Excretion: urinary. Dialysis: unknown.

Administration and dosage
Adult

PO—1 g 4 times daily for 1 to 2 weeks. For prolonged therapy administer 2 g daily after the initial treatment period.

Pediatric (3 months to 12 years of age)

NOTE: Do not administer to infants under 3 months of age.
PO—55 mg/kg/24 hr initially in 4 divided doses. For prolonged therapy the total daily dosage should be reduced to 33 mg/kg/24 hr.

Special remarks and cautions

The more common side effects of nalidixic acid include nausea and vomiting. Other side effects include drowsiness, headache, dizziness, and weakness.

Visual disturbances such as overbrightness of lights, change in color perception, difficulty in focusing, and double vision may occur with each dose during the first few days of therapy.

Toxic psychosis or convulsions have been reported. Predisposing factors include excessive dosage and patients with epilepsy or cerebral arteriosclerosis.

Patients receiving nalidixic acid therapy should avoid undue exposure to sunlight since photosensitivity may occur.

Nalidixic acid may cause false-positive urine glucose tests with Clinitest, but not with Tes-Tape or Clinistix.

Nalidixic acid may induce a hemolytic anemia in those patients with glucose-6-phosphate dehydrogenase deficiency. This deficiency is found in 10% of blacks and in a small percentage of ethnic groups of Mediterranean and Near Eastern origin.

Drug interactions

The dosage of oral anticoagulants (warfarin) may need to be reduced. Nalidixic acid may displace significant amounts of warfarin from serum protein-binding sites, resulting in hemorrhage.

NITROFURANTOIN
(*Furadantin, Macrodantin*)

AHFS 8:36
CATEGORY Urinary antibacterial agent

Action and use

Nitrofurantoin is an antibacterial agent for specific urinary tract infections. It is bacteriostatic in low concentrations and possibly bactericidal in higher concentrations. Its mechanism of action is thought to be based on its interference with several bacterial enzyme systems.

Nitrofurantoin is indicated for the treatment of pyelonephritis, pyelitis, and cystitis when caused by susceptible organisms. The drug does not appear to be effective on bacteria in blood or tissue outside the genitourinary tract.

Characteristics

Half-life: 20 min to 1 hr. Excretion: 40% unchanged in urine. Therapeutic level: 0.18 mg/100 ml; Dialysis: yes, H.

Administration and dosage
Adult

PO—50 to 100 mg 4 times daily for 10 to 14 days.

Pediatric (over 1 month of age)

NOTE: Do *not* use in infants under 1 month of age.
PO—5 to 7 mg/kg/24 hr in 4 divided doses.

Special remarks and cautions

Anorexia, nausea, and vomiting are the most frequent side effects of nitrofurantoin. Reduction of dosage and administration with food or milk may minimize gastric upset.

The clinically effective use of nitrofurantoin is dependent on adequate concentration of the drug in the urine. The agent is not recommended for use in patients with a creatinine clearance of less than 40 ml/min.

Severe peripheral neuropathies may result from use of nitrofurantoin. Predisposing conditions such as renal impairment, anemia, diabetes, electrolyte imbalance, vitamin B deficiency, and debilitating disease may enhance the risk of this side effect. The drug should be discontinued at the first sign of numbness or tingling in the extremities.

Metabolites of this agent may change the color of the urine to rust, yellow, or brown.

Allergic reactions manifested by dyspnea, chills, fever, erythematous rash, and pruritus have been reported. Acute reactions usually develop within 8 hr in previously sensitized patients and within 7 to 10 days in patients who develop sensitivity during the course of therapy.

Nitrofurantoin may induce a hemolytic anemia in those patients with glucose-6-phosphate dehydrogenase deficiency. This deficiency is found in 10% of blacks and in a small percentage of ethnic groups of Mediterranean and Near Eastern origin.

Nitrofurantoin may induce hemolytic anemia caused by immature enzyme systems in infants younger than 3 months of age. This caution includes mothers nursing these infants since the drug is excreted in breast milk.

Drug interactions

No clinically significant adverse reactions have been reported.

PHENAZOPYRIDINE HYDROCHLORIDE
(Pyridium)

AHFS 8:36
CATEGORY Urinary analgesic

Action and use

Phenazopyridine exerts an anesthetic effect on the mucosa of the urinary tract as it is excreted in the urine. It is used for symptomatic relief of pain, burning, urgency, and frequency arising from irritation of the lower urinary tract.

Administration and dosage
Adult

PO—200 mg 3 times daily.

Pediatric (6 to 12 years of age)

PO—100 mg 3 times daily.

Special remarks and cautions

Phenazopyridine produces a reddish orange discoloration of the urine.

A yellowish tinge to the sclera or the skin may indicate accumulation caused by diminished renal function. The drug should be discontinued if this manifestation results.

This agent is frequently used in combination with sulfonamides (Azo Gantanol and Azo Gantrisin). The same side effects apply, as well as those of the sulfonamides.

Drug interactions

No clinically significant adverse reactions have been reported.

Antifungal agents
AMPHOTERICIN B
(*Fungizone*)

AHFS 8:12.04
CATEGORY Antifungal agent

Action and use

Amphotericin B is a fungistatic agent that binds to sterols in the fungal cell membrane. Alterations in permeability result in the loss of cellular contents. Amphotericin B is primarily used in the treatment of systemic fungal infections and meningitis.

Characteristics

Protein binding: 90%. Half-life: 18 to 24 hr. Metabolism: unknown. Excretion: urine (inactive). Dialysis: No.

Administration and dosage
Adult

NOTE:
1. Amphotericin B must be reconstituted with sterile water for injection without bacteriostatic agent.
2. An in-line membrane filter must *not* be used during infusion.
3. The infusion must be protected from light during administration.
4. The recommended infusion concentration is 1 mg/10 ml of dextrose 5% in water.

IV—Initially 250 μg/kg over a 6-hr period. The daily dose is gradually increased as patient tolerance develops. Dosage may range up to 1 mg/kg daily or up to 1.5 mg/kg on alternate days. Under no circumstances should a single administration dosage exceed 1.5 mg/kg. Venous irritation may be diminished by the addition of 1200 to 1600 units of heparin and/or 10 to 15 mg of hydrocortisone or methylprednisolone to the infusion solution.

INTRATHECAL—25 to 50 μg diluted with 10 to 20 ml of cerebrospinal fluid. The drug is administered 2 or 3 times per week. This dosage is gradually increased to 500 μg to 1 mg, depending on tolerance.

TOPICAL—Amphotericin B is applied liberally to candidal lesions 2 to 4 times daily. Any staining from cream or lotion preparations may be removed by soap and warm water, and any staining from amphotericin ointment may be removed by standard cleaning fluids.

Special remarks and cautions

Side effects of this drug are usually dose related and may be minimized by slow infusion, reduction of dosage, and alternate-day administration. They include headache, chills, fever, malaise, muscle and joint pain, cramping, nausea, and vomiting. Antipyretics, antihistamines, and antiemetics may provide some symptomatic relief.

Amphotericin B is nephrotoxic. The BUN and serum creatinine levels elevate in nearly all patients and should be monitored routinely. Urinary excretion of uric acid, potassium, and magnesium increases, and proteinuria may occur. Other potentially nephrotoxic agents, such as aminoglycoside antibiotics, should be given with caution.

.　A reversible normochromic normocytic anemia is common.

Drug interactions

Corticosteroids may enhance the potassium excretion caused by amphotericin B. The patient's electrolyte status should be watched closely.

CLOTRIMAZOLE
(Lotrimin, Gyne-Lotrimin)

AHFS 84:04.08
CATEGORY Antifungal agent

Action and use

Clotrimazole is a synthetic topical fungicidal agent that apparently acts by altering cell membrane permeability, resulting in loss of intracellular electrolytes. It has been shown to be effective against tinea pedis (athlete's foot), tinea cruris (jock itch), and tinea corporis caused by *Tricophyton rubrum, T. mentagrophytes,* and *Epiderophyton floccosum.* It is also effective in the treatment of vulvovaginitis (candidiasis) caused by *Candida albicans.*

Administration and dosage

TOPICAL—Clotrimazole is commercially available as a 1% cream and lotion (Lotrimin). The cream or lotion should be gently rubbed on the affected areas and surrounding skin morning and evening. Clinical improvement should be evident (relief of pruritus) within a week. If there is no improvement within 4 weeks, rediagnosis should be considered. Both the cream and solution should be stored between 2 and 30 C.

INTRAVAGINAL—For the treatment of candidiasis insert 1 clotrimazole 100 mg tablet (Gyne-Lotrimin) into the vagina at bedtime for 7 consecutive days.

Special remarks and cautions

The only adverse reactions reported with clotrimazole are in those patients who have developed hypersensitivity reactions to any of the ingredients. Adverse effects are manifested by pruritus, urticaria, blistering, and erythema. Discontinue treatment if any adverse effects develop.

Therapy with clotrimazole during the first 3 months of pregnancy is not recommended. No adverse effects have been reported when used during the second and third trimesters of pregnancy.

Drug interactions

No specific drug interactions have been reported.

FLUCYTOSINE
(Ancobon)

AHFS 8:12.04
CATEGORY Antifungal agent

Action and use

Flucytosine is a nonantibiotic antifungal agent. Its mechanism of action is unknown, but it is effective against susceptible candidal septicemia, endocarditis, urinary tract infections, cryptococcal meningitis, and pulmonary infections.

Characteristics

Peak plasma levels: 2 hr. Protein binding: 50%; Half-life: 3 to 4 hr. Excretion: 90% unchanged in urine. Dialysis: yes, H, P.

Administration and dosage
Adult

NOTE: Close monitoring of hematologic, renal, and hepatic status is essential.

PO—50 to 150 mg/kg/day given at 6-hr intervals. Doses up to 250 mg/kg/day may be required in cryptococcal meningitis. Nausea may be reduced if the capsules are given a few at a time over 20 to 30 min. Dosage adjustment is required in patients with impaired renal function as a result of the high urinary content of unmetabolized drug.

Special remarks and cautions

Many of the potentially serious adverse effects of flucytosine are related to affects on rapidly proliferating tissues, especially in the bone marrow and mucosa of the gastrointestinal tract. Indications of this are leukopenia, pancytopenia, anemia, thrombocytopenia, nausea, vomiting, and diarrhea.

Decrease in hemoglobin levels and elevation of alkaline phosphatase, SGOT, SGPT, BUN, and serum creatinine levels are common. Elevations of liver function tests generally appear to be dose related and reversible.

Other side effects include confusion, hallucinations, headache, sedation, and vertigo.

Caution must be used prenatally and postnatally since flucytosine has produced birth defects in laboratory animals.

Use with caution in patients with impaired renal function.

Drug interactions

Flucytosine and amphotericin B display synergistic activity when used concomitantly. It is proposed that amphotericin B affects the fungal cell membrane, allowing greater penetration of flucytosine.

GRISEOFULVIN

(Grisactin, Grifulvin V, Fulvicin-U/F, Gris-PEG, Fulvicin P/G)

AHFS 8:12.04
CATEGORY Antifungal agent

Action and use

Griseofulvin is a fungistatic agent used to treat ringworm infections of skin, hair, and nails. Its proposed mechanism of action is destruction of the fungal cell's mitotic spindle structure, preventing cell division and multiplication. Since griseofulvin is only active against certain species of fungi and not against bacterial or yeast infection, the infecting organism should be identified as a dermatophyte before initiating therapy.

Characteristics

Half-life: 9 to 24 hr. Metabolism: minimal; Excretion: less than 1% in urine, primarily unchanged in feces.

Administration and dosage
Adult

PO—Depending on the specific organism and the location of the infection, 500 mg to 4 g in single or divided doses daily. Absorption from the gastrointestinal tract may be increased by giving the drug with a meal high in fat content.

Special remarks and cautions

The length of treatment depends on the time required for the replacement of infected skin, hair, or nails. Treatment of skin infections may require only a few weeks of therapy, while infections of toenails may require at least 6 months of continuous treatment.

Hypersensitivity reactions manifesting as skin rashes and urticaria are relatively common adverse effects of griseofulvin. Others include headaches especially in oral therapy, oral thrush, nausea, vomiting, diarrhea, dizziness, and confusion.

The patient should be advised concerning possible photosensitivity reaction to sunlight. Proper hygiene and continuation of therapy beyond remission of symptoms is essential.

During prolonged therapy, periodic laboratory tests should be completed to warn of changes in renal, hepatic, and hematopoietic function. Leukopenia and proteinuria have been reported. Acute attacks of intermittent porphyria have been related to the use of griseofulvin.

Use with caution in pregnancy. Embryogenic and teratogenic effects have been observed in laboratory animals.

Drug interactions

Griseofulvin may induce hepatic enzymes to increase metabolism of warfarin. Griseofulvin therapy must not be started or stopped while patients are taking oral anticoagulants without monitoring the prothrombin time.

Phenobarbital impairs the absorption of griseofulvin. If concomitant therapy is required, divided doses 3 times daily may be absorbed better than larger doses taken less often.

MICONAZOLE NITRATE
(Monistat, Micatin)

AHFS 84:04.08
CATEGORY Antifungal agent

Action and use

Miconazole nitrate is a topical antifungal agent that has been shown to be effective against tinea pedis (athlete's foot), tinea cruris (jock itch), and tinea corporis caused by *T. rubrum, T. mentagrophytes*, and *E. floccosum*. It is also effective in the treatment of vulvovaginitis (candidiasis) caused by *C. albicans*. Although the exact mechanism of action is unknown, miconazole alters cell membrane permeability, resulting in the loss of intracellular constituents.

Administration and dosage

TOPICAL—Miconazole nitrate is available as a 2% cream or lotion (Micatin). The cream should be gently rubbed on the affected areas and surrounding skin morning and evening. The lotion is recommended for use in intertriginous areas and is applied in the same manner. Clinical improvement should be evident (relief of pruritus) within 1 week. If no improvement is noted within 4 weeks, reexamination and diagnosis should be considered.

INTRAVAGINAL—For treatment of candidiasis insert 1 applicatorful (Monistat-7 vaginal cream) intravaginally once daily at bedtime for 7 days.

NOTE: Miconazole nitrate is not effective in treating vulvovaginitis caused by *Trichomonas* species or *Haemophilus vaginalis*.

Special remarks and cautions

Miconazole nitrate may cause irritation, burning, and erythema in a few patients. If a hypersensitivity reaction or chemical irritation occurs, discontinue use.

Avoid eye contact with any of the miconazole products. Wash eyes immediately if contact should occur.

Miconazole is effective in pregnant and nonpregnant women; however, intravaginal use of Monistat-7 is not recommended during the first trimester of pregnancy.

Drug interactions

No specific drug interactions have been reported.

NYSTATIN
(Mycostatin, Nilstat)

AHFS 8:12.04
CATEGORY Antifungal agent

Action and use

Nystatin is an antifungal antibiotic used in the treatment of monilial infections of the skin, oral cavity, vulvovaginal mucosa, and intestinal tract. It is not effective in the treatment of systemic monilial infections. Antifungal activity is derived from nystatin binding to sterols within the fungal cell membrane, resulting in the loss of selective permeability.

Administration and dosage

PO 1. Gastrointestinal tract: 500,000 to 1 million units 3 times daily.
2. Oral cavity: 400,000 to 600,000 units of suspension 4 times daily. The suspension should be retained in the mouth for several minutes before swallowing if possible.

Treatment of the oral cavity and gastrointestinal tract should be continued for at least 48 hr after remission of symptoms and after cultures have returned to normal flora.

Pediatric

Infants. Administer 200,000 units (2 ml) 4 times daily (1 ml in each side of the mouth). For premature and low birth weight infants administer 100,000 units (1 ml) 4 times daily.

Children. As for adult dosages.

Special remarks and cautions

Side effects are uncommon with nystatin, although administration of the tablets and suspension may produce transient nausea, vomiting, and diarrhea. Hypersensitivity to nystatin is quite rare; however, patients more commonly develop a contact dermatitis to the preservatives in the topical preparations.

When treating topical candidal infection the powder is recommended where the lesions are moist, such as in skin folds or on feet. The affected areas should be kept dry and exposed to air if possible. Concomitant therapy must include proper hygiene to prevent reinfection.

Drug interactions

No specific interactions have been reported.

TOLNAFTATE
(Tinactin)

AHFS 84:04.08
CATEGORY Antifungal agent

Action and use

Tolnaftate is a fungistatic and fungicidal agent effective against *T. rubrum, T. menta-grophytes, T. tonsurans,* and various *Microsporum* and *Aspergillus* species. Tolnaftate is commonly used to treat tinea pedis (athlete's foot), tinea cruris (jock itch), tinea corporis, and tinea manuum when caused by the above fungal pathogens. The mechanism of action is unknown. Tolnaftate is not effective against the yeastlike *C. albicans.*

Administration and dosage

TOPICAL—Tolnaftate is available in cream, solution, powder, and spray powder, all in 1% concentrations. All the products may be used interchangeably; however, the powder is most effective in intertriginous areas and in cases when a dry environment may enhance the therapeutic response. Only small amounts of the cream or solution are necessary for therapy. Dry the affected areas, apply, and gently massage in until the medication disappears. Apply the medication 2 times daily for 2 to 3 weeks. Clinical improvement should be observed within 2 to 3 days. Treatments may be required for 6 weeks or more with long-standing infections and in areas with thickened skin. If no improvement is evident after 4 weeks, the diagnosis should be reviewed.

Special remarks and cautions

Adverse effects with tolnaftate are quite infrequent. Local irritation and burning have been reported when the medication has been applied to excoriated skin or to lesions caused by multiple pathogens. Discontinue therapy if the lesions get worse or if there is evidence of hypersensitivity (pruritus, urticaria, erythema).

Avoid contact with the eyes. Wash the eyes immediately if contact occurs.

Drug interactions

No specific drug interactions have been reported.

Trichomonacidal agent
METRONIDAZOLE
(Flagyl)

AHFS 8:32
CATEGORY Trichomonacide

Actions and use

Metronidazole is used in the treatment of trichomoniasis of the urogenital tract and of amebic dysentery and amebic liver abscess. The mechanism of action is as yet unknown.

Administration and dosage
Adult

TRICHOMONIASIS   1. Females: 250 mg PO 3 times daily for 7 days.
2. Males: 250 mg PO 3 times daily for 7 days.
NOTE: Sexual partners should be treated concurrently to prevent reinfection.
3. Recent reports indicate that a single 2-g dose provides adequate treatment for trichomoniasis in both sexes.

AMEBIC DYSENTERY—750 mg 3 times daily for 5 to 10 days.

GIARDIASIS—250 mg PO 2 to 3 times daily for 5 to 10 days.

Pediatric

TRICHOMONIASIS—35 to 50 mg/kg/24 hr PO divided into 3 doses for 7 days.

GIARDIASIS—As for adult dosages.

Special remarks and cautions

The most common side effects are nausea, headache, anorexia, and occasionally vomiting, diarrhea, and abdominal cramping. An unpleasant metallic taste is also common.

Mild, reversible leukopenia is occasionally observed, and follow-up white cell counts with differential are recommended after therapy.

Overgrowth of oral and vaginal monilia may result in furry tongue, glossitis, stomatitis, vaginal itching and burning, and urethral irritation.

Metronidazole therapy may impart a reddish-brown discoloration to the urine, especially when higher doses are used.

Metronidazole crosses the placental barrier and passes rapidly into fetal circulation. The drug is also excreted in breast milk. Metronidazole should generally not be used in pregnant women.

Drug interactions

Consumption of alcoholic beverages during metronidazole therapy may result in abdominal cramping, vomiting, and flushing (antabuse-like reaction).

Antitubercular agents
ETHAMBUTOL HYDROCHLORIDE
(*Myambutol*)

AHFS 8:16
CATEGORY Antitubercular agent

Action and use

Ethambutol is a bacteriostatic agent used in combination with other chemotherapy in the treatment of pulmonary tuberculosis. Its mode of action is inhibition of RNA synthesis and phosphate metabolism, resulting in inhibition of cellular multiplication.

Characteristics

Peak plasma level: 2 to 4 hr (PO). Half-life: 8 hr. Excretion: 50% unchanged and 15% as metabolites in urine in 24 hr. Dialysis: yes, H, P.

Administration and dosage

NOTE: Ethambutol should not be used alone, but in combination with other antitubercular agents. Ethambutol is not recommended for use in patients under 13 years of age.

PO 1. Patients who have received no previous antitubercular therapy: 15 mg/kg as a single dose every 24 hr.
  2. Retreatment: 25 mg/kg as a single daily dose. After 60 days reduce the dose to 15 mg/kg and administer as a single dose every 24 hr.
  3. Patients with renal insufficiency should be observed for cumulative effects of the drug. The dosage for those patients with a creatinine clearance of less than 10 ml/min should be 6 to 10 mg/kg.

Special remarks and cautions

Approximately 6% of patients receiving therapy exhibit decreased visual acuity and reduction of green color vision. These effects usually appear within 7 months after starting therapy and generally disappear within several weeks after therapy is discontinued.

Other side effects include dermatitis, pruritus, anorexia, nausea, vomiting, headache, dizziness, mental confusion, disorientation, and hallucinations.

Elevated serum uric acid levels occur, and precipitation of acute gout has been reported.

Transient elevations of liver function tests are a common observation.

Patients should be warned that omission or interrupted intake may result in drug resistance, reversal of clinical improvement, and increased susceptibility of family members to tuberculosis.

Ethambutol is not recommended in pregnant women.

Drug interactions

No specific interactions have been reported.

ISONIAZID
(Hyzyd, Nydrazid)

AHFS 8:16
CATEGORY Antitubercular agent

Action and use

Isoniazid is both a tuberculostatic and tuberculocidal agent effective against *Mycobacterium tuberculosis* as well as other organisms of this genus. The bactericidal effects are exerted only against actively growing tubercle bacilli and do not affect those cells in a resting state. Although the mechanism of action is unknown, isoniazid penetrates sensitive cells well and is effective against intracellularly located bacilli as well as those growing in vitro.

Characteristics

Peak plasma levels: 1 to 2 hr (PO). Half-life: 50 to 110 min in "rapid inactivators," 140 to 250 minutes in "slow inactivators." Metabolism: acetylation in liver. Excretion: 75% to 95% in urine as metabolites; Dialysis: yes, H, P.

Administration and dosage
Adult

PO 1. For treatment of active tuberculosis isoniazid should be used in conjunction with other effective antitubercular agents, 5 mg/kg to a maximum of 300 mg daily.
   2. Prophylactic therapy: 300 mg daily in single or divided doses.
   3. Concurrent administration of pyridoxine, 25 to 50 mg daily, is recommended for prevention of peripheral neurophathies.

IM—As for PO administration.

Pediatric

Infants and children tolerate larger doses than adults and may be given 10 to 30 mg/kg/24 hr PO in single or divided doses. Maximum dose is 500 mg daily.

Special remarks and cautions

Approximately 50% of blacks and whites are slow inactivators, while the majority of Eskimos, American Indians, and Orientals are rapid inactivators. This does not significantly alter the effectiveness of the medication; however, slow inactivators may have higher blood levels and may manifest more toxic symptoms.

Peripheral neuropathy, often preceded by numbness and tingling of the hands or feet, nausea, vomiting, dizziness, and ataxia are relatively common side effects of isoniazid and are dose related.

The incidence of hepatotoxicity increases with age to about 2.3% of those patients over 50 years of age. This reaction often occurs within the first 3 months of therapy and is suspected of being an allergic manifestation. Early symptoms include fatigue, weakness, anorexia, and malaise. Serum transaminase levels are not a good indicator of this toxic reaction, since they may already be elevated.

Hematologic reactions include agranulocytosis, eosinophilia, thrombocytopenia, hemolytic anemia, and methemoglobinemia.

Patient counseling must emphasize that omission or interrupted intake may result in drug resistance, reversal of clinical improvement, and increased susceptibility of family members to tuberculosis.

Drug interactions

Combined therapy with disulfiram (Antabuse) and isoniazid may result in changes in affect and behavior as well as incoordination.

Concomitant use of meperidine (Demerol) and isoniazid is not recommended because of the interaction of meperidine and MAO inhibitors. Isoniazid does display some MAO inhibition.

Clinical evidence indicates that concomitant use of isoniazid and rifampin may result in hepatotoxicity, especially in patients with previous liver impairment and/or those patients who are slow acetylators. Either agent when used alone may result in abnormal liver function tests.

Isoniazid inhibits the metabolism of phenytoin (Dilantin), resulting in elevated phenytoin levels. The reaction is usually significant only in slow acetylators, but may result in excessive sedation and incoordination.

RIFAMPIN
(*Rifadin*)

AHFS 8:16
CATEGORY Antitubercular agent

Action and use

Rifampin is a bacteriostatic and bactericidal antibiotic used with other chemotherapy in the treatment of pulmonary tuberculosis. Rifampin exerts its therapeutic effect by interacting with bacterial DNA-dependent RNA polymerase.

Characteristics

Peak plasma levels: 2 to 4 hr. Protein binding: 75% to 90%. Half-life: 1½ to 5 hr; the half-life diminishes by up to 40% during the first 14 days of treatment as a result of increased biliary excretion. Excretion: up to 30% in urine, unchanged and as metabolites. Dialysis: unknown.

Administration and dosage

NOTE: Rifampin should not be used alone, but in combination with other antitubercular agents. Administer 1 hr before or 2 hr after meals.

Adult

PO—600 mg once daily.

Pediatric

PO—10 to 20 mg/kg/24 hr with a maximum daily dose of 600 mg.

Special remarks and cautions

Gastrointestinal disturbances such as heartburn, anorexia, nausea, vomiting, cramps, gas, and diarrhea are some of the more common side effects. Other adverse reactions include headache, dizziness, mental confusion, visual disturbances, and generalized numbness.

Transient elevations in serum bilirubin, alkaline phosphatase, SGOT, SGPT, BUN, and uric acid levels have been noted. Rifampin may produce liver dysfunction and should be used with caution in patients with liver disease.

Rare hematologic side effects include thrombocytopenia, leukopenia, hemolytic anemia, hemoglobinuria, and hematuria.

The patient should be informed of the possibility of red-orange urine, feces, saliva, sputum, sweat, and tears.

Patient counseling must emphasize that omission or interrupted intake may result in drug resistance, reversal of clinical improvement, and increased susceptibility of family members to tuberculosis.

Although birth defects have not been reported, caution must be used prenatally and postnatally, since rifampin diffuses across the placental barrier and is secreted in breast milk.

Drug interactions

Rifampin may decrease the prothrombin time and increase the dosage of warfarin.

Increased liver dysfunction may result from the combined use of isoniazid and rifampin, especially in patients with previous liver impairment and/or in those who are slow isoniazid inactivators.

The contraceptive efficacy of oral contraceptives when taken with rifampin may be impaired. Alternative contraceptive methods should be considered.

Anthelmintic agents
MEBENDAZOLE
(*Vermox*)

AHFS 8:08
CATEGORY Anthelmintic agent

Action and use

Mebendazole is an oral anthelmintic agent that apparently works by inhibiting carbohydrate transport and metabolism by the intestinal cells of worms. The intestinal cells die, resulting in the death of the parasite. There does not appear to be any alteration of carbohydrate metabolism in humans. Mebendazole is used in the treatment of *Trichuris trichiura* (whipworm), *Enterobius vermicularis* (pinworm), *Ascaris lumbricoides* (roundworm), *Ancylostoma duodenale* (common hookworm), and *Necator americanus* (American hookworm).

Administration and dosage
Adult and pediatric (over 2 years of age)

PO   1. Pinworm: 1 tablet (100 mg) 1 time, well mixed with food and chewed.
2. Roundworm, whipworm, and hookworm: 1 tablet (100 mg) morning and evening on 3 consecutive days. If evidence of infestation persists beyond 3 to 4 weeks, another course of therapy may be administered.

Special diets, fasting, enemas, or laxatives are not necessary prior to therapy.

The safe use of mebendazole in children under 2 years of age has not been established. The risk versus the benefit of therapy must be considered in these patients.

Special remarks and cautions

Side effects are usually minimal; however, patients may experience nausea, diarrhea, and abdominal pain.

Hygienic procedures should be explained to patients to help prevent reinfection. Precautions should include wearing shoes, washing hands with soap and cleaning under fingernails especially before eating and after defecation, and washing all fruits and vegetables thoroughly before eating them.

The use of mebendazole is *contraindicated* in pregnant women. Teratogenic effects have been reported in pregnant rats after a single dose of this agent.

Drug interactions

No specific drug interactions have been reported.

PIPERAZINE CITRATE
(Antepar, Multifuge, Vermizine)

AHFS 8:08
CATEGORY Anthelmintic agent

Action and use

Piperazine is an oral anthelmintic agent that acts by blocking the effects of acetylcholine at the neuromuscular junctions of worms, resulting in paralysis. The paralyzed parasites are then expelled from the gastrointestinal tract by normal peristalsis. Piperazine is effective against *E. vermicularis* (pinworm) and *A. lumbricoides* (roundworm).

Administration and dosage
Adult

PO 1. Roundworm: a single daily dose of 3.5 g PO for 2 consecutive days.
2. Pinworm: a single daily dose of 65 mg/kg (maximum daily dose: 2.5 g) for 7 consecutive days.

Pediatric

PO 1. Roundworm: a single daily dose of 75 mg/kg (maximum daily dose: 3.5 g) for 2 consecutive days.
2. Pinworm: as for adult dosages.
Special diets, fasting, enemas, or laxatives are not necessary prior to therapy.

Special remarks and cautions

Hygienic procedures should be explained to patients to help prevent reinfection. Precautions should include wearing shoes, washing hands with soap and cleaning under fingernails especially before eating and after defecation, and washing all fruits and vegetables thoroughly before eating them.

Side effects are usually minimal and transient. Complaints of nausea, vomiting, diarrhea, cramps, dizziness, and headache occur occasionally.

Hypersensitivity reactions consisting of skin rashes, pruritus, fever, joint pain, purpura, fever, and chills have been reported. Discontinue therapy immediately if these symptoms develop.

Piperazine may cause central nervous system effects in some patients (especially children). If ataxia, muscle spasticity, nystagmus, muscle weakness, or numbness develops, discontinue therapy immediately. Patients with a history of neurologic disorders such as epilepsy should not be given piperazine.

Safe use of piperazine in pregnant or lactating patients has not been established.

Drug interactions

Pyrantel pamoate (Antiminth) and piperazine have antagonistic mechanisms of action. Courses of therapy should not be administered concurrently.

PYRANTEL PAMOATE
(Antiminth)

AHFS 8:08
CATEGORY Anthelmintic agent

Action and use

Pyrantel is also a neuromuscular blocking agent, but in contrast to piperazine citrate, pyrantel acts by stimulating acetylcholine release at the neuromuscular junction. It also inhibits acetylcholinesterase, the enzyme necessary for metabolism of acetylcholine. The paralyzed worms are then expelled from the gastrointestinal tract by normal peristalsis. Pyrantel may be used to treat *E. vermicularis* (pinworm) and *A. lumbricoides* (roundworm).

Administration and dosage
Adult and pediatric

PO—Administer 11 mg/kg (maximum dose: 1 g) once only. The suspension may be given with food or milk at any time of the day.

Special diets, fasting, enemas, or laxatives are not necessary prior to therapy.

The safe use of pyrantel pamoate in children under 2 years of age has not been established. The risk versus the benefit of therapy must be considered in these patients.

Special remarks and cautions

Hygienic procedures should be explained to patients to help prevent reinfection. Precautions should include wearing shoes, washing hands with soap and cleaning under fingernails especially before eating and after defecation, and washing all fruits and vegetables thoroughly before eating them.

Side effects are usually minimal and transient. Complaints of nausea, vomiting, diarrhea, and headache occur most frequently.

Pyrantel pamoate should be used with caution in patients with liver disease.

Safe use of pyrantel pamoate in pregnant or lactating patients has not been established.

Drug interactions

Piperazine Citrate (Antepar, Multifunge, Vermizine) and pyrantel pamoate have antagonistic mechanisms of action. Courses of therapy should not be administered concurrently.

PYRVINIUM PAMOATE
(Povan)

Action and use

Pyrvinium pamoate is an organic dye that exerts its anthelmintic effects in worms by altering carbohydrate absorption and by inhibiting respiration. Pyrvinium pamoate is used to treat *E. vermicularis* (pinworm).

Administration and dosage
Adult and pediatric

PO—Administer a single dose of 5 mg/kg (maximum dose: 350 mg). Tablets should be swallowed without chewing to prevent staining of teeth.

Special diets, fasting, enemas, or laxatives are not necessary prior to therapy.

If the infestation persists after 2 to 3 weeks, the treatment may be repeated.

Special remarks and cautions

Pyrvinium pamoate is a bright red dye that will stain clothing, stools, and vomitus. The staining is harmless to patients but may be unremovable if spilled on most materials.

Hygienic procedures should be explained to patients to help prevent reinfection. Precautions should include wearing shoes, washing hands with soap and cleaning under fingernails especially before eating and after defecation, and washing all fruits and vegetables thoroughly before eating them.

Nausea, vomiting, cramping, and diarrhea are the most frequently reported side effects. Vomiting occurs more commonly in adults who receive large doses; it is also more common with the suspension than with the tablets.

Do not use in patients with conditions such as inflammatory bowel disease. Gastrointestinal absorption is enhanced, and toxic effects may result.

Safe use in pregnant and lactating patients has not been established.

Drug interactions

No specific drug interactions have been reported.

QUINACRINE HYDROCHLORIDE
(*Atabrine hydrochloride*)

AHFS 8:08
CATEGORY Anthelmintic agent

Action and use

The mechanism of action of quinacrine hydrochloride is unknown except that it causes detachment of the parasite from the intestinal wall, allowing it to be removed by purging. Quinacrine may be effective against *Taenia saginata* (beef tapeworm), *T. solium* (pork tapeworm), *Diphyllobothrium latum* (fish tapeworm), and *Hymenolepis nana* (dwarf tapeworm). Quinacrine may also be used to treat malaria and giardiasis.

Administration and dosage

For tapeworm:
Restrict the patient to a bland, nonfat, liquid, or semisolid diet for 24 to 48 hours.
The patient should not eat or drink anything after the last evening meal.
A saline cathartic and/or cleansing enema may be given before treatment.

Adult

PO—Administer 4 doses of 200 mg, 10 min apart (total dose: 800 mg) accompanied by 600 mg of sodium bicarbonate with each dose to reduce vomiting.

Pediatric

Ages 5 to 10 years. Administer 2 doses of 200 mg 10 min apart (total dose: 400 mg) followed by 300 mg of sodium bicarbonate with each dose.
Ages 11 to 14 years. Administer 3 doses of 200 mg 10 min apart (total dose: 600 mg) followed by 300 mg of sodium bicarbonate after each dose.
Over 14 years of age. As for adult dosages.
A saline cathartic should be administered 1 to 2 hr after administration of quinacrine to expel the tapeworm.
The worm will be stained yellow and should be examined carefully for the presence of the scolex (head). If the scolex is not found, the patient may be considered cured only if segments do not reappear in the stool over the next 3 to 6 months.
Episodes of nausea and vomiting are frequent, especially when large doses are administered in the treatment of tapeworm. Use of a duodenal tube may reduce emesis. If a tube is used, administer the saline cathartic about 30 min after quinacrine.

For giardiasis:

Adult

PO—100 mg 3 times daily for 5 to 7 days.

Pediatric

PO—7 mg/kg daily in 3 divided doses (maximum dose: 300 mg/day) for 5 days.
Repeat in 2 weeks if stool specimens still indicate the presence of giardia.

Special remarks and cautions

Other side effects noted with chronic administration for malaria include headaches, anorexia, and diarrhea. CNS stimulation manifested by restlessness, nightmares, anxiety, emotional changes, aggressive behavior, and acute psychoses have been reported.
Patients should be informed that the drug imparts a yellowish color to skin and urine. This color change is reversible on discontinuation of therapy.
The drug should be used with great caution in patients with liver disease, alcoholism, renal disease, and glucose-6-phosphate dehydrogenase deficiency. Patients receiving

prolonged therapy should periodically have an ophthalmologic examination and a complete blood count.

Use with caution in patients with psoriasis. Quinacrine may seriously exacerbate the disease.

Because of possible teratogenic effects, quinacrine must not be administered to pregnant women.

Drug interactions

Toxic levels of primaquine may result if quinacrine and primaquine are administered concurrently.

THIABENDAZOLE
(Mintezol)

AHFS 8:08

CATEGORY Anthelmintic agent

Action and use

Thiabendazole has a spectrum of activity against a large variety of helminths, making it quite useful as in the treatment of mixed helminthic infestations. The exact mechanism of action of thiabendazole has not been determined; however, it is an enzyme inhibitor in the parasitic worm. Thiabendazole is effective in the treatment of *E. vermicularis* (pinworm), *A. lumbricoides* (roundworm), strongyloidiasis (threadworm), cutaneous larva migrans (creeping eruption), *A. duodenale* (common hookworm), and *N. americanus* (American hookworm).

Characteristics

Onset: rapid. Peak levels: 1 to 2 hr. Duration: 7 to 8 hr. Metabolism: hepatic to glucuronide and sulfate conjugates. Excretion: 90% in urine as inactive metabolites. Dialysis: unknown.

Administration and dosage
Adult

PO—25 mg/kg for patients under 70 kg; 1.5 g for patients over 70 kg. Maximum daily dose: 3 g.

Pediatric

PO—22 mg/kg.

Administer preferably after meals.

For pinworms, the dose is given once in the morning and once in the evening on 1 day only. Repeat regimen in 7 days.

For roundworm, hookworm, threadworm, and creeping eruption, the dosage is given once in the morning and once in the evening on 2 successive days. Special diets, fasting, enemas, or laxatives are not necessary prior to therapy.

The safe use of thiabendazole in children under 2 years of age has not been established. The risk versus the benefit of therapy must be considered in these patients.

Special remarks and cautions

Hygienic procedures should be explained to patients to help prevent reinfection. Precautions should include wearing shoes, washing hands with soap and cleaning under fingernails especially before eating and after defecation, and washing all fruits and vegetables thoroughly before eating them.

About one third of patients treated with thiabendazole complain of some side effects from therapy. Most are mild and transient, occurring 3 to 4 hr after administration and lasting for 2 to 8 hr. The most frequent adverse effects are nausea and dizziness. Diarrhea, lethargy, drowsiness, and headache are less common. Patients should be warned not to attempt tasks requiring mental alertness.

Hypersensitivity reactions consisting of skin rashes, fever, chills, and facial flushing have been reported. Discontinue therapy immediately if these symptoms develop.

Because of significant hepatic metabolism and renal excretion, thiabendazole should be used with caution in patients with hepatic or renal impairment.

Safe use in pregnancy and lactation has not been established.

Drug interactions

No specific drug interactions have been reported.

Antiparasitic agents
BENZYL BENZOATE

AHFS 84:04.12
CATEGORY Antiparasitic agent

Action and use

Benzyl benzoate is an organic compound toxic to arthropods such as *Sarcoptes scabiei* (scabies), *Pediculus humanis* var. *capitis* (head lice), and *Phthirus pubis* (crab lice). The mechanism of action is not known. Although gamma benzene hexachloride 1% (pp. 66 and 67) is considered the drug of choice for the treatment of scabies in adults, benzyl benzoate is most frequently used in infants and young children because of its lower potential for toxicity.

Administration and dosage

NOTE: For external use only. Do not administer orally; do not apply to inflamed or raw, weeping skin. Benzyl benzoate lotion is available as a 28% and a 50% solution. Dilute the 50% solution with an equal volume of water before using.

For scabies:
1. Have the patient bathe with soap and water to scrub and remove scaly skin. Towel dry.
2. While skin is still slightly damp, apply a thin layer of 28% lotion over the entire body from neck to toes (cover all extremities, including soles of feet). Gently rub into all skin surfaces, especially between fingers, toes, and skin folds. Avoid contact with the face, eyes, mucous membranes, and urethral meatus.
3. Apply a second coat after the first layer has dried. Some clinicians recommend that 2 more coats be applied the next day.
4. The drug should be removed by bathing 24 to 48 hours after the last application.
5. Repeat treatment in 7 to 10 days if mites appear or new lesions develop.

For head or pubic (crab) lice:
1. Bathe as above.
2. Rub 28% benzyl benzoate lotion into the affected hairy areas. Avoid exposure to eyes.
3. Remove with soap and water after 12 to 24 hours.
4. Comb hair with a fine-toothed comb to remove nit shells.
5. Repeat in 1 week if the first application was not adequate.

Special remarks and cautions

The first manifestations of scabies infestation may not occur until 2 to 6 weeks after contact. During this period scabies is highly contagious. All family members and close social contacts should be carefully examined and treated if necessary. Pruritus from scabies and their by-products may last for several weeks after treatment. Unless new lesions develop or the patient is recontaminated, there is no indication for further treatment.

All clothing and bedding should be machine-washed or dry-cleaned to prevent reinfestation. Combs and brushes should be washed with gamma benzene hexachloride shampoo and then rinsed thoroughly to remove the drug.

Even when applied in appropriate quantities, topical benzyl benzoate may cause minor local irritation with itching and burning. If major irritation or a rash develops, discontinue therapy.

Drug interactions

No specific drug interactions have been reported.

GAMMA BENZENE HEXACHLORIDE
(Kwell)

AHFS 84:04.12
CATEGORY Antiparasitic agent

Action and use

Gamma benzene hexachloride is a synthetic, chlorinated hydrocarbon insecticide. It is particularly effective topically against *S. scabiei* (scabies), *P. humanis* var. *capitis* (head lice), *P. corporis* (body lice), and *P. pubis* (crab lice). Gamma benzene hexachloride acts as a central nervous system (CNS) stimulant to arthropods, resulting in convulsions and death.

Administration and dose

NOTE: For external use only. Do not administer orally. Do not apply to inflamed or raw, weeping skin. Gamma benzene hexachloride is available as a 1% cream, lotion, or shampoo. Shake well before use.

For scabies:
1. Have the patient bathe with soap and water to scrub and remove scaly skin. Towel dry.
2. Apply a thin layer of cream or lotion uniformly over the body from neck to toes (cover all extremities, including soles of feet). Gently rub into all skin surfaces, especially between fingers, toes, and skin folds. Avoid contact with face, eyes, mucous membranes, and urethral meatus.
3. After 12 to 24 hr bathe and remove the drug.
4. Dress with freshly laundered clothing.
5. One application is usually adequate; however, 1 or 2 more applications may be required at weekly intervals.

For body lice:
1. Bathe as above.
2. Apply a thin layer of cream or lotion to hairy infested areas and adjacent skin (avoid contact with the face, mucous membranes, and urethral meatus).
3. Bathe thoroughly after 12 to 24 hr to remove all medication. Dress in freshly laundered clothing.
4. Repeat in 4 days if necessary.

For head or pubic (crab) lice:
1. Bathe as above.
2. Apply 15 to 30 ml of shampoo (long hair may require 60 ml) to head or pubic hair and lather well for 5 min.
3. Rinse the hair thoroughly and rub with a dry towel.
4. Comb hair with a fine-toothed comb to remove nit shells.
5. Repeat in 24 hr if needed. Do not apply more than twice in 1 week.
6. Dress in freshly laundered clothing.

Special remarks and cautions

The first manifestations of scabies infestation may not occur until 2 to 6 weeks after contact. During this period scabies is highly contagious. All family members and close social contacts should be carefully examined and treated if necessary. Pruritus from scabies and their by-products may last for several weeks after treatment. Unless new lesions develop or the patient is recontaminated, there is no indication for further treatment. Repeated application frequently causes contact dermatitis.

All clothing and bedding should be machine-washed or dry-cleaned to prevent reinfestation. Combs and brushes should be washed with gamma benzene hexachloride shampoo and then rinsed thoroughly to remove the drug.

This product is not effective as a prophylactic agent against scabies or lice. Do not use the shampoo routinely.

Avoid contact with the eyes. If accidently contaminated, wash eyes immediately with water.

Use cautiously and sparingly in infants and small children. Avoid ingestion via hand-to-mouth (thumbsucking) or hand-to-eye contact.

Oral ingestion or chronic exposure may result in serious CNS, renal, and hepatic toxicities. If ingested orally, treat immediately with gastric lavage and follow with saline cathartics. Do not use oil laxatives such as castor or mineral oil since absorption may be enhanced.

Drug interactions

No specific drug interactions have been reported.

CHAPTER TWO

Cardiovascular agents

Cardiac glycosides
   General information
   Digoxin
   Digitoxin
Adrenergic agents
   Dopamine hydrochloride
   Epinephrine
   Isoproterenol
   Isoxsuprine hydrochloride
   Levarterenol (norepinephrine)
   Metaraminol
   Phenylephrine hydrochloride

Antiarrhythmic agents
   Bretylium tosylate
   Disopyramide phosphate
   Lidocaine hydrochloride
   Phenytoin
   Procainamide hydrochloride
   Propranolol hydrochloride
   Quinidine
"Coronary vasodilators"
   General information
   Nitroglycerin

Cardiac glycosides
GENERAL INFORMATION

Digitalis glycosides have played an active role in medicine for more than 200 years. The glycosides are a recurrent topic in the literature and are perhaps the most frequently discussed class of compounds in the armamentarium of therapeutic medication.

Digitalis glycosides have two primary pharmacologic actions on the heart. The exact mechanisms of action have been difficult to determine, partially as a result of differences in compensatory extracardiac activity in patients with a normal heart versus those with impaired cardiac function.

Digitalis provides an increased force of contraction (positive inotropy) by acting on cellular structures of the heart to increase the quantity of intracellular free calcium. Calcium ions potentiate the binding of proteins (actin and myosin) necessary for myocardial contraction, thus increasing the force of contraction and cardiac output in the failing heart.

Digitalis slows the heart rate (negative chronotropy) by directly suppressing the conduction of electric impulses at the atrioventricular (AV) node. As cardiac output increases and peripheral circulation improves, mechanisms needed to compensate for the failing heart are no longer required, further decreasing the heart rate.

The most frequent use of digitalis is in the treatment of congestive heart failure. By improving contractility, digitalis helps restore circulatory function. Another major use of digitalis is slowing the ventricular rate in atrial fibrillation, atrial flutter, supraventricular tachycardia, and premature extrasystoles. This is effected by increasing block of the AV node, so that fewer atrial beats will be followed by a ventricular beat.

Although it may be used, digitalis is usually less effective in heart failure secondary to respiratory insufficiency, infection, and hyperthyroidism (so called high-output failures).

Characteristics

Although there are structural similarities between the digitalis glycosides, the small structural dissimilarities make a significant difference in the characteristics of the individual digitalis preparations. Compare the characteristics on the monographs for digoxin and digitoxin (pp. 70 to 72).

Administration and dosage

As a result of a more complete understanding of the pharmacokinetics of the digitalis glycosides, more precise dosage adjustments may be made with a lower incidence of toxicity. It is important to realize that in most patients the optimal dose is considerably below that of digitalis intoxication. Patients do not need to receive large doses to produce toxic nausea and vomiting to determine the maintenance level.

The most appropriate dosage is obviously that which provides the greatest recovery in cardiac efficiency with maximal reduction in initial symptomatology. The most effective way to determine this optimal dosage is by careful and frequent observation of the patient.

See the individual monographs on digoxin and digitoxin for administration and dosage (pp. 70 to 72).

Special remarks and cautions

Hypokalemia, hypomagnesemia, and hypercalcemia sensitize the heart to digitalis intoxication. Attempts must be made to restore and maintain electrolyte balance prior to initiation of digitalis therapy. Lower doses of digitalis should be used initially, and patients should be placed on ECG monitors if possible (see Table 4-1, p. 130).

Clinical conditions other than electrolyte imbalance that may require lower doses of digitalis glycosides include myxedema (hypothyroidism), acute myocardial infarction, renal disease, severe respiratory disease, and far-advanced heart failure. Those that may require higher than average doses include hyperthyroidism and atrial arrhythmias. Remember, however, that it is essential to treat the patient and the clinical symptomatology and that individual variation is frequently observed with the digitalis glycosides.

The most common toxic manifestations are fatigue, anorexia, nausea, vomiting, blurred vision, mental confusion, and arrhythmias. Many of the arrhythmias for which digitalis is used are also observed in digitalis intoxication. If the arrhythmias occur while a patient is receiving digitalis, it is often difficult to determine whether the arrhythmias are secondary to digitalis treatment or an indication of inadequate treatment. Clinical judgment is certainly required, but if the possibility of intoxication cannot be ruled out, digitalis should be temporarily withheld. Monitoring of both serum electrolyte and specific digitalis (digoxin or digitoxin) levels may be beneficial in formulating a clinical impression.

Drug interactions

Drugs that may alter digitalis response and the incidence of toxicities by alteration of electrolyte imbalance include:

Hypokalemia	*Hyperkalemia*	*Hypomagnesemia*
Amphotericin B (Fungizone)	Potassium chloride	Chlorthalidone (Hygroton)
Chlorthalidone (Hygroton)	Potassium supplements—	Ethacrynic acid (Edecrin)
Ethacrynic acid (Edecrin)	K-Lyte, Kaon, K-Lor, and others	Furosemide (Lasix)
Furosemide (Lasix)	Spironolactone (Aldactone)	Metolazone (Zaroxolyn)
Metolazone (Zaroxolyn)	Triamterene (Dyrenium)	Ethanol
Thiazide diuretics		Thiazide diuretics
Corticosteroids		Neomycin (Mycifradin)

Parenteral calcium gluconate and chloride administration may potentiate the therapeutic and arrhythmic effects of any of the digitalis preparations. If used concomitantly the calcium should be given slowly and in low doses, accompanied by careful electrocardiographic monitoring.

Succinylcholine (Anectine, Quelicin) may enhance arrhythmias in the digitalized myocardium.

Concomitant use of propranolol and digitalis may potentiate the bradycardia associated with either agent.

Cholestyramine (Questran) decreases intestinal absorption of digitalis glycosides, altering expected response.

DIGOXIN
(Lanoxin)

AHFS 24:04
CATEGORY Cardiac glycoside

Action and use

See General information on cardiac glycosides (pp. 68 and 69).

Characteristics

Absorption: 80% to 90% (PO, liquids), 50% to 85% (PO, tablets). Onset: 5 to 30 min (IV), 30 to 60 min (PO). Peak activity: 5 to 6 hr. Protein binding: 23%. Half-life: 36 hr with normal renal function. Metabolism: liver, minimal, inactive; enterohepatic recirculation: 7%. Excretion: 35% of total amount in body in 24 hr, 20% in urine unchanged, 14% primarily fecal. Therapeutic level: 0.7 to 1.6 ng/ml. Toxic level: 2 ng/ml. Fatal level: 4 ng/ml. Dialysis: no, H, P.

Administration and dosage

A baseline ECG is recommended prior to initiation of therapy.

Assuming the patient has not ingested digoxin for the previous week or other digitalis preparations for the previous 2 weeks:

Adult

PO 1. Digitalizing: 0.50 to 0.75 mg initially, followed by 0.25 mg every 6 hr until adequate digitalization is achieved.
2. Maintenance: 0.125 to 0.25 mg daily for inotropic therapy. Some patients may require 0.375 to 0.5 mg daily for chronotropic effects.

IV 1. Digitalizing: 0.25 to 0.5 mg initially, followed by 0.25 mg every 6 hr until adequate digitalization is achieved. Administer at a rate of 0.5 to 1 ml/min.
2. Maintenance: as for PO administration.

Pediatric
Premature

IM or IV 1. Digitalizing: 0.015 to 0.02 mg/kg initially, followed by 0.01 mg every 6 to 8 hr for 2 doses (total digitalizing dose: 0.03 to 0.05 mg/kg).
2. Maintenance: 0.003 to 0.006 mg/kg every 12 hr.

Ages 2 weeks to 2 years

PO 1. Digitalizing: 0.03 to 0.04 mg/kg initially, followed by 0.02 mg/kg every 6 to 8 hr for 2 doses (total digitalizing dose: 0.06 to 0.08 mg/kg).
2. Maintenance: 0.006 to 0.01 mg/kg every 12 hr.

IM or IV 1. Digitalizing: 0.02 to 0.03 mg/kg initially, followed by 0.01 to 0.015 mg/kg every 6 to 8 hr for 2 doses (total digitalizing dose: 0.04 to 0.06 mg/kg).
2. Maintenance: 0.003 to 0.006 mg/kg every 12 hr.

Over 2 years of age

PO 1. Digitalizing: 0.02 to 0.03 mg/kg initially, followed by 0.01 to 0.015 mg every 6 to 8 hr for 2 doses (total digitalizing dose: 0.04 to 0.06 mg/kg).
2. Maintenance: 0.004 to 0.009 mg/kg every 12 hr.

IM or IV 1. Digitalizing: 0.01 to 0.02 mg/kg initially, followed by 0.005 to 0.01 mg/kg every 6 to 8 hr for 2 doses (total digitalizing dose: 0.02 to 0.04 mg/kg).
2. Maintenance: 0.002 to 0.004 mg/kg every 12 hr.

NOTE: Elderly patients and those with impaired renal function tend to accumulate the drug.

These patients often require reduced dosage. Also note the differences in absorption, depending on the route and preparation for administration.

Routine safety precautions require that a patient's pulse be monitored prior to administration of each dose. Usually the medication administration should be withheld if the patient's heart rate is less than 60 beats/min (less than 90 beats/min for infants) (an early sign of increasing AV block).

Special remarks and cautions

See General information on cardiac glycosides (pp. 68 and 69).

Drug interactions

See General information on cardiac glycosides (pp. 68 and 69).

Gastrointestinal absorption of digoxin is inhibited by neomycin and antacids. Patients should be observed more closely for clinical effect or the lack of it. Monitoring digoxin serum levels may also be particularly useful.

Quinidine, by unknown mechanisms, may cause an increase in digoxin serum levels, resulting in increased gastrointestinal and cardiac toxicity. Monitor serum digoxin levels, ECG readings, and the clinical course of the patient closely.

DIGITOXIN
(Crystodigin)

AHFS 24:04
CATEGORY Cardiac glycoside

Action and use

See General information on cardiac glycosides (pp. 68 and 69).

Characteristics

Absorption: 100% (PO). Onset: 1 to 2 hr. Peak activity: 4 to 12 hr. Protein binding: 90% to 95%. Half-life: 5⁷/₁₀ days with normal renal function. Metabolism: liver—92% inactive, 8% digoxin (active); enterohepatic recirculation: 26%. Excretion: 11% of total amount in body in 24 hr, 4% urinary, 7% nonurinary. Therapeutic level: 20 to 30 ng/ml. Toxic level: 45 ng/ml. Dialysis: no, H, P.

Administration and dosage

A baseline ECG is recommended prior to initiation of therapy.

Assuming the patient has not ingested a digitalis preparation in the preceding 3 weeks:

Adult

PO 1. Digitalizing: 0.6 mg initially, followed by 0.4 mg and then 0.2 mg at intervals of 4 to 6 hr.
2. Maintenance: 0.05 to 0.3 mg once daily. The average dose is 0.1 to 0.15 mg daily.

IV 1. Digitalizing: 0.6 mg initially followed by 0.4 mg 4 to 6 hr later and by 0.2 mg every 4 to 6 hr thereafter until therapeutic effects are apparent. These effects are usually observed within 8 to 12 hr.
2. Maintenance: As for PO maintenance therapy.

Pediatric

PO 1. Digitalizing
   a. Premature, full-term, and infants with impaired renal function: 0.022 mg/kg.
   b. Ages 2 weeks to 1 year: 0.045 mg/kg.
   c. Over 2 years of age: 0.03 mg/kg.

NOTE: Divide total digitalizing dose into 3 or more doses administered at least 6 hr apart.
2. Maintenance: Give one tenth the total digitalizing dose daily.

IV—As for PO therapy.

NOTE: Elderly patients and those with impaired renal function tend to accumulate digitoxin. These patients often require reduced dosage.

Routine safety precautions require that a patient's pulse be measured prior to administration of each dose. Usually the medication administration should be withheld if the patient's heart rate is less than 60 beats/min (less than 90 beats/min for infants) (an early sign of increasing AV block).

Special remarks and cautions

See General information on cardiac glycosides (pp. 68 and 69).

Drug interactions

See General information on cardiac glycosides (pp. 68 and 69).

Phenobarbital, phenylbutazone (Butazolidin), and phenytoin (Dilantin) have been reported to enhance the metabolism of digitoxin to digoxin, possibly as a result of enzyme induction. This has resulted in decreased digitoxin serum levels, shortened half-life, and diminished therapeutic effect caused by underdigitalization.

Cholestyramine (Questran) may bind digitoxin in the gastrointestinal tract, preventing reabsorption after enterohepatic recirculation. The half-life of digitoxin will be shortened, possibly leading to a diminished therapeutic effect.

Adrenergic agents
DOPAMINE HYDROCHLORIDE
(Intropin)

AHFS 12:12
CATEGORY Adrenergic stimulant

Action and use

Dopamine is a precursor in the synthesis of norepinephrine in the body and acts on alpha- and beta-adrenergic receptors. It also acts on specific dopamine receptors to cause vasodilatation of the renal and mesenteric vascular beds. It produces an inotropic and chronotropic effect on the myocardium, resulting in an increased cardiac output. It usually produces an increased systolic and pulse pressure with either no effect or a slight increase in diastolic pressure. Dopamine is indicated in shock caused by myocardial infarction, trauma, renal failure, and endotoxic septicemia.

Administration and dosage

The central venous pressure should be 10 to 15 cm of H_2O, or the pulmonary wedge pressure should be 14 to 18 mm Hg (see Table 2-1).

Begin administration of the diluted solution at doses of 2 to 5 μg/kg/min. Increase gradually using 5 to 10 μg/kg/min increments up to 20 to 50 μg/kg/min. Dosage should be adjusted according to the patient's response. Observe particularly for diminished urine output, increasing tachycardia, or the development of arrhythmias.

Do not add dopamine to sodium bicarbonate since the drug is inactivated in alkaline solution.

NOTE: Safety in children has not been established.

Special remarks and cautions

The most frequent adverse reactions are ectopic beats, nausea, vomiting, tachycardia, anginal pain, dyspnea, hypotension, and headache.

If a disproportionate rise in the diastolic pressure (a marked decrease in pulse pressure) is noted, the infusion rate should be decreased and the patient watched for further evidence of vasoconstrictor activity such as decreased urine output.

In overdosage, as noted by elevated blood pressure, reduce the administration rate or discontinue infusion. Dopamine's duration of action is quite short (1 to 5 min), and usually no other action is needed. If blood pressure remains elevated, the short-acting alpha-adrenergic blocking agent, phentolamine (Regitine), should be considered.

Extravasation of large amounts may cause ischemia and tissue necrosis. Gangrene of fingers and toes has been reported after prolonged infusion.

Drug interactions

Propranolol antagonizes the cardiac activity of dopamine.

Patients who have been treated with MAO inhibitors (isocarboxazid [Marplan], pargyline hydrochloride [Eutonyl], tranylcypromine sulfate [Parnate]) require a substantially reduced dosage of dopamine. The starting dose in such patients should be reduced to at least one tenth the usual dose. MAO inhibitors block the metabolism of dopamine.

Table 2-1. Dopamine administration*

amps/500 ml	1	2	4	8
mg/ml	200/500 ml	400/500 ml	800/520 ml	1600/540 ml
μg/ml	400	800	1538	2962
50 kg μgtts/min	μg/kg/min	μg/kg/min	μg/kg/min	μg/kg/min
10	1.3	3	5	10
20	2.6	5	10	20
30	4	8	15	30
40	5.3	11	20	39
50	6.6	13	26	49
60	8	16	31	59
60 kg μgtts/min				
10	1.1	2	4	8
20	2.2	4	8	16
30	3.3	7	13	25
40	4.4	8	17	33
50	5.5	11	21	41
60	6.6	13	26	49
70 kg μgtts/min				
10	0.9	2	3	7
20	1.9	4	7	14
30	2.8	6	11	21
40	3.8	8	15	28
50	4.7	10	18	35
60	5.7	11	22	42

*Using a microdrip administration set—60 gtts/ml.

Table 2-1. Dopamine administration—cont'd

amps/500 ml	1	2	4	8
mg/ml	200/500 ml	400/500 ml	800/520 ml	1600/540 ml
μg/ml	400	800	1538	2962
80 kg μgtts/min				
10	0.8	2	3	6
20	1.6	3	6	12
30	2.5	5	10	18
40	3.3	7	13	24
50	4.2	8	16	31
60	5	10	19	37
90 kg μgtts/min				
10	0.7	1	3	5
20	1.4	3	6	11
30	2.2	4	9	16
40	2.9	6	11	22
50	3.7	7	14	27
60	4.4	9	17	33
100 kg μgtts/min				
10	0.6	1	3	5
20	1.3	3	5	10
30	2	4	8	15
40	2.6	5	10	20
50	3.3	7	13	25
60	4	8	15	30

EPINEPHRINE

(Adrenalin)

AHFS 12:12
CATEGORY Cardiac stimulant

Action and use

Epinephrine is one of the primary catecholamines of the body, stimulating both alpha- and beta-receptor cells. It is a very potent cardiac stimulant, acting directly on the beta receptors of the myocardium, pacemaker cells, and conducting tissue. Stimulation results in increased spontaneous contractions (automaticity), heart rate (positive chronotropic effect), myocardial contraction (positive inotropic effect), cardiac output, coronary blood flow, and oxygen consumption.

Administration and dosage
Adult

IV—Cardiac resuscitation: epinephrine 1:1000, 0.2 to 1 ml (0.2 to 1 mg); epinephrine 1:10,000, 2 to 10 ml (0.2 to 1 mg).
INTRACARDIAC—As for IV administration.
ENDOTRACHEAL TUBE—As for IV administration.

Pediatric

IV—Cardiac resuscitation: epinephrine 1:1000, 0.01 ml/kg/dose; epinephrine 1:10,000, 0.1 ml/kg/dose.
NOTE: Dosages are given in milliliters rather than in milligrams.

Epinephrine conversion chart

Epinephrine	1:1000	1:10,000
1 ml	1 mg	0.1 mg
10 ml	10 mg	1.0 mg

NOTE: Do not use if discolored (red to brown) or if sediment is present. Do not mix with solutions containing aminophylline, phenytoin (Dilantin), or sodium bicarbonate.

Special remarks and cautions

Be extremely cautious with dosage calculations and administration.

Isoproterenol and epinephrine should not be administered simultaneously, since both drugs are potent cardiac stimulants. They may be given alternately, however.

Palpitation, tachycardia, headache, tremor, weakness, and dizziness are common side effects. Serious arrhythmias, ventricular fibrillation, anginal pain, nausea, respiratory difficulty, and cerebral hemorrhage may also occur.

Dosage should be adjusted carefully in the elderly, in patients with coronary insufficiency, diabetes, hyperthyroidism, hypertension, and in psychoneurotic individuals. These patients are particularly sensitive to sympathomimetic amines.

Drug interactions

Tricyclic antidepressants (doxepin, nortriptyline, amitriptyline, protriptyline, imipramine, desipramine) strongly potentiate the actions of epinephrine. If they must be used concurrently, start with significantly lower doses of epinephrine.

Use epinephrine with caution in patients receiving propranolol. Vagal reflex has resulted in marked bradycardia.

Epinephrine causes hyperglycemia. Diabetics may require increased doses of insulin or oral hypoglycemic agents.

Epinephrine may produce arrhythmias in patients anesthetized with cyclopropane.

ISOPROTERENOL HYDROCHLORIDE
(*Isuprel*)

AHFS 12:12
CATEGORY Beta-adrenergic stimulant

Action and use

Isoproterenol is a beta-receptor stimulant. Cardiac output is raised by inotropic and chronotropic action combined with an increase in venous return to the heart. Usual doses maintain or raise the systolic pressure, although the mean pressure is reduced. Peripheral vascular resistance is lowered in skeletal muscle and renal and mesenteric vascular beds. Diastolic pressure falls.

Isoproterenol is used primarily in cardiac standstill (arrest), AV block, carotid sinus hypersensitivity, ventricular arrhythmias—especially those occurring during the course of AV block—and bronchospasm. For its use as a bronchodilator see pp. 150 and 151.

Administration and dosage
Adult and pediatric

Infusion rates of 0.5 to 5 μg/min have been recommended. The rate of infusion should be adjusted on the basis of heart rate, central venous pressure, systemic blood pressure, and urine output. Rates over 30 μg/min have been used in advanced stages of shock (Table 2-2).

Table 2-2. Isoproterenol administration for cardiac standstill and arrhythmias in adults*

1. *Intravenous infusion*

5 ml amps/500 ml		2	4	8	12	16
mg/500 ml		2	4	8	12	16
μg/ml		4	8	16	24	32
μgtts/min	ml/min	μg/min	μg/min	μg/min	μg/min	μg/min
5	0.08	0.3	0.6	1.2	1.9	2.5
10	0.16	0.6	1.2	2.4	3.8	5.3
15	0.25	1	2	4	6	8
20	0.33	1.3	2.6	5.3	8	11
25	0.41	1.6	3.3	6.5	9.8	13.1
30	0.5	2	4	8	12	16
35	0.58	2.3	4.6	9.3	13.9	18.5
40	0.66	2.6	5.3	10.5	15.8	21.1
45	0.75	3	6	12	18	24
50	0.83	3.3	6.6	13.3	20	26.5
55	0.91	3.6	7.3	14.5	21.8	29.1
60	1.0	4	8	16	24	32

	Preparation	Initial dose	Subsequent dosage range
2. *Intramuscular*	Use solution 1:5000 undiluted	0.2 mg (1 ml)	0.02 to 1 mg (0.1 to 5 ml)
3. *Subcutaneous*	Use solution 1:5000 undiluted	0.2 mg (1 ml)	0.15 to 0.2 mg (0.75 to 1 ml)
4. *Intracardiac*	Use solution 1:5000 undiluted	0.2 mg (1 ml)	

*Using a microdrip administration set—60 gtts/ml. Each milliliter of the sterile 1:5000 solution contains 0.2 mg isoproterenol (Isuprel). The drug is available in 5 ml (1 mg) ampules and should be diluted in dextrose 5% before administration. Normal saline solution is not a recommended diluent.

Special remarks and cautions

Administration of isoproterenol is contraindicated in patients with tachycardia caused by digitalis intoxication.

Isoproterenol and epinephrine should not be administered simultaneously, since both drugs are direct cardiac stimulants. They may be given alternately, however.

Dosage should be adjusted carefully in patients with coronary insufficiency, diabetes, and hyperthyroidism, and in patients sensitive to sympathomimetic amines.

If the cardiac rate increases sharply, patients with angina pectoris may experience anginal pain until the cardiac rate decreases.

Palpitation, tachycardia, headache, and flushing of the skin are common side effects. Serious arrythmias, anginal pain, nausea, tremor, dizziness, weakness, and sweating occasionally occur.

Although there have been no teratogenic effects reported, safe use in pregnant or lactating women has not been established.

Drug interactions

The beta-adrenergic stimulant effects of isoproterenol are blocked by propranolol, a beta-adrenergic blocker.

Isoproterenol may produce arrhythmias in patients anesthetized with cyclopropane.

ISOXSUPRINE HYDROCHLORIDE
(Vasodilan)

AHFS 24:12
CATEGORY Beta-adrenergic stimulant

Action and use

Isoxsuprine has beta-receptor stimulant properties that result in dilatation of blood vessels of skeletal muscle and cardiac stimulation. Increased circulation in skeletal muscle and lowered peripheral vascular resistance is present. As a result of increased cardiac output the mean blood pressure stays about the same, but there appears to be improved circulation to skeletal muscle and cerebral circulation. Isoxsuprine may be effective in relieving symptoms of cerebral vascular insufficiency, Buerger's disease, and Raynaud's disease. Because of its ability to relax uterine musculature, it may also be used in cases of premature labor and threatened abortion.

Administration and dosage

For peripheral vasodilatation:

PO—10 to 20 mg 3 to 4 times daily.

IM—5 to 10 mg (1 to 2 ml) 2 to 3 times daily. IM administration may result in hypotension and tachycardia.

IV—Not recommended because of increased incidence of side effects.

Guidelines for use in premature labor:

1. Initiate a control IV of dextrose 5%, Ringer's lactate, or saline solution and administer 400 to 500 ml in 15 to 20 min prior to initiation of the medication. Then decrease dosage to 100 to 125 ml/hr.
2. Add 400 mg of isoxsuprine to 1000 ml of dextrose 5% (400 µg/ml).
3. An initial loading dose used in premature labor is 0.5 to 1 mg/min (see Table 2-3). This rate is continued for the first ½ hr to 1 hr of therapy until control of contractions has been established or tachycardia (pulse over 120), hypotension (systolic below 100, diastolic below 60), or vomiting results. The initial uterine response should occur within the first 15 min.
4. A maintenance infusion of 0.25 to 0.75 mg/min can be given for 2 to 12 hr or more.
5. After control of uterine activity is established, the IV dose is tapered while control is maintained by PO isoxsuprine, 20 mg every 4 to 6 hr.
6. The maintenance PO dosage ranges from 10 to 20 mg 4 to 6 times daily, depending upon clinical response.
7. If labor begins again, restart the IV infusion as above.

Table 2-3. Isoxsuprine administration for premature labor*

ml/hr	ml/min	mg/min
15	0.25	0.11
20	0.33	0.13
25	0.42	0.17
50	0.82	0.33
75	1.25	0.5
100	1.67	0.67
125	2.08	0.83
150	2.5	1
175	2.91	1.16
200	3.33	1.33

*Administer 400 mg/1000 ml or 400 µg/ml.

Special remarks and cautions

When isoxsuprine is used for premature labor a sometimes significant drop in blood pressure (due to the vasodilatory effect), can be seen in the first 10 to 15 min of the infusion. Blood pressure and pulse monitoring should be done prior to and every 5 min after the infusion has been started until the patient's condition is stable. Use continuous electronic fetal monitoring. If maternal pulse exceeds 120 beats/min and does not decrease with an increase in fluids or if there is any evidence of a decrease in uterine perfusion, discontinue the infusion.

Other dose-related side effects include tachycardia, dizziness, nausea, and vomiting.

Long-term PO administration has resulted in severe skin rashes. If a rash should develop, the drug should be discontinued.

Drug interactions

Patients who have been taking antihypertensive agents (hydralazine hydrochloride, diuretics, methyldopa) may be more susceptible to the hypotensive effects of isoxsuprine.

LEVARTERENOL (NOREPINEPHRINE)
(*Levophed*)

AHFS 12:12
CATEGORY Adrenergic stimulant

Action and use

Levarterenol acts predominantly on alpha receptors and has little action on beta receptors, except in the heart. As a result of general peripheral vasoconstriction (alpha stimulation) and beta stimulation of the heart, systolic, diastolic, and usually, pulse pressure levels are increased. Compensatory vagal reflex activity slows the heart, overcoming the direct cardioaccelerator action, thus increasing the stroke volume. The peripheral vasoconstriction reduces blood flow through the kidney, brain, liver, and usually skeletal muscle. Glomerular filtration rate is maintained unless the decrease in renal blood flow is quite marked. Coronary circulation is increased probably because of both indirect coronary dilatation and elevated blood pressure. Levarterenol is used to restore blood pressure after an acute hypotensive episode such as myocardial infarction, cardiac arrest, drug reaction, septicemia, blood transfusions, and surgical procedures.

Administration and dosage

NOTE: Levarterenol infusions must *never* be left unattended. Monitor blood pressure and infusion rate continuously.

IV—See Table 2-4.

Extravasation ischemia: Care must be taken that necrosis and sloughing do not occur at the site of IV infusion as a result of extravasation of the drug. Blanching along the course of the infused vein may be an early indication of extravasation. The area will later develop a cold, hard, and pallid appearance. Whenever possible, levarterenol should be administered through a large vein. To prevent sloughing and necrosis in areas where extravasation has taken place, the area should be infiltrated as soon as possible with 10 to 15 ml of saline solution containing from 5 to 10 mg of phentolamine (Regitine), an alpha-adrenergic blocking agent. Administration with whole blood or plasma is not recommended. If these fluids are required, use separate infusion sites or Y tubing with the connections as close to the infusion site as possible.

Special remarks and cautions

Severe hypotension may result if levarterenol is suddenly discontinued. Plasma volumes must be adequate and the dosage reduced in increments while the blood pressure response is monitored.

Other side effects include severe hypertension, reflex bradycardia, and hyperglycemia. Violent headache, photophobia, stabbing chest and neck pain, pallor, intense sweating, and vomiting may be indications of overdose.

A decrease in urinary output should be expected. Monitor fluid intake and output to avoid overhydration.

Use of levarterenol in pregnant women must be used on a risk-versus-benefit basis. Levarterenol increases the frequency of contraction of the gravid uterus.

Drug interactions

General anesthetics such as cyclopropane and halothane increase cardiac autonomic irritability. Patients receiving levarterenol during or immediately after anesthesia have an increased risk of ventricular tachycardia or fibrillation. The same type of arrhythmias may result from the use of levarterenol in patients with profound hypoxia or hypercarbia.

Levarterenol should be used with extreme caution in patients receiving MAO inhibitors (pargyline [Eutonyl, Eutron], tranylcypromine sulfate [Parnate]), tricyclic antidepressants (imipramine, amitriptyline, Triavil), and guanethidine (Ismelin) because severe, prolonged hypertension may result.

Table 2-4. Levarterenol administration*

amps/500 ml		1	2	4
mg base/500 ml		4	8	16
μg base/ml		8	16	32
μgtts/ml	ml/min	μg base/min	μg base/min	μg base/min
5	0.08	0.64	1.3	2.5
10	0.16	1.3	2.6	5.2
15	0.25	2.0	4	8
20	0.33	2.6	5.3	10.5
25	0.41	3.3	6.6	13.2
30	0.5	4.0	8	16
35	0.58	4.6	9.3	18.5
40	0.66	5.3	10.6	21.2
45	0.75	6	12	24
50	0.83	6.6	13.3	26.5
55	0.91	7.3	14.6	29.2
60	1.0	8.0	16	32

*Using a microdrip administration set—60 gtts/ml.

Each 1 ml of the 0.2% solution contains 2 mg of levarterenol bitartrate or the equivalent of 1 mg levarterenol base (1 ml solution = 1 mg of base). Dilute in dextrose 5%. Saline solution is not recommended. Adding one 4 ml ampule of 0.2% levarterenol to 1000 ml of dextrose 5% gives a concentration of 4 μg levarterenol base/ml of final solution.

Although the clinical condition of the patient must be a major determinant, the recommended initial dosage is 8 to 12 μg of base/min. The average maintenance dose ranges from 2 to 4 μg of base/min. Great individual variation occurs in the dose required to attain and maintain normotension. Dosage must be titrated to the response of the patient. The pressor response can readily be controlled since the drug is rapidly metabolized. Activity-response is insignificant 1 to 2 min after the infusion is stopped.

Overdoses may cause severe hypertension with violent headache, photophobia, stabbing chest and neck pain, pallor, intense sweating, and vomiting.

Levarterenol infusions must never be left unattended. Blood pressure must be monitored at least every 5 min and more frequently when the dosage is being adjusted.

METARAMINOL
(Aramine)

AHFS 12:12
CATEGORY Adrenergic stimulant

Action and use

Metaraminol is a sympathomimetic amine that acts indirectly by stimulating the release of stored norepinephrine from nerve ending storage granules and directly by stimulating the sympathetic receptor. There are both alpha- and beta-receptor effects, causing cardiac stimulation and peripheral arteriolar vasoconstriction in all vascular beds, resulting in a rise in both systolic and diastolic pressure. Metaraminol may be used to treat paroxysmal atrial tachycardia and acute hypotensive states induced by spinal anesthesia, drug reactions, and shock.

Administration and dosage

IM—2 to 10 mg (0.2 to 1 ml).

IV 1. Direct injection: 0.5 to 5 mg (0.05 to 0.5 ml undiluted). Administration by direct injection is recommended only in a life-threatening emergency.
   2. Infusion: Initially, 15 to 100 mg (1.5 to 10 ml) in 500 ml of dextrose 5% or saline solution. Adjust the rate of infusion to maintain the blood pressure at the desired level. More concentrated solutions may be used to restrict fluid intake. Concentrations of 150 to 500 mg/500 ml of dextrose 5% or saline solution may be used. When IV infusions are discontinued the dosage should be gradually tapered with close observation of the blood pressure. Avoid abrupt withdrawal.

Extravasation ischemia: Injections and infusions may occasionally result in abscess formation, tissue necrosis, and sloughing. Administer with caution in patients with peripheral vascular disease or shock. Blanching along the course of the infused vein may be an early indication of extravasation. The area will later develop a cold, hard, and pallid appearance. To prevent sloughing and necrosis in mottled, cold tissue, infiltrate the area as soon as possible with 10 to 15 ml of saline solution containing 5 to 10 mg of phentolamine (Regitine), an alpha-adrenergic blocking agent.

Special remarks and cautions

Metaraminol may cause tachycardia or arrhythmias, particularly in patients with previous myocardial injury. Other side effects include severe hypertension, reflex bradycardia, headache, anginal pain, nausea, and vomiting.

Patients potentially more sensitive to metaraminol are those with impaired hepatic function, thyroid disease, hypertension, heart disease, hyperthyroidism, and diabetes. Therefore use with caution in these patients.

After discontinuation of therapy, prolonged hypertension may occur due to cumulative effects of metaraminol. However, the converse is more likely to occur. Hypotension, partially due to depletion of norepinephrine stores, may require the administration of levarterenol to replace tissue stores of norepinephrine.

Use with extreme caution in pregnant patients. Metaraminol may cause uterine contractions and decreased uterine blood flow, resulting in fetal hypoxia and bradycardia.

Drug interactions

Patients who have been treated with MAO inhibitors (isocarboxazid [Marplan], pargyline [Eutonyl], tranylcypromine sulfate [Parnate]) require much smaller doses of metaraminol. MAO inhibitors block the metabolism of norepinephrine, prolonging and intensifying the activity of metaraminol.

Metaraminol may produce arrhythmias in patients anesthetized with halothane or cyclopropane.

Phentolamine (Regitine) decreases but does not completely block the vasoconstriction of metaraminol.

Atropine sulfate blocks the reflex bradycardia caused by metaraminol.

Guanethidine (Ismelin) and tricyclic antidepressants (imipramine, amitriptyline) potentiate the pressor effects of metaraminol.

PHENYLEPHRINE HYDROCHLORIDE
(Neo-Synephrine)

AHFS 12:12
CATEGORY Alpha-adrenergic stimulant

Action and use

Phenylephrine is a sympathomimetic agent that acts predominantly by direct stimulation of alpha-adrenergic receptors. There is also a minor indirect component of activity due to release of norepinephrine from nerve ending storage granules. Most vascular beds are constricted, and renal, splanchnic, cutaneous, and limb blood flow is reduced. In contrast to levarterenol and metaraminol, there are essentially no direct effects on receptors within the heart. A reflex bradycardia is frequently seen, however, secondary to peripheral vasoconstriction.

Phenylephrine may be used to maintain systolic and diastolic blood pressure during spinal and inhalation anesthesia and shock. It is also used to terminate episodes of paroxysmal supraventricular tachycardia by induction of reflex bradycardia.

Administration and dosage

For mild to moderate hypotension:

Adult

sc—Usual dose: 2 to 5 mg (0.2 to 0.5 ml). Range: 1 to 10 mg (0.1 to 1 ml). Initial dose should not exceed 5 mg (0.5 ml).

im—As for SC administration.

iv—Usual dose: 0.2 mg. Range: 0.1 to 0.5 mg. Initial dose should not exceed 0.5 mg. Dilute 1 ml of phenylephrine with 9 ml of saline solution to make a concentration of 0.1 mg phenylephrine/0.1 ml, or 1 mg/ml, for ease of administration.

iv infusion—See Table 2-5.

Pediatric

sc—0.1 mg/kg.

im—As for SC administration.

NOTE: Injections should not be repeated more often than every 10 to 15 min. (A 5 mg dose IM should raise blood pressure for 1 to 2 hr; a 0.5 mg dose IV should raise blood pressure for about 15 min.)

For paroxysmal supraventricular tachycardia:

Adults

iv—0.5 mg over 20-30 sec. Further doses may be increased by increments of 0.1 to 0.2 mg depending on blood pressure response. The systolic blood pressure should generally not rise above 160 mm Hg. The maximum single dose should not exceed 1 mg.

Extravasation ischemia: Injections and infusions may occasionally result in abscess formation, tissue necrosis, and sloughing. Administer with caution in patients with peripheral vascular disease or shock. Blanching along the course of the infused vein may be an early indication of extravasation. The area will later develop a cold, hard, and pallid appearance. To prevent sloughing and necrosis in mottled, cold tissue, infiltrate the area as soon as possible with 10 to 15 ml of saline solution containing 5 to 10 mg of phentolamine (Regitine), an alpha-adrenergic blocking agent.

Special remarks and cautions

Side effects of phenylephrine include restlessness, anxiety, nervousness, respiratory distress, arrhythmias, anginal pain, and numbness and/or cool sensations of the extremities. Overdosage may result in hypertension, palpitations, cerebral hemorrhage, and convulsions. Headache may be an early indication of hypertension and overdose.

Phenylephrine should be administered with extreme caution to the elderly and to patients with hyperthyroidism, bradycardia, partial heart block, myocardial disease, or hypertension.

A decrease in urinary output should be expected. Monitor fluid intake and output to avoid overhydration.

Use with caution in patients with peripheral circulatory insufficiency. Vasoconstriction produced by phenylephrine may cause further necrosis.

Use with extreme caution in late pregnancy and during delivery. Phenylephrine increases uterine contractility and reduces uterine blood flow, which may result in fetal hypoxia and bradycardia.

Drug interactions

Phentolamine (Regitine) may be used to reduce vasoconstriction and hypertension induced by phenylephrine.

Atropine sulfate blocks the reflex bradycardia induced by phenylephrine.

Propranolol (Inderal) may be used to treat cardiac arrhythmias arising from phenylephrine therapy.

Arrhythmias may result from concurrent administration of halothane or cyclopropane anesthesia and phenylephrine. This reaction is much less likely to occur with phenylephrine than with levarterenol or metaraminol therapy.

Patients who have been treated with MAO inhibitors (isocarboxazid [Marplan], pargyline [Eutonyl], tranylcypromine sulfate [Parnate]) require much smaller doses of phenylephrine. MAO inhibitors diminish the metabolism of phenylephrine.

Guanethidine (Ismelin) and tricyclic antidepressants (imipramine, amitriptyline) potentiate the vasoconstriction induced by phenylephrine.

Table 2-5. Phenylephrine administration*

amps/500 ml		1	2	4	6	8	10	12
mg/500 ml		10	20	40	60	80	100	120
μg/ml		20	40	80	120	160	200	240
μgtts/min	ml/min	μg/min	μg/min	μg/min	μg/min	μg/min	μg/min	μg/min
5	0.08	1.6	3.2	6.4	9.6	12.8	16	19
10	0.16	3.2	6.4	12.8	19.2	25.6	32	38
15	0.25	5	10	20	30	40	50	60
20	0.33	6.6	13.2	26.4	39.6	52.8	66	79
25	0.41	8.2	16.4	32.8	49.2	65.6	82	98
30	0.5	10	20	40	60	80	100	120
35	0.58	11.6	23.2	46.4	69.6	92.8	116	139
40	0.66	13.2	26.4	52.8	79.2	105.6	132	158
45	0.75	15	30	60	90	120	150	180
50	0.83	16.6	33.2	66.4	99.6	132.8	166	200
55	0.91	18.2	36.4	72.8	109.2	145.6	182	218
60	1.0	20	40	80	120	160	200	240

*Using a microdrip administration set—60 gtts/ml. Each 1 ml of the 1% solution contains 10 mg of phenylephrine (1 ml = 10 mg). Dilute in dextrose 5% or saline solution.

Although the clinical condition of the patient must be a primary determinant, the recommended initial dosage is 100 to 180 μg/min. After the blood pressure stabilizes, 40 to 60 μg/min is usually adequate. There is great patient variation in the dosage required to attain and maintain the desired blood pressure. Dosage must be titrated to the response of the patient.

Antiarrhythmic agents
BRETYLIUM TOSYLATE
(Bretylol)

AHFS 24:04
CATEGORY Antiarrhythmic; adrenergic blocking agent

Action and use

Bretylium tosylate is an antiarrhythmic adrenergic blocking agent indicated for use in patients with life-threatening arrhythmias, ventricular tachycardia, or ventricular fibrillation uncontrollable by other antiarrhythmic agents or electrical cardioversion. The mechanism of action has not been established, but pharmacologic actions observed include inhibition of the release of norepinephrine from adrenergic nerve terminals, positive inotropic and chronotropic effects on the heart, and restoration of the resting membrane potential toward normal in damaged myocardial cells.

Characteristics

Onset: Ventricular fibrillation, 5 to 10 min (IV), 20 to 60 min (IM). ventricular tachycardia, 20 to 120 min (IM and IV). Duration: 6 to 8 hr (IM and IV). Half-life: about 10 hr (range: 4 to 17 hr). Metabolism: no apparent metabolites. Excretion: unchanged in urine, 70% to 80% in 24 hr.

Administration and dosage

For ventricular fibrillation:

After failure of electrical cardioversion, 5 mg/kg IV undiluted. Repeat cardioversion. If fibrillation persists, the dosage may be increased to 10 mg/kg and repeated every 15 to 30 min. Maximum total dosage should not exceed 30 mg/kg.

For other ventricular arrhythmias:

Administer 5 to 10 mg/kg IV over 8 to 10 min. Dilute the solution at least fivefold (500 mg/10ml diluted in at least 50 ml with dextrose 5% or saline solution). If nausea or vomiting occurs, reduce the rate of infusion. The dose may be repeated in 1 to 2 hr if the arrhythmia persists.

IV—Continuous infusion: recommended dosage is 1 to 2 mg/min (Table 2-6).

IM—5 to 10 mg/kg. Do *not* dilute prior to IM injection. Dosage may be repeated in 1 to 2 hr if the arrhythmia still persists. Thereafter repeat every 6 to 8 hr.

For routine bretylium administration add 2 ampules (1000 mg/20 ml) of bretylium to dextrose 5% as shown in Table 2-6.

For bretylium administration in patients with restricted fluid intake add bretylium to 500 mg of dextrose 5% as shown in Table 2-7.

NOTE: The dosage of bretylium should be tapered and discontinued within 3 to 5 days under electrocardiographic monitoring.

Special remarks and cautions

When bretylium therapy is initiated, transient hypertension followed by postural hypotension may be observed. Patients may complain of dizziness, light-headedness, vertigo, or syncope. Symptoms may be reduced by keeping the patient in a supine position. Avoid the use of subtherapeutic dosages (that is, less than 5 mg/kg), since hypotension may occur at dosages lower than those needed to suppress arrhythmias. Hypotension with systolic blood pressure readings consistently below 75 mm Hg may be treated with infusions of dopamine or levarterenol. Initiate catecholamine therapy at low dosages, since the pharmacologic effects of bretylium may enhance the pressor activity of these agents. Transient tachycardia, increased frequency of arrhythmias, bradycardia, and precipitation of anginal attacks have been reported in a few patients.

Table 2-6. Bretylium administration*

Add 2 ampules of 1000 mg/20 ml bretylium to any of the following volumes of dextrose 5%

Dextrose 5% (ml)		150	250	500	1000
Final volume (ml)		170	270	520	1020
mg/ml		5.88	3.70	1.92	1
μgtts/min	ml/min	mg/min	mg/min	mg/min	mg/min
5	0.08	0.47	0.3	0.15	0.08
10	0.16	0.94	0.6	0.30	0.16
15	0.25	1.47	0.92	0.48	0.25
20	0.33	1.94	1.22	0.63	0.33
25	0.41	2.4	1.51	0.78	0.41
30	0.5	2.94	1.85	0.96	0.5
35	0.58	3.41	2.14	1.11	0.58
40	0.66	3.88	2.44	1.26	0.66
45	0.75	4.41	2.77	1.44	0.75
50	0.83	4.88	3.07	1.6	0.83
55	0.91	5.35	3.36	1.75	0.91
60	1.0	5.88	3.70	1.92	1.0

*Using a microdrip administration set—60 gtts/ml. The drug is available in 10 ml ampules containing 500 mg of bretylium.

Drug interactions

Bretylium therapy may aggravate digitalis glycoside toxicity. Use only in digitalized patients if the arrhythmia does not appear to be induced by digitalis and if other antiarrhythmic agents are not effective.

Table 2-7. Bretylium administration: patients with restricted fluid intake*

amp/500ml		1	2	4	6
	mg/ml	500/500 ml	1000/520 ml	2000/540 ml	2500/560 ml
	mg/ml	1	1.92	3.7	4.46
μgtts/min	ml/min	mg/min	mg/min	mg/min	mg/min
5	0.08	0.08	0.15	0.3	0.35
10	0.16	0.16	0.3	0.6	0.71
15	0.25	0.25	0.48	0.9	1.11
20	0.33	0.33	0.63	1.2	1.47
25	0.41	0.41	0.78	1.5	1.82
30	0.5	0.5	0.96	1.85	2.23
35	0.58	0.58	1.11	2.14	2.60
40	0.66	0.66	1.26	2.44	2.94
45	0.75	0.75	1.44	2.77	3.34
50	0.83	0.83	1.6	3.07	3.70
55	0.91	0.91	1.75	3.36	4.05
60	1.0	1.0	1.92	3.7	4.46

*Using a microdrip administration set—60 gtts/ml. The drug is available as 10 ml ampules containing 500 mg of bretylium.

DISOPYRAMIDE PHOSPHATE
(Norpace)

AHFS 24:04
CATEGORY Antiarrhythmic agent

Action and use

Disopyramide is a new antiarrhythmic agent with properties similar to those of quinidine and procainamide. It is indicated for the suppression and treatment of ventricular arrhythmias, especially in patients refractory to procainamide or quinidine therapy or in patients in whom the side effects of other antiarrhythmic therapy are unacceptable.

Characteristics

Peak plasma levels: less than 2 hr. Protein binding: 50%. Half-life: 5 to 10 hr. Excretion: 50% unchanged, 30% as metabolites, in urine, 10% in feces. Therapeutic level: 2 to 4 µg/ml. Toxic level: more than 9 µg/ml. Dialysis: unknown.

Administration and dosage

PO
1. Normal renal function:
   a. Initial: 300 mg.
   b. Maintenance: Initially, 150 mg every 6 hr. Individual dosage adjustments must be made; some patients may require as much as 400 mg every 6 hr.
2. Moderately impaired renal function (creatinine clearance greater than 40 ml/min), hepatic insufficiency, or severe cardiac disease:
   a. Initial: 200 mg.
   b. Maintenance: Initially, 100 mg every 6 hr.
3. Severe renal impairment (creatinine clearance less than 40 ml/min):
   a. Initial: 200 mg.
   b. Maintenance: 100 mg according to the following chart:

Creatinine clearance (ml/min)	40-15	15-5	5-1
Dosage interval (hr)	10	20	30

Special remarks and cautions

Disopyramide is a myocardial depressant. Myocardial toxicity may be manifested by premature ventricular contractions (PVCs), bradycardia, AV block, ventricular tachycardia, ventricular fibrillation, or an increase in congestive heart failure. Electrocardiographic changes may include prolongation of the PR interval, widened QRS interval (greater than 25%), widened QT interval (greater than 25%), ST segment depression, idioventricular rhythm, SA block, AV block, and asystole.

More common adverse effects of therapy include dry mouth, nose, and throat, urinary hesitancy and retention, constipation with bloating and gas, and occasional diarrhea.

Use disopyramide with *extreme* caution in heart block and digitalis intoxication.

Complete effects of disopyramide therapy during pregnancy and delivery have not been evaluated. It is not known as yet whether disopyramide is excreted in human breast milk. Studies on lactating rats indicate that milk concentrations may be 1 to 3 times greater than maternal plasma concentration. Therefore nursing during disopyramide therapy is not recommended.

Drug interactions

Disopyramide may potentiate the hypotensive effects of the thiazides, other diuretics, and antihypertensive agents.

Disopyramide may be additive with procainamide (Pronestyl), quinidine, digitalis, and propranolol (Inderal), resulting in further myocardial depression.

Other drug interactions may be observed as more clinical experience is gained. Patients receiving disopyramide with other medications should be monitored closely for potential multiple drug toxicity.

LIDOCAINE HYDROCHLORIDE
(Xylocaine hydrochloride)

AHFS 24:04
CATEGORY Antiarrhythmic agent

Action and use

Lidocaine exerts its antiarrhythmic effect by increasing the electric stimulation threshold of the ventricles without depressing the force of ventricular contractions. Lidocaine is the drug of choice for the treatment of ventricular arrhythmias associated with acute myocardial infarction and ventricular tachycardia.

Characteristics

Onset: 1 to 2 min (IV bolus), 5 to 15 min (IM). Duration of antiarrhythmic effect: 10 to 20 min (IV bolus), 60 to 90 min (IM). Distribution: after bolus administration lidocaine is rapidly distributed to almost all body tissues. The serum half-life of the initial (active) phase of distribution is 8 to 9 min. To maintain serum blood levels initiated by the bolus, a continuous infusion must be started within about 10 min (see p. 94). The half-life of the second phase is 1½ to 2 hr. Metabolism: primarily liver. Excretion: <5% unchanged in urine. Therapeutic level: 1 to 5 µg/ml. Toxic level: 6 to 10 µg/ml. Dialysis: unknown.

Administration and dosage

NOTE: Lidocaine should not be used in patients with complete heart block.

Adult

IM—200 to 300 mg in the deltoid muscle. IM administration is recommended only in emergency conditions when IV facilities are not available and when the potential benefits outweigh the risks.

NOTE: IM injections may result in increased creatine phosphokinase levels, invalidating the use of this enzyme determination, without isoenzyme separation, in diagnosing acute myocardial infarction.

IV—The initial dose (bolus) is 50 to 100 mg (1 mg/kg) at a rate of 25 to 50 mg/min. Boluses of 50 to 100 mg may be given every 3 to 5 min until the desired effect is achieved or side effects appear. Do not exceed 300 mg by intermittent bolus. To maintain the antiarrhythmic effect an IV infusion must be initiated. The usual rate of administration is 1 to 4 mg/min (see Table 2-8).

Pediatric

IV   1. Initial (bolus): 1 mg/kg up to 15 mg if under 25 kg (55 lb); up to 25 mg if over 25 kg (55 lb).
   2. Continuous infusion: 20 to 40 µg/kg/min (maximum total dose: 5 mg/kg).

For routine lidocaine administration for cardiac arrhythmias add 50 ml of 40 mg/ml (2 g) of lidocaine hydrochloride to dextrose 5% as shown in Table 2-8.

For lidocaine administration for cardiac arrhythmias in patients with restricted fluid intake add lidocaine hydrochloride to 500 ml of dextrose 5% as shown in Table 2-9.

Special remarks and cautions

Most side effects are dose related and of short duration when the administration rate is decreased. Minor side effects include lightheadedness, tinnitus, muscle twitches, and blurred or double vision. Adverse effects mediated through the central nervous system are depression, stupor, restlessness, euphoria, hypotension, and convulsions. Infrequently, lidocaine may produce bradycardia and/or aggravate arrhythmias.

Safe use in pregnancy has not been established. Lidocaine does cross the placental barrier.

Drug interactions

Large IV doses of lidocaine have been shown to enhance the neuromuscular blocking action of succinylcholine. Use the combination with caution particularly if large doses of lidocaine are used.

Table 2-8. Routine lidocaine administration*

Add 50 ml of 40 mg/ml (2 g) lidocaine to any of the following volumes of dextrose 5%

Dextrose 5% (ml)	100	250	450	500	1000
Final volume (ml)	150	300	500	550	1050
mg/ml	13.3	6.6	4	3.6	2
μgtts/min	mg/min	mg/min	mg/min	mg/min	mg/min
10	2.2	1.1	0.66	0.6	0.33
20	4.4	2.1	1.3	1.2	0.66
30	6.6	3.3	2	1.8	1.0
40	8.8	4.4	2.6	2.4	1.3
50	11.0	5.5	3.3	3	1.6
60	13.3	6.6	4	3.6	2

*Using a microdrip administration set—60 gtts/ml.
NOTE: If the infusion rate is to be increased, a loading bolus of 25 to 50 mg of lidocaine should also be administered. Toxicity is usually seen at administration rates greater than 5 mg/min or with prolonged administration rates greater than 4 mg/min. There will be variation, especially in patients with shock, hypovolemia, congestive heart failure, and hepatic insufficiency. Serum levels accumulate, since the volume of distribution and/or metabolism is diminished.

Table 2-9. Lidocaine administration: patients with restricted fluid intake*

Lidocaine (g)	1	2	3	4	5	6
Final volume (ml)	525	550	575	600	625	650
mg/ml	1.9	3.6	5.2	6.6	8	9.2
μgtts/min	mg/min	mg/min	mg/min	mg/min	mg/min	mg/min
10	0.3	0.6	0.8	1	1.3	1.5
20	0.6	1.2	1.7	2.2	2.6	3
30	0.9	1.8	2.6	3.3	4	4.6
40	1.2	2.4	3.4	4.3	5.3	6
50	1.6	3	4.3	5.5	6.6	7.6
60	1.9	3.6	5.2	6.6	8	9.2

*Using a microdrip administration set—60 gtts/ml.
NOTE: If the infusion rate is to be increased, a loading bolus of 25 to 50 mg of lidocaine should also be administered. Toxicity is usually seen at administration rates greater than 5 mg/min or with prolonged administration rates greater than 4 mg/min. There will be variation, especially in patients with shock, hypovolemia, congestive heart failure, and hepatic insufficiency. Serum levels accumulate, since the volume of distribution and/or metabolism is diminished.

PHENYTOIN
(*Dilantin*)

AHFS 28:12
CATEGORY Antiarrhythmic agent

Action and use

Phenytoin is generally thought of as an anticonvulsant, but it may also be effective in the treatment of ventricular arrhythmias, particularly those produced by overdoses of digitalis. Phenytoin depresses automaticity as do quinidine and procainamide, but improves conduction in depressed myocardial tissue. Reduction in automaticity helps control arrhythmias, while enhanced conduction of electric impulses through previously depressed conduction tissue (such as that seen in digitalis intoxication) may improve cardiac function.

Characteristics

Onset: Within 1 hr following an IV loading dose of 1 to 1.5 g, 2 to 24 hr following a PO loading dose of 1 g. Protein binding: 95%. Half-life: 18 to 24 hr. Metabolism: liver to inactive metabolites. Excretion: 1% unchanged in urine, 75% in urine as metabolites. Therapeutic level: 7.5 to 20 μg/ml. Toxic level: 10 to 50 μg/ml. Dialysis: yes, H.

Administration and dosage

For treatment of arrhythmias:

Adult

PO—250 mg 4 times during the first day, 500 mg daily on days 2 and 3, and 300 to 400 mg on subsequent days.

IM—Not recommended as a result of erratic absorption and pain on injection.

IV—250 mg initially, at a rate no faster than 50 mg/min until the arrhythmia is abolished, a total of 1000 mg has been given, or side effects appear.

Pediatric

IV—1 to 5 mg/kg slow IV push. Repeat as needed. Maximum total dose: 500 mg in a 4-hr interval.

NOTE: If given too rapidly by the IV route, bradycardia and severe hypotension may result. The diluent, propylene glycol, will also potentiate the hypotensive effect of phenytoin and cause ECG changes. Cardiac and respiratory arrest may occur with excessive dosage and speed of administration. Blood pressure and the ECG should be monitored carefully, especially during administration.

Phenytoin should not be mixed with any drugs or added to any IV infusion solutions. The solubility is very pH dependent, and use with other medications or solutions will result in a white precipitate.

Each IV injection should be followed by an injection of sterile saline through the same needle or IV catheter to avoid local venous irritation.

Special remarks and cautions

Frequent side effects include nystagmus, ataxia, slurred speech, and mental confusion. Dizziness and transient nervousness may also occur. These side effects are usually dose related and disappear at reduced administration rates. If these symptoms appear before the arrhythmias are controlled, it is less likely that phenytoin will be effective, and therapy may have to be altered.

Phenytoin may elevate blood glucose levels, especially if larger doses are used. Patients with diabetes mellitus or renal insufficiency may be more susceptible to hyperglycemia.

Fatal dermatologic manifestations sometimes accompanied by fever, blood dyscrasias, toxic hepatitis, and liver damage have been attributed to phenytoin.

Gingival hyperplasia occurs frequently, but the incidence may be reduced by good oral hygiene including gum massage, frequent brushing, and proper dental care.

Phenytoin will occasionally discolor urine with shades from pink to red to red-brown.

There have been reports suggesting a correlation between birth defects and the administration of anticonvulsant drugs. Use of phenytoin must be based on risk versus benefit.

Drug interactions

Barbiturates may enhance the rate of metabolism of phenytoin.

Warfarin (Coumadin), disulfiram (Antabuse), phenylbutazone (Butazolidin), chloramphenicol (Chloromycetin), and isoniazid (INH) inhibit the metabolism of phenytoin, resulting in signs of phenytoin toxicity (nystagmus, ataxia, lethargy, and confusion).

Complex relationships exist between folic acid, phenytoin, and anticonvulsant activity. Phenytoin may induce folic acid deficiency, while folic acid replacement may result in partial loss of seizure control.

Phenytoin stimulates microsomal enzyme activity that enhances the metabolism of corticosteroids.

PROCAINAMIDE HYDROCHLORIDE

(Pronestyl)

AHFS 24:04
CATEGORY Antiarrhythmic agent

Action and use

The actions and uses of procainamide are similar to those of quinidine. Procainamide increases the threshold to electric stimulation in both the atria and the ventricles. Conduction in the atria and the ventricles is diminished, while the refractory period of the atria is prolonged.

Procainamide is most commonly used for the treatment of PVCs and ventricular tachycardia. Procainamide is used in atrial arrhythmias, but usually after quinidine has failed.

Characteristics

Peak plasma level: 15 to 60 min (IM), 60 min (PO). Protein binding: 15%. Half-life: 3 to 4 hr. Metabolism: liver to active N-acetylprocainamide, other inactive metabolites. Excretion: 2% to 10% unchanged drug, 50% as metabolites, in urine. Therapeutic level: 0.4 mg/100 ml to 0.8 mg/100 ml. Toxic level: 1 mg/100 ml. Dialysis: yes, H.

Administration and dosage

NOTE: Do not use in complete AV block, and use with extreme caution in partial AV block.

Adult

PO   1. Loading: 1 to 1.25 g.
     2. Second: 750 mg 1 hr after the loading dose if the arrhythmia is still present.
     3. Maintenance: 0.5 to 1 g every 4 to 6 hr. As a result of the short half-life, some patients may require maintenance doses every 3 to 4 hr to maintain adequate control of arrhythmias. Patients should be advised of the importance of adhering to the administration schedule.

IM—0.5 to 1 g every 6 hr until PO therapy is possible.

IV—100 mg every 5 min at 25 to 50 mg/min until arrhythmias are suppressed, a maximum of 1 g has been administered, or side effects develop. Once arrhythmias are suppressed, a continuous infusion may be started at 25 to 30 µg/kg/min. If arrhythmias recur, suppress the arrhythmias with bolus therapy as above and increase the rate of infusion (see Table 2-10).

Pediatric

PO—50 mg/kg divided in 4 to 6 doses for treatment of cardiac arrhythmias.

IV—2 mg/kg diluted in dextrose 5% and given over 5 min. Repeat the dose every 10 to 15 min until arrhythmias are controlled. Maximum total dosage is 1 g. Normal sinus rhythm may then be maintained by an infusion of 20 to 80 µg/kg/min.

NOTE: Cardiovascular toxicities include hypotension, particularly with IV administration. The blood pressure, the apical-radial pulses, and the electrocardiogram must be monitored. If the fall in blood pressure exceeds 15 mm Hg, the infusion should be discontinued. Other manifestations of cardiotoxicity include bradycardia, partial or complete heartblock, extrasystole, asystole, ventricular tachycardia, or fibrillation. If the QRS complex widens beyond 50% or if the PR interval widens, the drug should be discontinued.

Psychoses with hallucinations, giddiness, confusion, CNS stimulation, and convulsions have been reported.

If the infusion is continued for more than 8 to 10 hr, the infusion rate should be reduced as tolerated. Procainamide as well as an active metabolite, N-acetylprocainamide, may accumulate, particularly in those patients with congestive heart failure, hepatic insufficiency, or

Table 2-10. Procainamide administration*

g/500 ml	1.25		1.5		1.75		2.00		2.25		2.50	
mg/ml	2.5		3		3.5		4		4.5		5	
µg/ml	2500		3000		3500		4000		4500		5000	
50 kg µgtts/min	µg/kg/min	mg/min	µg/kg/min	mg/min	µg/kg/min	mg/min	µg/kg/min	mg/min	µg/kg/min	mg/min	µg/kg/min	mg/min
10	8.3	0.4	9.96	0.5	11.6	0.6	13.3	0.66	14.4	0.75	16.6	0.83
20	16.5	0.8	19.8	1.0	23	1.2	26.4	1.3	29.7	1.5	33	1.65
30	25	1.2	30	1.5	35	1.7	40	2.0	45	2.2	50	2.5
40	33	1.65	39.6	2	46.2	2.3	52.8	2.6	59.4	3	66	3.3
50	41.5	2.0	49.8	2.5	58.1	2.9	66.4	3.3	74.7	3.7	83	4.1
60	50	2.5	60	3	70	3.5	80	4.0	90	4.5	100	5
60 kg µgtts/min												
10	6.9	0.4	8.3	0.5	9.7	0.6	11.0	0.66	12.5	0.75	13.8	0.83
20	13.7	0.8	16.5	1.0	19.2	1.2	21.9	1.3	24.7	1.5	27.5	1.65
30	20.8	1.2	24	1.5	29.1	1.7	33.3	2.0	37.5	2.2	41.6	2.5
40	27.5	1.65	33	2	38.5	2.3	43.9	2.6	49.5	3	55	3.3
50	34.5	2.0	41.5	2.5	48.4	2.9	55.3	3.3	62.2	3.7	69.1	4.1
60	41.6	2.5	50	3	58.3	3.5	66.6	4.0	75	4.5	83.3	5
70 kg µgtts/min												
10	5.9	0.4	7.1	0.5	8.3	0.6	9.5	0.66	10.7	0.75	11.8	0.83
20	11.7	0.8	14.14	1.0	16.5	1.2	18.8	1.3	21.2	1.5	23.5	1.65
30	17.8	1.2	21.4	1.5	25	1.7	28.5	2.0	32.1	2.2	35.7	2.5
40	23.5	1.65	28.3	2	33	2.3	37.7	2.6	42.4	3	47.1	3.3
50	29.6	2.0	35.5	2.5	41.5	2.9	47.4	3.3	53.4	3.7	59.3	4.1
60	35.7	2.5	42.8	3	50	3.5	57.1	4.0	64.3	4.5	71.4	5

80 kg

μgtts/min												
10	0.4	5.2	0.5	6.22	0.6	7.2	0.66	8.3	0.75	9.3	0.83	10.3
20	0.8	10.3	1.0	12.3	1.2	14.4	1.3	16.5	1.5	18.5	1.65	20.6
30	1.2	15.6	1.5	18.7	1.7	21.8	2.0	25	2.2	28.1	2.5	31.2
40	1.65	20.6	2	24.7	2.3	28.8	2.6	33	3	37.1	3.3	41.2
50	2.0	25.9	2.5	31.1	2.9	36.3	3.3	41.5	3.7	46.7	4.1	51.8
60	2.5	31.2	3	37.5	3.5	43.7	4.0	50	4.5	56.2	5	62.5

90 kg

μgtts/min												
10	0.4	4.6	0.5	5.53	0.6	6.4	0.66	7.37	0.75	8.3	0.83	9.2
20	0.8	9.14	1.0	11	1.2	12.8	1.3	14.6	1.5	16.5	1.65	18.3
30	1.2	13.85	1.5	16.6	1.7	19.4	2.0	22.2	2.2	25	2.5	27.7
40	1.65	18.28	2	22	2.3	25.6	2.6	29.3	3	33	3.3	36.6
50	2.0	23	2.5	27.6	2.9	32.2	3.3	36.8	3.7	41.5	4.1	46.1
60	2.5	27.7	3	33.3	3.5	38.8	4.0	44.4	4.5	50	5	55.5

100 kg

μgtts/min												
10		4.15		4.98		5.8		6.64		7.5		8.3
20		8.25		9.9		11.5		13.2		14.9		16.5
30		12.5		15		17.5		20		22.5		25
40		16.5		19.8		23.1		26.4		29.7		33
50		20.75		24.9		29		33.2		37.3		41.5
60		25		30		35		40		45		50

110 kg

μgtts/min												
10	0.4	3.77	0.5	4.5	0.6	5.3	0.66	6.0	0.75	6.8	0.83	7.5
20	0.8	7.5	1.0	9	1.2	10.5	1.3	12	1.5	13.5	1.65	15
30	1.2	11.3	1.5	13.6	1.7	15.9	2.0	18.18	2.2	20.5	2.5	22.7
40	1.65	15	2	18	2.3	21	2.6	24	3	27	3.3	30
50	2.0	18.8	2.5	22.6	2.9	26.3	3.3	30.17	3.7	33.9	4.1	37.7
60	2.5	22.72	3	27.2	3.5	31.8	4.0	36.36	4.5	40.9	5	45.5

*Using a microdrip administration set—60 gtts/ml.

renal impairment. Dosage adjustments are best guided by monitoring of the serum procain-amide concentrations.

Special remarks and cautions

When the drug is taken orally, the most common side effects are anorexia, nausea, vomiting, flushing, bitter taste, and diarrhea.

Hypersensitivity reactions including chills, fever, joint and muscle pain, pruritus, urticarial or maculopapular skin rashes, photosensitivity, and anaphylaxis have been reported.

Patients on long-term therapy are more susceptible to blood dyscrasias, including agranulocytosis and thrombocytopenia, and clinical manifestations of systemic lupus erythematosus. These conditions are usually reversible, but the symptoms may last for weeks or months.

Drug interactions

Procainamide may potentiate the hypotensive effects of the thiazides, other diuretics, and antihypertensive agents.

Procainamide may be additive with quinidine, digitalis, and propranolol (Inderal), resulting in further myocardial depression.

Procainamide may potentiate neuromuscular blockade in patients recovering from the effects of surgical muscle relaxants (tubocurarine, succinylcholine, gallamine triethiodide [Flaxedil]) and aminoglycoside antibiotics (gentamicin, streptomycin, kanamycin).

PROPRANOLOL HYDROCHLORIDE
(*Inderal*)

AHFS 24:04
CATEGORY Beta-adrenergic blocking agent

Action and use

Propranolol blocks the beta-adrenergic stimulating action of the catecholamines (isoproterenol, epinephrine, and norepinephrine). It causes lowered heart rate, reduced cardiac output, reduced resting stroke volume, reduced oxygen consumption, and increased left ventricular end diastolic pressure.

It is indicated in the treatment of angina pectoris caused by coronary atherosclerosis, supraventricular arrhythmias, and ventricular tachycardias. Propranolol is also being used for antihypertensive therapy, various types of tremors, anxiety, migraine, and arrhythmias associated with acute myocardial infarction and overdoses of tricyclic antidepressants.

Characteristics

Onset: 30 min (PO), immediate (IV). Peak plasma levels: 60 to 90 min (PO). Peak response: 15 min (IV). Duration: 3 to 6 hr (IV). Protein binding: 90%. Half-life: 10 min (IV) caused by distribution, 3⅖ to 6 hr (PO) after chronic administration. Metabolism: liver, active, and inactive metabolites. Excretion: several metabolites in urine, 1% to 4% in feces as unchanged drug and metabolites. Dialysis: no, H.

Administration and dosage

PO—10 to 80 mg 3 to 4 times daily. When the drug is to be discontinued after chronic administration, therapy should be reduced slowly as tolerated.

IV—The usual dose is from 1 to 5 mg at a rate not to exceed 1 mg/min every 2 to 3 min under close monitoring of ECG.

NOTE: To treat overdose or exaggerated response:
Bradycardia: atropine 0.3 to 1 mg IV or IM
Hypotension: levarterenol (Levophed)
Bronchospasm: isoproterenol (Isuprel) and/or aminophylline
Cardiac failure: digitalization and/or diuretics

Special remarks and cautions

The pharmacologic activity of propranolol may produce hypotension and/or marked bradycardia. This is the most common cardiovascular side effect; it may be accompanied by syncope, shock, and angina pectoris.

Other side effects include exacerbation of congestive heart failure, confusion, giddiness, visual disturbances, hallucinations, mental depression, skin rashes, and hematologic effects (eosinophilia, thrombocytopenia, agranulocytosis).

Propranolol produces bronchoconstriction. Use with extreme caution in patients with bronchial asthma or allergic rhinitis during the pollen season.

Use with caution in diabetic patients and patients subject to hypoglycemia. Because of its beta-adrenergic blocking activity, propranolol may induce relative hypoglycemia by blocking epinephrine-induced glycogenolysis. Propranolol may also prevent the appearance of signs and symptoms (tachycardia, sweating) of acute hypoglycemia.

The risk to the human fetus during propranolol therapy is unknown. Propranolol readily crosses the placental barrier and may appear in breast milk.

Drug interactions

Propranolol is not a potent antihypertensive agent, but the additive hypotensive effect with agents such as guanethidine sulfate (Ismelin), methyldopa (Aldomet), and hydralazine hydrochloride (Apresoline) may be large enough to be clinically significant.

Propranolol may potentiate bradycardia caused by digitalis.

Propranolol blocks the effects of isoproterenol (Isuprel), a beta-adrenergic stimulant.

Propranolol and phenothiazines may have additive hypotensive effects.

Use epinephrine with caution in patients receiving propranolol. Vagal reflex has resulted in marked bradycardia.

Propranolol may prolong the activity of neuromuscular blocking agents (tubocurarine).

QUINIDINE

AHFS 24:04
CATEGORY Antiarrhythmic agent

Action and use

Quinidine has been used clinically for its antiarrhythmic effects for several decades. It is a myocardial depressant having both direct and indirect effects on the heart. Directly, quinidine decreases the excitability of the cardiac muscle to electric stimulation, depresses conduction velocity, prolongs the refractory period, and depresses myocardial contractility. The direct depressant actions of quinidine are complicated by a "vagolytic effect" that in some patients may result in a paradoxic increased heart rate. Quinidine also exhibits alpha- and beta-adrenergic blocking activity as well as anticholinergic properties.

Quinidine is used for the prevention and treatment of cardiac arrhythmias. Those arrhythmias most frequently suppressed are atrial fibrillation, atrial flutter, paroxysmal supraventricular and ventricular tachycardia, and PVCs.

Characteristics

Peak activity: 30 to 90 min (IM), 1 to 3 hr (PO). Duration: 6 to 8 hr. Protein binding: 60%. Half-life: 5 hr. Metabolism: liver, active and inactive. Excretion: kidney, 10% to 50% unchanged in urine in 24 hr. Therapeutic level: 0.3 mg/100 ml to 0.6 mg/100 ml. Toxic level: 1 mg/100 ml. Fatal levels: 3 mg/100 ml to 5 mg/100 ml. Dialysis: yes, H, P.

Administration and dosage

NOTE: As a result of the variable effects of quinidine, dosage must be individualized and patients monitored closely, particularly when initiating therapy.

Adult

PO—Quinidine sulfate: 200 to 400 mg 3 to 5 times daily. Higher doses may be used, but the maximum single dose should not exceed 600 to 800 mg.

IM—Quinidine gluconate: 600 mg initially, then 400 mg every 2 hr as needed.

IV—Quinidine gluconate: 800 mg diluted to 40 ml with dextrose 5% and infused at a rate of 1 ml/min. (IV administration is extremely hazardous. Blood pressure and ECG readings should be monitored continuously as hypotension and arrhythmias may occur.)

Pediatric

PO—Quinidine sulfate: 30 mg/kg/24 hr divided into 4 to 6 doses.

IM—Quinidine gluconate: As for PO administration.

Special remarks and cautions

Myocardial toxicity may be manifested by PVCs, bradycardia, AV block, ventricular tachycardia, ventricular fibrillation, or an increase in congestive heart failure. Electrocardiographic changes include notched P waves, widened QRS complex interval, (greater than 25%—0.14 sec indicates impending toxicity) widened QT interval, ST segment depression, development of U waves, idioventricular rhythm, SA block, AV block, and cardiac arrest.

The most common side effects are diarrhea, nausea, and vomiting. Other symptoms of cinchonism (salivation, tinnitus, vertigo, headache, visual disturbances, confusion) may occur but will diminish if the dosage is lowered.

Hypersensitivity reactions include skin rash, hemolytic anemia, thrombocytopenia, agranulocytosis, or drug fever. Vascular collapse is manifested by severe hypotension, restlessness, cold sweat, pallor, and fainting.

Use quinidine only with *extreme* caution in heart block and digitalis intoxication.

Quinidine should be used with caution during pregnancy and in nursing mothers.

Drug interactions

Quinidine may potentiate the hypotensive effects of the thiazides, other diuretics, and antihypertensive agents.

Quinidine may be additive with procainamide (Pronestyl), digitalis, and propranolol (Inderal) resulting in further myocardial depression.

Quinidine may cause an increase in digoxin serum levels, resulting in increased gastrointestinal and cardiac toxicity. Monitor serum digoxin levels, ECG readings, and the clinical course of the patient closely.

Phenothiazines may have an additive effect when administered with quinidine, increasing myocardial depression, ventricular tachycardia, and/or hypotension.

Quinidine may potentiate neuromuscular blockade in patients recovering from the effects of surgical muscle relaxants (tubocurarine, succinylcholine, gallamine triethiodide [Flaxedil]) and aminoglycoside antibiotics (gentamicin, kanamycin).

Patients receiving both quinidine and warfarin derivatives may be more susceptible to increased anticoagulation and bleeding caused by suppression of vitamin K–dependent coagulation factors.

"Coronary vasodilators"
GENERAL INFORMATION

The nitrites (organic nitrites and nitrates) have long been the treatment of choice for angina pectoris. The primary action of these agents is dilatation of vascular smooth muscle, causing decreased peripheral vascular resistance and a decrease in venous blood return to the heart. The net result is a decreased workload on the heart with a reduction in myocardial oxygen consumption. The nitrites may also allow a redistribution of coronary blood flow, improving the supply of oxygen to the hypoxic areas. For various preparations see Table 2-11.

Characteristics

The nitrites (amyl nitrite) and the nitrates (nitroglycerin, pentaerythritol tetranitrate) appear to act through release of the nitrite ion. The parent nitrate compounds appear to be very rapidly metabolized to nitrite ions at specific "nitrate" receptors located in smooth muscle, resulting in relaxation of the smooth muscle.

Amyl nitrite is administered via inhalation while the nitrates are absorbed quite rapidly through the sublingual mucosa and the gastrointestinal tract. The sublingual route is clinically much more preferable, however, because degradation by the liver is so rapid and complete that little of the active drug reaches systemic circulation. Nitroglycerin may also be readily absorbed through the skin (as evidenced by the use of nitroglycerin 2% ointment).

Special remarks and cautions

All nitrites and nitrates may cause cutaneous vasodilatation and flushing, along with a severe or persistant headache. Patients may complain of transient episodes of dizziness, weakness, and faintness as well as other signs of cerebral ischemia associated with vasodilatation and postural hypotension that may develop.

Table 2-11. Preparations of nitrites and organic nitrates

Generic name	Trade name	Doses, routes of administration	Preparations
Short-acting			
Amyl nitrite	Vaporole	0.18 ml or 0.3 ml inhalation	Pearls: 0.18 and 0.3 ml
Nitroglycerin (glyceryl trinitrate)	Nitrostat	0.15 to 0.6 mg sublingual	Tablets: 0.15, 0.3, 0.4, and 0.6 mg
	Nitrobid	2.5 mg PO every 12 hr	Tablets: 2.5 and 6.5 mg
	Nitrol	Topical to skin every 3 to 4 hr and at bedtime	Ointment: 2%
Long-acting			
Erythrityl tetranitrate	Cardilate	5 to 15 mg, sublingual 15 to 60 mg PO	Tablets: 5, 10, 15 mg PO and sublingual
Pentaerythritol tetranitrate	Peritrate	10 to 40 mg PO	Tablets: 10 and 20 mg
	SK-PETN Duotrate*	30 to 80 mg PO every 12 hr*	30 to 80 mg*
Isosorbide dinitrate	Isordil Sorbitrate	2.5 to 10 mg sublingual 10 to 60 mg PO	Tablets: 2.5, 5 mg sublingual 5 and 10 mg PO
Mannitol hexanitrate	Nitranitol	32 to 64 mg PO	Tablets: 32 mg

*Sustained-release preparations.

An occasional patient may show marked sensitivity to the hypotensive effects of nitrites with normal therapeutic doses. Severe hypotensive episodes may occur, manifested by nausea and vomiting, weakness, restlessness, pallor, cold sweat, and collapse.

Drug rash and/or exfoliative dermatitis is produced by all the organic nitrates, but appears most commonly with pentaerythritol tetranitrate.

Insufficient data has been accumulated to establish the safety of the use of nitrates during the acute phase of a myocardial infarction.

Drug interactions

Ethanol accentuates the vasodilatation and postural hypotension of the nitrites and nitrates. Patients should be cautioned about vasodilatation and hypotension with the ingestion of alcohol while on nitrite therapy.

NITROGLYCERIN (GLYCERYL TRINITRATE)
(Numerous brands)

AHFS 24:12
CATEGORY Vasodilator

Action and use

See General information on the "coronary vasodilators" (pp. 105 and 106).

Administration and dosage

SUBLINGUAL
1. Sit or lie down at the first sign of oncoming anginal attack.
2. Place a tablet under the tongue and allow to dissolve; do not swallow saliva.
3. Do not take more than 3 tablets in 15 min.
4. 1 or 2 tablets may be taken prophylactically a few minutes before engaging in activities that may trigger an anginal attack.

PO—Sustained-release tablets or capsules: 1.3, 2.5, or 6.5 mg 2 to 3 times daily at 8- and 12-hr intervals.

TOPICAL OINTMENT—This dosage form is more for prophylactic use, especially for patients
(nitroglycerin 2%) who suffer from the fear of nocturnal attacks of angina pectoris. If the dosage is adjusted properly, the ointment may be used every 3 to 4 hr and at bedtime.
1. Lay the dose-measuring applicator with the printed side down.
2. Squeeze the proper amount of ointment onto the applicator.
3. Place the measuring applicator on the skin, ointment down, spreading in a thin, uniform layer. Do not massage or rub in. The applicator allows measuring of the proper dose and also prevents absorption through the fingertips.
4. Close the tube tightly and store in a cool place.

NOTE: A chronic headache is a sign of overdosage, requiring the dose to be reduced. Sudden dizziness and faintness (postural hypotension) may result from sudden changes in position. Patients should be cautioned to change positions slowly when arising from a recumbent or sitting position. When terminating the use of the topical ointment, gradually reduce the dose and frequency of application over 4 to 6 weeks.

Special remarks and cautions

Nitroglycerin tablets are inactivated by light, heat, air, and moisture. The tablets should be stored at room temperature in amber glass containers with a tight-fitting screw-on cap. Patients should be warned not to store nitroglycerin tablets within other containers, such as pill boxes, or with other medications, so as to maintain maximum potency.

It should be explained that even though only a few tablets may have been used from a bottle, the patient should test the tablets once a month, and if found subpotent, to discard the bottle and replace it with a fresh supply. A new, potent nitroglycerin tablet should produce a headache or a burning sensation under the tongue when administered sublingually.

See General information on "coronary vasodilators" (pp. 105 and 106).

Drug interactions

See General information on "coronary vasodilators" (pp. 105 and 106).

CHAPTER THREE

Antihypertensive agents

General information on treatment of	*Methyldopa*
hypertension	*Metoprolol tartrate*
Clonidine hydrochloride	*Phentolamine*
Diazoxide	*Prazosin hydrochloride*
Guanethidine sulfate	*Reserpine*
Hydralazine hydrochloride	*Sodium nitroprusside*

GENERAL INFORMATION ON TREATMENT OF HYPERTENSION

Hypertension is a disease characterized by an elevation of the blood pressure above values considered normal for patients of similar environmental and racial backgrounds. In North America statistics indicate that blood pressures above 149/90 to 150/90 mm Hg are associated with premature death resulting from accelerated vascular disease of the brain, heart, and kidneys.

Clinical classification usually divides this disease into primary (essential) hypertension and secondary hypertension. Secondary hypertension may be caused by renal or endocrine dysfunction or a number of other miscellaneous causes such as coarctation of the aorta, toxemia of pregnancy, and CNS disorders. Treatment of secondary hypertension is often unnecessary after controlling the underlying disorder.

Primary hypertension accounts for 80% to 90% of all clinical cases of high blood pressure. Its etiology is basically unknown; it is incurable at the present time, but certainly controllable. A vast array of statistical data indicates that 20 to 25 million Americans have hypertension. The prevalence rises steadily with advancing age; however, in every age group the incidence is higher for blacks than for whites of both sexes. In addition to the age-sex-race patterns, other factors associated with high blood pressure include a family history of hypertension, spikes of high blood pressure in young adult years, obesity, cigarette smoking, hypercholesterolemia, hyperglycemia, abnormal renal function, retinopathies, preexisting cardiovascular disease (that is, angina, congestive heart failure), and a previous history of stroke.

The landmark Veteran's Administration Cooperative Study on hypertension provided dramatic indications of the influence of adequate therapy on morbidity and mortality. Treatment of hypertension requires a multifaceted approach to delay progression of the disease. The ultimate goal of antihypertensive therapy is prolongation of a useful life by preventing cardiovascular complications. To accomplish this the blood pressure must be reduced and maintained at acceptable levels. *Acceptable levels* are variable, since they imply achieving and maintaining an acceptable blood pressure without the patient's neglecting therapy because of the side effects of treatment. Treatment regimens should be established that interfere as little as possible with the patient's life-style.

Patient education is extremely important in treating hypertension and maintaining compliance with the treatment regimen. Patients must be advised that their disease is progressive and that they cannot rely on symptoms to alert them of a higher blood pressure, since hypertension is notoriously asymptomatic until complications occur. Drug therapy is a mainstay of antihypertensive therapy, but ancillary measures are also important. Reduction of dietary sodium intake and weight (if necessary), regular times of relaxation, developing hobbies, and a plan of moderate exercise to improve the patient's physical condition should also be encouraged. Cigarette smoking should be stopped since it is an added risk factor in coronary artery disease.

Prior to initiation of therapy the patient should undergo a thorough physical examination in an attempt to determine the cause and the severity of the hypertension as well as to establish baseline data to monitor both the benefits and the side effects of therapy. If no cause for the hypertension is found, it is assumed that the patient has essential hypertension.

Despite the large number of antihypertensive agents available, there are only three general classes of drugs: (1) diuretics—thiazides, furosemide (Lasix), ethacrynic acid (Edecrin), (2) direct vasodilators—hydralazine (Apresoline), and (3) sympathetic nervous system inhibitors—reserpine, methyldopa (Aldomet), guanethidine (Ismelin), clonidine (Catapres), propranolol (Inderal). All of the above agents act either directly or indirectly to reduce the peripheral vascular resistance, therefore lowering blood pressure. Combination therapy using two or more antihypertensive agents is routine practice. (See Table 3-2 for the ingredients of combination antihypertensive products.) Using drugs that act by different mechanisms to reduce peripheral vascular resistance provides the benefit of using lower doses of each agent so that the patient suffers fewer adverse effects from the therapy.

A patient is classified as having mild hypertension if the diastolic blood pressure is between 90 and 105 mm Hg and if there is no indication of tissue damage (for example, retinopathies). Mild hypertension is usually treated with a thiazide diuretic, and, if necessary, reserpine, clonidine, or methyldopa may be added to the regimen.

Moderate hypertension exists when the diastolic pressure is between 105 and 130 mm Hg. Tissue damage may or may not be present. Treatment usually consists of methyldopa, hydralazine, clonidine, and/or propranolol in combination with an oral diuretic.

A patient may have severe hypertension if the diastolic blood pressure is above 130 mm Hg. These patients are symptomatic and do display tissue damage. The treatment regimen is initiated with an oral diuretic, hydralazine, and propranolol. Inadequate response might require the addition of guanethidine. Other combinations using clonidine and methyldopa may also be successful.

Patients who suddenly develop hypertensive encephalopathy, indicated by neurologic signs and symptoms, require more rapid control of blood pressure. Boluses of diazoxide or a sodium nitroprusside infusion may be indicated to control the symptomatology.

Considerations in the treatment of hypertension

Recognize that the patient's cooperation in redirecting much of his or her life-style is a difficult task to achieve. Adherence to the treatment objectives will be more successful if the goals are realistic for the patient. Patient education with periodic encouragement and reinforcement will increase the patient's ability to maintain therapy.

Request the assistance of the patient and the spouse or a family member in planning a coordinated treatment guide that includes a dietary plan, a reduction in smoking, and a plan to lower stressful, emotional activities.

If feasible, teach the patient to monitor blood pressure at home. Inform the patient of the blood pressure readings that should be reported to the physician.

Plan a schedule so that medications are taken regularly at a proper but yet convenient time. Inform the patient of the side effects of the therapeutic medications and offer assistance in coping with these effects. The frequency of orthostatic hypotension is higher in the morning on arising, and the patient should be taught to get up slowly to offset the feeling of dizziness or to lie down immediately if feeling faint. Other bothersome side effects include nasal congestion, anorexia, loss of strength, and fatigue.

Inform the patient of conditions that will minimize an increased arterial pressure. Situations with associated feelings of anxiety, anger, or annoyance aggravate hypertension. Alterations in normal, ordinary functions such as eating, sleeping, and elimination also increase the physiologic stress response.

To effectively monitor the antihypertensive agents, consult the monographs on those specific medications.

CLONIDINE HYDROCHLORIDE
(*Catapres*)

AHFS 24:08

CATEGORY Antihypertensive agent

Action and use

Clonidine is a potent antihypertensive agent that acts within the central nervous system to reduce both systolic and diastolic blood pressure. It also causes bradycardia, resulting in decreased cardiac output. After prolonged therapy the lowered blood pressure results primarily from reduced peripheral vascular resistance. Clonidine is now used in the treatment of mild to moderate hypertension. Its effectiveness is generally improved when used in combination with diuretics and/or other antihypertensive agents.

Characteristics

Onset: 30 to 60 min (PO). Peak activity: 2 to 4 hr (PO). Duration: 8 hr (PO); Half-life: 12 to 16 hr with normal renal function, 25 to 37 hr with impaired renal function. Metabolism: liver, to 4 metabolites. Excretion: 20% in feces, 32% unchanged in urine, 33% as metabolites in urine.

Administration and dosage
Adult

PO   1. Initial: 0.1 mg 2 times daily.
2. Maintenance: Add 0.1 to 0.2 mg daily until desired effect is achieved. Average daily doses range from 0.2 to 0.8 mg in divided doses. Maximum recommended daily dose is 2.4 mg.

Pediatric

No dosage recommendations are available.

Special remarks and cautions

Patients must be informed of the need for continuity of therapy. Abrupt discontinuance of therapy may result in a rapid increase in systolic and diastolic pressure. Patients may display such symptoms as nervousness, restlessness, agitation, tremor, headache, nausea, and increased salivation. These symptoms are more pronounced after 1 to 2 months of therapy and begin to appear a few hours after a dose is missed. Blood pressure rises significantly within 8 to 24 hr. When clonidine therapy is to be discontinued, dosage should be gradually reduced over 2 to 4 days, depending on the patient's response.

The most frequent adverse effects reported with clonidine are dry mouth, drowsiness, and sedation (caution patients about performing hazardous tasks). Other side effects include constipation, dizziness, and headache. Numerous other gastrointestinal, metabolic, cardiovascular, dermatologic, and genitourinary effects have also been reported.

Diuretic therapy is often beneficial in diminishing sodium and water retention, especially during the first few days of clonidine therapy.

Periodic ophthalmologic examinations are recommended for patients on long-term clonidine therapy. Laboratory animals have developed degenerative retinal changes, although none have been reported in humans.

Patients suffering from mental depression may be more susceptible to further depressive activity.

Reproduction studies have found no teratogenic activity, but embryo toxicities have been found at doses within the normal therapeutic range. Clonidine should therefore not be used in pregnant women unless the potential benefit outweighs the potential risk. It is not known whether clonidine is found in breast milk.

Drug interactions

The sedative effects of clonidine may enhance the CNS depressant effects of alcohol, barbiturates, tranquilizers, and antihistamines.

Desipramine (Norpramin, Pertofrane) blocks the antihypertensive effects of clonidine. Other tricyclic antidepressants may also result in loss of hypertensive control.

Clonidine may be administered together with hydralazine, guanethidine, methyldopa, reserpine, spironolactone, furosemide, and the thiazide diuretics without interactions. However, the antihypertensive effects of all these agents will be enhanced, requiring careful adjustment of dosages.

The bradycardic effects of clonidine may be enhanced by guanethidine, propranolol, and the digitalis glycosides.

DIAZOXIDE
(Hyperstat I.V.)

AHFS 24:08
CATEGORY Antihypertensive agent

Action and use

Diazoxide lowers blood pressure by a direct vasodilatory action on the smooth muscle of peripheral arterioles, thus reducing peripheral vascular resistance. Diazoxide is used for emergency reduction of blood pressure in hospitalized patients with severe hypertension when a rapid decrease in diastolic pressure is required.

Characteristics

Onset and peak: less than 5 min (IV). Duration: 4 to 12 hr. Protein-binding: more than 90%. Half-life: 28 hr. Metabolism: questionable. Excretion: urine, primarily unchanged. Dialysis: yes, H, P.

Administration and dosage
Adult

IV—300 mg in 30 sec or less. Monitor the blood pressure closely. A second dose may be required for a satisfactory reduction in blood pressure if the first injection fails to give an adequate response within 30 min.

Pediatric

IV—5 mg/kg in 30 sec or less. Monitor the blood pressure closely. A second dose may be needed within 30 min.

NOTE: Administer undiluted in a peripheral vein. As a result of the alkalinity of the solution, extravascular injection or leakage may be quite irritating and should be avoided.

Special remarks and cautions

Blood pressure must be monitored at frequent intervals, particularly during the first hour after administration. If hypotension occurs, it will usually respond to the administration of dopamine or levarterenol.

Diazoxide may caused marked sodium and water retention, particularly after repeated injections, resulting in edema and congestive heart failure. Potent diuretics such as furosemide (Lasix) or ethacrynic acid (Edecrin) may be required to diminish the water retention. The diuretics may also potentiate the hypotensive and hyperglycemic properties of diazoxide.

Hyperglycemia is a frequent adverse effect of diazoxide therapy. Treatment with insulin is occasionally required, especially in those patients with diabetes mellitus.

Diazoxide must be used with caution during pregnancy. Fetal abnormalities have been observed in animals. Diazoxide crosses the placental barrier, but its presence and content in human breast milk is not known.

Drug interactions

The anticoagulant activity of warfarin (Coumadin) may be increased as a result of the displacement from protein-binding sites by diazoxide.

The hyperglycemic potential of diazoxide may be enhanced by patients concurrently receiving diuretics, phenytoin (Dilantin), propranolol (Inderal), corticosteroids such as prednisone, and oral contraceptives.

GUANETHIDINE SULFATE
(Ismelin)

AHFS 24:08
CATEGORY Antihypertensive agent

Action and use

Guanethidine sulfate acts both by blocking the release of norepinephrine from nerve endings in response to nerve stimulation and by depleting norepinephrine from storage sites at adrenergic nerve endings. The effects of PO administration are cumulative over 10 days to 2 weeks and result in gradual reduction of both systolic and diastolic blood pressure. Guanethidine sulfate is a potent agent used in combination therapy with other antihypertensive agents to treat sustained moderate to severe hypertension.

Characteristics

Gastrointestinal absorption varies from 3% to 27% of the administered PO dose. Onset and duration: cumulative over several days. Metabolism: hepatic microsomal enzymes. Excretion: via urine as active and inactive metabolites.

Administration and dosage
Adult

PO 1. Initial: 10 mg daily. Increase the dose 10 mg every 5 to 7 days if the blood pressure measurements so indicate and side effects are tolerable.
2. Maintenance: 25 to 50 mg daily; however, much higher doses are occasionally required. The dose may be given once daily.

Pediatric

PO 1. Initial: 0.2 mg/kg/day.
2. Maintenance: increase every 7 to 10 days by 0.2 mg/kg. A final dose 6 to 8 times the initial dose may be required for optimal therapy.
NOTE: Take the blood pressure with the patient in the supine position and after standing for 10 min. The dosage should be reduced if there is a normal supine pressure or an excessive fall in pressure on standing or if severe diarrhea is present.

Special remarks and cautions

Orthostatic hypotension occurs frequently, especially with sudden changes in posture. Patients must be taught to rise slowly from a horizontal position to a sitting position and then flex the arms and legs several times before standing. Orthostatic symptoms are more apparent in the morning and may also be aggravated by heavy exercise, hot weather, and ingestion of alcohol. Standing for prolonged periods may also make the patient feel dizzy and weak. The patient should be forewarned to sit or lie down with the onset of weakness and dizziness.

Frequent adverse reactions include bradycardia, fluid retention, increased numbers of bowel movements and diarrhea. The diarrhea may be severe enough to result in discontinuance of the drug.

Other side effects include fatigue, nausea, muscle tremor, mental depression, nasal congestion, blurred vision, dry mouth, angina, and asthma in susceptible patients. Genitourinary symptoms include impotence, nocturia, urinary incontinence, and retrograde ejaculation.

Safe use has not been established in pregnancy.

Drug interactions

The following drugs may enhance the hypotensive effects of guanethidine:

Ethanol
Propranolol hydrochloride (Inderal)
Quinidine*
Diuretics
Methotrimeprazine (Levoprome)
Reserpine

The following drugs may antagonize the hypotensive effects of guanethidine:

Amphetamines (Dexadrine, Benzadrine)
Methylphenidate (Ritalin)
Ephedrine
Tricyclic antidepressants
    Desipramine (Norpramin, Pertofrane)
    Imipramine (Tofranil)
    Protriptyline hydrochloride (Vivactil)
    Nortriptyline (Aventyl)
    Amitriptyline hydrochloride (Elavil)
    Doxepin (Sinequan)
Phenothiazines
Haloperidol (Haldol)
Monamine oxidase inhibitors
Oral contraceptives

The response from the following drugs would be expected to be enhanced by guanethidine as a result of increased sensitivity of receptor sites (initial therapy with very low doses):

Levarterenol bitartrate (Levophed)
Dopamine hydrochloride (Intropin)
Phenylephrine (Neo-Synephrine)

Guanethidine may potentiate the hypoglycemic effects of oral hypoglycemic agents and insulin.

---

*More hypotension observed after parenteral administration.

HYDRALAZINE HYDROCHLORIDE
(Apresoline)

AHFS 24:08
CATEGORY Antihypertensive agent

Action and use

Hydralazine is a hypotensive agent that acts on the smooth muscle in arteries and veins, causing vasodilatation. Hydralazine is used to treat moderate to severe hypertension, usually in combination with other agents. Propranolol is often used in combination with hydralazine to prevent the adverse hemodynamic effects of hydralazine.

Characteristics

Peak blood levels: 3 to 4 hr (PO). Duration: 24 hr. Metabolism: liver, by conjugation and acetylation. Excretion: urine as metabolites.

Administration and dosage
Adult

PO 1. Initial: 10 mg 4 times daily for the first 2 to 4 days, then 25 mg 4 times daily. The second week, increase the dosage to 50 mg 4 times daily as the patient tolerates the dosage and the blood pressure is brought under control.
    2. Maintenance: adjust the dosage to the lowest effective levels.

IM or IV—20 to 40 mg repeated as necessary. Monitor blood pressures frequently. Results usually become evident within 10 to 20 min.

Pediatric

PO 1. Initial: 0.75 mg/kg/24 hr in 4 divided doses.
    2. Maintenance: increase over 3 to 4 weeks to 10 times the initial dosage.

IM or IV—1.7 to 3.5 mg/kg/24 hr in 4 to 6 divided doses.

NOTE: Some patients may require 300 mg or more daily. Combination therapy with thiazides, reserpine, propranolol, or clonidine may allow a reduction in dosage of hydralazine. At these higher doses there is a greater incidence of an arthritis-like syndrome that may lead to a syndrome indistinguishable from disseminated lupus erythematosus. The syndrome is reversible on discontinuance of hydralazine and may require months of corticosteroid therapy before elimination of the symptoms.

Special remarks and cautions

As with any antihypertensive therapy, patients should be advised concerning orthostatic hypotension.

Headache, palpitations, tachycardia, angina pectoris, nausea, vomiting, and diarrhea are common side effects of hydralazine.

During prolonged therapy, complete blood count determinations are indicated, as well as LE cell preparations and antinuclear antibody titer determination. Blood dyscrasias and rheumatoid disease have been reported during prolonged therapy.

Peripheral neuritis, characterized by numbness and tingling, has been reported. Pyridoxine may be effective in treating these symptoms.

Hydralazine may cause sodium and water retention. Diuretic therapy may be required to control the edema.

Drug interactions

Hydralazine is often used in combination with other antihypertensive medications to enhance the hypotensive activity and allow a reduction in the dosages of the antihypertensive agents. Propranolol is particularly useful in this respect.

METHYLDOPA
(Aldomet)

AHFS 24:08

CATEGORY Antihypertensive agent

Action and use

Methyldopa is a hypotensive agent whose mechanism of action has not been completely determined. It has several proposed mechanisms, but the major antihypertensive effects now appear to be caused by the formation of a metabolite, α-methylnorepinephrine, which acts predominantly within the central nervous system. There are some unexplained discrepancies in activity, however, and other mechanisms yet to be explained are involved. Methyldopa is recommended for sustained moderate to severe hypertension, usually in combination with other agents.

Characteristics

Fifty percent absorbed from GI tract. Onset: 6 to 12 hr. Peak plasma levels: 3 to 6 hr. Duration: 8 to 12 hr. Elimination: biphasic. Normal renal function: first half-life: approximately 100 min, 90% of unchanged drug in urine, second half-life: 5 to 8 hr. Severely impaired renal function: first half-life: 3½ hr, with only 50% excreted in early phase. Accumulation occurs with chronic administration. Metabolism: liver. Dialysis: yes, H, P.

Administration and dosage
Adult

PO 1. Initial: 250 mg 3 times daily for the first 48 hr. Add 250 to 500 mg every 2 to 3 days as indicated by blood pressure measurement and patient's tolerance.
2. Maintenance: the minimum effective dose. Combination therapy with thiazide diuretics often allows the use of lower doses of methyldopa with fewer side effects. The maximum daily dose is 3.0 g.

IV—250 to 500 mg every 6 hr as needed. Hypotensive effects are noted in 4 to 6 hr with a duration of 10 to 16 hr. Add the desired dose of methyldopa (50 mg/ml) to 100 ml of dextrose 5% and infuse IV over 30 to 60 min.

Pediatric

PO— 10 to 20 mg/kg/24 hr in 2 to 4 divided doses. Adjust maintenance doses every 2 to 3 days for optimal effect. Maximum dosage is 65 mg/kg/24 hr or 3.0 g (whichever is less).
IV—20 to 40 mg/kg/24 hr in 4 divided doses.

Special remarks and cautions

Sedation, lethargy, and dizziness commonly occur when methyldopa therapy is initiated or during adjustment to higher doses. These effects are most notable during the first 2 to 3 days and tend to dissipate with time.

Between 1% and 3% of patients develop a drug-induced fever during the first 2 to 3 weeks of therapy. It is often associated with muscle pain, malaise, nausea, vomiting, and diarrhea. Occasionally abnormal liver function tests, eosinophilia, and skin rashes have been reported. The symptoms are reversible on discontinuance of the drug, but the fever will redevelop 6 to 12 hr after a challenge dose.

An average of about 20% of patients on methyldopa therapy for 6 to 12 months develop a positive reaction to the direct Coombs' test. The incidence is dose related. Which patients with a positive direct Coomb's test who may develop true hemolytic anemia secondary to methyldopa therapy cannot be predicted, but data indicate that only 0.1% to 0.2% of the patients will develop an autoimmune hemolytic anemia. It takes another 6 to 12 months after methyldopa is discontinued for the Coombs' test to revert to normal. Periodic blood counts should be determined during therapy to detect hemolytic anemia.

Other adverse effects that occur with methyldopa therapy include angina pectoris, bradycardia, nasal stuffiness, dry mouth, constipation, weight gain, and edema.

Methyldopa or its metabolites may discolor the urine, causing it to darken on exposure to air.

Methyldopa may cause a false-positive Clinitest reaction for urine glucose. It does not affect Tes-tape or Diastix, however.

Methyldopa crosses the placental barrier and is not recommended in pregnancy. Excretion in breast milk is unknown.

Drug interactions

The following drugs may enhance the hypotensive activity of methyldopa:

Diuretics
Propranolol (Inderal)
Procainamide (Pronestyl)
Quinidine
Levodopa (Dopar, Larodopa)
Phenothiazines

The following tricyclic antidepressants may antagonize the hypotensive effects of methyldopa:

Doxepin (Sinequan)
Imipramine (Tofranil)
Desipramine (Pertofrane, Norpramin)
Amitriptyline (Elavil)
Protriptyline hydrochloride (Vivactil)

METOPROLOL TARTRATE
(Lopressor)

AHFS unclassified
CATEGORY Antihypertensive, beta-adrenergic blocking agent

Action and use

Metoprolol is a synthetic antihypertensive agent that acts by selectively blocking $beta_1$-adrenergic receptors. As a $beta_1$-adrenergic blocking agent it has an inhibitory effect on cardiac muscle, resulting in a reduction of heart rate and cardiac output both at rest and during exercise. At higher doses metoprolol also blocks $beta_2$-adrenergic receptors, which are located in bronchial and vascular smooth muscle. Metoprolol is now used in the treatment of mild to moderate hypertension. Its effectiveness is generally improved when used in combination with thiazide diuretics and/or other antihypertensive agents.

Characteristics

Onset: 60 min (PO). Peak activity: 1½ hr (PO). Duration: dose related. Half-life: 3 to 4 hr. Metabolism: liver to several metabolites. Excretion: 95% excreted in urine, 3% to 10% unchanged.

Administration and dosage
Adult

PO   1. Initial: 50 mg 2 times daily. Increase the dosage by 50 mg every 7 to 10 days until desired blood pressure is obtained.
2. Maintenance: usually 100 mg 2 times daily. Dosage range: 100 to 450 mg daily.

Pediatric

Safety in children has not been established.

NOTE: Bradycardia may occur. Therefore do not administer to patients with heart disease or a heart rate of less than 60 beats/min unless the patient uses a pacemaker.

Special remarks and cautions

The pharmacologic activity of metoprolol may produce hypotension, congestive heart failure, and/or marked bradycardia if dosages are not adjusted properly. The most common side effects noted include tiredness, headache, and diarrhea.

Metoprolol should be administered with caution to patients with respiratory conditions such as bronchitis, bronchial asthma, or allergic rhinitis. Metoprolol may produce broncho-constriction and may aggravate wheezing, especially during the pollen season.

Use with caution in diabetic patients and patients subject to hypoglycemia. Because of its adrenergic blocking activity, metoprolol may induce relative hypoglycemia by blocking epinephrine-induced glycogenolysis. Metoprolol may also prevent the appearance of signs and symptoms (tachycardia) of acute hypoglycemia.

The risk to the human fetus during metoprolol therapy is unknown. It is not known whether metoprolol is excreted in breast milk.

Drug interactions

Metoprolol may potentiate bradycardia induced by digitalis glycosides.

Metoprolol partially blocks the effects of isoproterenol (Isuprel), a beta-adrenergic stimulant.

Metoprolol and phenothiazines may have additive hypotensive effects.

Metoprolol may have additive cardiovascular effects when used with such agents as guanethidine (Ismelin), hydralazine (Apresoline), methyldopa (Aldomet), reserpine, and propranolol (Inderal).

PHENTOLAMINE
(Regitine)

AHFS 24:08
CATEGORY Alpha-adrenergic blocking agent

Action and use

Phentolamine acts on vascular smooth muscle, blocking alpha-stimulated vasoconstriction. The resulting dilatation decreases the peripheral vascular resistance, usually causing a drop in blood pressure.

Phentolamine is used as an adjunct in the diagnosis of pheochromocytoma, in the control of hypertensive episodes before and during surgical removal of a pheochromocytoma, and in the prevention and treatment of skin necrosis following IV administration or extravasation of levarterenol (Levophed).

Administration and dosage

PO—Control of hypertensive episodes prior to surgery, 50 mg 4 to 6 times daily. Higher doses may be required.

IM—Preoperative and operative reduction of blood pressure, 5 mg 1 to 2 hr prior to surgery and repeated as necessary.

IV—5 mg as needed.

NOTE: Prolonged hypotensive episodes may result, especially after parenteral use.

For dermal necrosis and sloughing following IV administration or extravasation of levarterenol (Levophed):

PREVENTION—Add 10 mg of phentolamine to each liter of solution containing levarterenol.

TREATMENT—Inject 5 to 10 mg of phentolamine diluted in 10 ml saline into the area of extravasation as soon as possible.

Special remarks and cautions

Phentolamine, both as an indirect cardiac stimulant and as a result of hypotensive episodes, may cause tachycardias, cardiac arrhythmias, anginal pain, myocardial infarction, cerebrovascular spasm, and cerebrovascular occlusion.

Other adverse effects include nausea, vomiting, diarrhea, and exacerbation of peptic ulcer caused by gastrointestinal stimulation; weakness; dizziness; flushing; and nasal stuffiness.

Safe use during pregnancy and lactation has not been established.

Drug interactions

No specific drug interactions have been reported with phentolamine.

PRAZOSIN HYDROCHLORIDE
(Minipress)

AHFS 24:08
CATEGORY Antihypertensive agent

Action and use

Prazosin is an antihypertensive medication structurally unrelated to other antihypertensive agents. Although the exact mechanism of action is unknown, prazosin is an alpha blocker that may also act directly on smooth muscle to produce peripheral dilation and a reduction in diastolic blood pressure. There is no significant change in heart rate or renal blood flow. Prazosin is now used in the treatment of mild to moderate hypertension. Prazosin's effectiveness is generally improved when the drug is used in combination with diuretics and/or other antihypertensive agents.

Characteristics

Onset: 2 hr. Peak activity: 2 to 3 hr. Duration: less than 24 hr. Protein binding: 97%. Half-life: 2 to 4 hr. Metabolites: hepatic, to several active and inactive metabolites. Excretion: 5% to 10% unchanged in urine, remainder in feces. Dialysis: unknown.

Administration and dosage

PO
1. Initial: 1 mg 3 times daily.
2. Maintenance: dosage may be gradually increased to 20 mg daily. For maintenance therapy, prazosin may be administered twice daily. Maximum recommended dosage is 40 mg daily.

When adding other antihypertensive agents, reduce the dose of prazosin to 1 to 2 mg 3 times daily, add other agents, and then readjust the prazosin dosage.

Special remarks and cautions

The initial doses of prazosin may cause tachycardia, followed by syncope and unconsciousness. This adverse effect occurs in about 1% of patients starting on the drug; symptoms develop 15 to 90 min after the initial dose. This effect may be minimized by giving the first dose with food and limiting it to 1 mg. Patients should be warned that this side effect may occur, that it is transient, and that they should lie down immediately if symptoms develop.

The most frequent adverse effects reported with prazosin include dizziness, headache, drowsiness, nausea, weakness, and lethargy. All are transient and rarely require discontinuation of therapy.

Reproduction studies have not reported teratogenetic activity; however, prazosin is not recommended in pregnant women unless the potential benefit outweighs the potential risk. It is not known whether prazosin is secreted in breast milk.

Drug interactions

The sedative effects of prazosin may enhance the CNS depressant effects of alcohol, barbiturates, tranquilizers, and antihistamines.

The hypotensive effects of prazosin are enhanced by the concomitant administration of other antihypertensive agents and diuretics.

RESERPINE
(Serpasil)

AHFS 24:08
CATEGORY Antihypertensive agent

Action and use

Reserpine acts to lower blood pressure by depleting stores of catecholamines at nerve endings. It also prevents the reuptake of norepinephrine at storage sites, allowing enzymatic destruction of the neuronal transmitter. There is a gradual reduction over a few days to several weeks in peripheral vasoconstriction, resulting in a drop in blood pressure. Reserpine is used to treat mild essential hypertension and may be an effective adjunct to the treatment of more severe hypertension.

Administration and dosage

PO 1. Initial: 0.5 mg daily for 1 to 2 weeks.
    2. Maintenance: 0.1 to 0.25 mg daily.
IM—Hypertensive crises:
    1. Initial: 0.5 to 1 mg.
    2. Maintenance: 2 to 4 mg every 3 hr as needed.

Special remarks and cautions

Severe mental depression is the most dangerous side effect of reserpine. The onset of depression may be quite insidious and often difficult to relate to initiation of reserpine therapy. Chronic administration of low doses (0.25 mg) can produce nightmares and mental depression that may require hospitalization or result in suicide. It is recommended that therapy be discontinued at the first sign of despondency, early morning insomnia, loss of appetite, impotence, or self-deprecation. These effects may continue for several weeks after discontinuance, depending on the dosage used and the duration of therapy.

A pharmacologic action of reserpine is the stimulation of gastric hydrochloric acid. Although the doses required are usually higher than those used routinely for hypertension, patients should be observed for the development of gastric ulcers, and reserpine should be used with caution in patients with a history of ulcer disease.

Other side effects include nausea, vomiting, diarrhea, abdominal cramps, bradycardia, angina-like symptoms, arrhythmias, (particularly when used concurrently with digitalis or quinidine), nasal stuffiness, and dryness of the mouth.

Reserpine is not recommended for pregnant or lactating women. It crosses the placental barrier and is secreted in breast milk. Increased respiratory tract secretions, nasal congestion, and cyanosis have been reported in neonates and nursing infants whose mothers had been treated with reserpine.

Drug interactions

The following drugs may add to the hypotensive effects of reserpine:

Diuretics	Quinidine
Phenothiazines	Thiothixene (Navane)
Procainamide (Pronestyl)	Methotrimeprazine (Levoprome)

The following tricyclic antidepressants may antagonize the antihypertensive effects of reserpine:

Doxepin (Sinequan)	Imipramine (Tofranil)
Amitriptyline hydrochloride (Elavil)	Desipramine (Norpramin)
Nortriptyline (Aventyl)	

SODIUM NITROPRUSSIDE
(Nipride)

AHFS 24:08
CATEGORY Antihypertensive agent

Action and use

Nitroprusside is a potent vasodilator that acts directly on vascular smooth muscle to produce a peripheral vasodilation. It has been approved for use as an antihypertensive in hypertensive crisis. The drug is also being investigated for possible use in treating dissecting

Table 3-1. Nitroprusside administration*

amps/500 ml	1	2	4	6	8
mg/500 ml	50	100	200	300	400
μg/1 ml	100	200	400	600	800
50 kg μgtts/min	μg/kg/min	μg/kg/min	μg/kg/min	μg/kg/min	μg/kg/min
10	0.33	0.66	1.32	1.98	2.64
20	0.66	1.3	2.64	3.96	5.28
30	1.00	2.0	4.0	6	8
40	1.32	2.6	5.28	7.92	10.56
50	1.66	3.3	6.64	9.96	13.28
60	2.0	4.0	8	12	16
60 kg μgtts/min					
10	0.27	0.55	1.1	1.66	2.21
20	0.55	1.1	2.2	3.3	4.4
30	0.83	1.6	3.33	5.0	6.6
40	1.1	2.2	4.4	6.6	8.8
50	1.36	2.7	5.53	8.3	11.0
60	1.66	3.3	6.6	10	13.3
70 kg μgtts/min					
10	0.23	0.47	95	1.42	1.9
20	0.47	0.94	1.88	2.82	3.77
30	0.71	1.4	2.85	4.3	5.7
40	0.94	1.9	3.77	5.65	7.5
50	1.16	2.4	4.74	7.11	9.5
60	1.4	2.8	5.7	8.57	11.4
80 kg μgtts/min					
10	0.2	0.41	0.83	1.24	1.66
20	0.41	0.82	1.65	2.5	3.3
30	0.62	1.25	2.5	3.75	5
40	0.82	1.6	3.3	4.95	6.6
50	1.0	2.0	4.15	6.22	8.3
60	1.25	2.5	5	7.5	10

*Using a microdrip administration set—60 gtts/ml.

aneurysms, acute myocardial infarction, and low-output syndromes combined with increased peripheral resistance.

Characteristics

Onset: immediate. Duration: within minutes of discontinuance. Metabolism: in erythrocytes and tissues to cyanogen, which is then converted to thiocyanate in the liver (see Special remarks and cautions).

Table 3-1. Nitroprusside administration—cont'd

amps/500 ml	1	2	4	6	8
mg/500 ml	50	100	200	300	400
μg/1 ml	100	200	400	600	800
90 kg μgtts/min	μg/kg/min	μg/kg/min	μg/kg/min	μg/kg/min	μg/kg/min
10	0.18	0.36	0.73	1.10	1.5
20	0.36	0.74	1.46	2.2	2.93
30	0.55	1.1	2.2	3.3	4.4
40	0.73	1.5	2.93	4.4	5.86
50	0.92	1.8	3.7	5.5	7.37
60	1.11	2.2	4.4	6.6	8.88
100 kg μgtts/min					
10	0.16	0.33	0.66	1	1.33
20	0.33	0.66	1.32	2	2.64
30	0.5	1.0	2	3	4
40	0.66	1.3	2.64	4	5.32
50	0.83	1.6	3.3	5	6.64
60	1.0	2.0	4	6	8
110 kg μgtts/min					
10	0.15	0.3	0.6	0.9	1.2
20	0.3	0.6	1.2	1.8	2.4
30	0.45	0.9	1.81	2.7	3.6
40	0.6	1.2	2.4	3.6	4.8
50	0.75	1.5	3	4.5	6.0
60	0.9	1.8	3.6	5.4	7.3
120 kg μgtts/min					
10	0.14	0.27	0.55	0.83	1.1
20	0.27	0.55	1.1	1.65	2.2
30	0.41	0.83	1.65	2.5	3.3
40	0.55	1.1	2.2	3.3	4.4
50	0.69	1.38	2.76	4.15	5.5
60	0.83	1.66	3.33	5	6.6

Administration and dosage

IV—The usual initial infusion rate is between 0.5 to 1.5 μg/kg/min. The dosage must be carefully titrated with close monitoring of blood pressure in each patient. A dose of 1 μg/kg/min usually produces a prompt drop in pressure, although a dose required to produce a given hypotensive effect is variable. The average dose of nitroprusside is 3 μg/kg/min with a range of 0.5 to 8 μg/kg/min. For dosage adjustment see Table 3-1. Nitroprusside is highly light sensitive. A paper bag or foil wrap should be placed over the IV fluid container to protect against degradation. At slow infusion rates the translucent plastic tubing should also be taped. Solutions over 4 hr old should be discarded. With cessation of the drip, blood pressure promptly begins to rise, reaching control levels usually in 10 min or less.

NOTE: Safe use in children has not been established.

Special remarks and cautions

Adverse effects include nausea, retching, abdominal pain, diaphoresis, restlessness, apprehension, headache, muscle twitching, palpitations, and retrosternal discomfort. These symptoms are usually dose related and may be further minimized by keeping the patient supine.

Thiocyanate is a metabolite of nitroprusside. Toxic symptoms (fatigue, anorexia, weakness, skin rashes, tinnitus, and mental confusion) begin to appear at thiocyanate plasma levels of 5 to 10 mg/100 ml, with fatalities occurring at 20 mg/100 ml. The half-life of thiocyanate in patients with normal renal function is 7 days, but is prolonged in patients with impaired hepatic or renal function. Peritoneal dialysis and hemodialysis may be used to treat thiocyanate toxicities.

The distribution of nitroprusside and its metabolites across the placenta and into breast milk has not been studied. Thus its safety for pregnant and lactating women has not been established.

Drug interactions

Thiocyanate inhibits both the uptake and binding of iodine. Symptoms of hypothyroidism have been reported after several days of nitroprusside therapy.

Table 3-2. Ingredients of antihypertensive combination products

Product	Diuretic (mg)											Antihypertensive (mg)							Other (mg)
	Bendroflumethiazide	Benzthiazide	Chlorothiazide	Chlorthalidone	Cyclothiazide	Flumethiazide	Hydrochlorothiazide	Hydroflumethiazide	Methyclothiazide	Polythiazide	Trichlormethiazide	Clonidine	Deserpidine	Guanethidine	Hydralazine	Methyldopa	Rauwolfia	Reserpine	
Aldochlor-150			150													250			
Aldochlor-250			250													250			
Aldoril-15							15									250			
Aldoril-25							25									250			
Apresazide 25/25							25								25				
Apresazide 50/50							50								50				
Apresazide 100/50							50								100				
Apresoline-Esidrix							15								25				
Butiserpazide-25							25											0.1	Butabarbital, 30
Butiserpazide-50							50											0.1	Butabarbital, 30
Combipres 0.1 mg				15								0.1							
Combipres 0.2 mg				15								0.2							
Demi-Regroton				25														0.125	

Continued.

Table 3-2. Ingredients of antihypertensive combination products—cont'd

Product	Diuretic (mg) Bendroflumethiazide	Benzthiazide	Chlorothiazide	Chlorthalidone	Cyclothiazide	Flumethiazide	Hydrochlorothiazide	Hydroflumethiazide	Methyclothiazide	Polythiazide	Trichlormethiazide	Antihypertensive (mg) Clonidine	Deserpidine	Guanethidine	Hydralazine	Methyldopa	Rauwolfia	Reserpine	Other (mg)
Diupres-250			250															0.125	
Diupres-500			500															0.125	
Diutensen									2.5										Cryptenamine, 2
Diutensen-R									2.5									0.1	
Dralserp															25			0.1	
Enduronyl									5				0.25						
Enduronyl Forte									5				0.5						
Esimil							25							10					
Eutron Filmtab									5										Pargyline, 25
Exna-R		50																0.125	
Hydropres-25							25											0.125	
Hydropres-50							50											0.125	

Product									
Hydrotensin-25		25							0.125
Hydrotensin-50		50							0.125
Hydrotensin-Plus		15				25			0.1
Hystol		15				25			
Metatensin					2/4				0.1
Naquival					4				0.1
Naturetin W/K	25/5							Potassium chloride, 500	
Oreticyl		25/50							0.125
Oreticyl Forte		25							0.25
Rautrax		400					50	Potassium chloride, 400	
Rautrax-N	4						50	Potassium chloride, 400	
Rautrax-N Modified	2						50	Potassium chloride, 400	
Rauzide	4						50		
Regroton			50						0.25
Renese-R					2				0.25
Ro-Chloro-Serp 250				250					0.125
Ro-Chloro-Serp 500				500					0.125

Continued.

Table 3-2. Ingredients of antihypertensive combination products—cont'd

	Diuretic (mg)											*Antihypertensive (mg)*							
Product	*Bendroflumethiazide*	*Benzthiazide*	*Chlorothiazide*	*Chlorthalidone*	*Cyclothiazide*	*Flumethiazide*	*Hydrochlorothiazide*	*Hydroflumethiazide*	*Methyclothiazide*	*Polythiazide*	*Trichlormethiazide*	*Clonidine*	*Deserpidine*	*Guanethidine*	*Hydralazine*	*Methyldopa*	*Rauwolfia*	*Reserpine*	*Other (mg)*
Salutensin								50										0.125	
Ser-Ap-Es							15								25			0.1	
Serpasil-Apresoline #1															25			0.1	
Serpasil-Apresoline #2															50			0.2	
Serpasil-Esidrix #1							25											0.1	
Serpasil-Esidrix #2							50											0.1	
Thia-Serp-25							25											0.125	
Thia-Serp-50							50											0.125	
Thia-Serpa-Zine							15								25			0.1	
Thia-zine							15								25				
Unipres							15								25			0.1	

CHAPTER FOUR

Diuretic agents

General information on diuretics   *Mannitol*
Ethacrynic acid   *Spironolactone*
Furosemide   *Triamterene*
Hydrochlorothiazide

GENERAL INFORMATION ON DIURETICS

Diuretics act primarily on the kidneys to promote excretion of excess fluid. Appropriate selection of a diuretic agent to treat edema (excessively increased fluid volume in the interstitial compartment) or hypertension (elevated blood pressure) depends on the pathophysiology of the disease creating the edema or hypertension, the mechanism of action and characteristics of the diuretics, and the physiologic side effects that the diuretics may produce. Diuretics act primarily by enhancing sodium excretion, but they may also alter electrolyte balance, acid-base equilibrium, renal perfusion, and the effect of hormones on the kidneys. See Fig. 1 for the sites of actions of diuretics and Tables 4-2 and 4-3 for the characteristics and dosages of diuretic agents.

Special remarks on monitoring diuretics

Weigh the patient before drug therapy begins and daily during therapy. Maintain consistency of measurement by calibrating and using the same scales. Weigh the patient at the same time daily and with the same type of clothing. Measuring the circumference of edematous extremities or an abdomen filled with ascitic fluid is also a worthwhile parameter for fluid control. Use guideline marks to ensure measurement in the same location.

Record the daily input and output. Be conscious of output from wounds and drainage and insensible losses by perspiration and respiration.

Dehydration, possibly secondary to overzealous diuretic therapy, may be monitored by decreased skin turgor, thirst, hypotension, and elevated hemoglobin, hematocrit, and BUN levels.

Diuretics, as a result of multiple mechanisms, have hypotensive properties. Patients should be advised of orthostatic hypotension and how to avoid excessive dizziness. Blood pressure should be monitored routinely and vital signs taken, especially during dosage adjustment periods.

Signs of possible hypokalemia include weakness, hyporeflexia, tingling or numbness in extremities, arrhythmias (particularly with those patients on digitalis), irritability, stupor, increased thirst, anorexia, and vomiting (Table 4-1). Supplemental potassium chloride intake may be required.

Patients particularly susceptible to the clinical effects of hypokalemia and hypochloremia include the elderly; the debilitated; those patients losing body fluids through gastric suction, drainage, diaphoresis, vomiting, or diarrhea; and those patients receiving digitalis, diuretics, and adrenocorticosteroids.

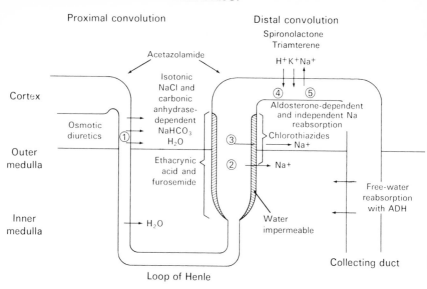

Fig 1. Sites of actions of diuretics.

Table 4-1. Indications of electrolyte imbalance

	Excess	Deficit
Extracellular fluid volume	Puffy eyelids Peripheral edema Ascites Acute weight gain Pleural effusion Moist rales in lungs ↑ CVP Pulmonary edema	Dry skin and mucous membranes Fatigue Systolic BP 10 mm ↓ standing than supine Rapid pulse Subnormal temperature Elevated respiration ↓ CVP Body weight loss Urine flow rate under 20 to 40 ml/hr Longitudinal wrinkles in tongue Depressed fontanel (infant)
Sodium (hyponatremia, hypernatremia)	Agitation→mania→convulsions Dry, sticky mucous membranes; rough, dry tongue Oliguria → anuria Firm rubbery tissue turgor Thirst → fever	"Heat prostration," apprehension, feeling of "impending doom," weak, confused, stuporous, convulsions Abdominal cramps, muscle twitching Diarrhea
Potassium (hypokalemia, hyperkalemia)	Irritability, nausea, diarrhea Oliguria progressing to anuria Weakness and flaccid paralysis Cardiac conduction disturbances leading to ventricular fibrillation and cardiac arrest	Muscular flaccidity and weakness, malaise Cardiac arrhythmias, ↓ BP, weak pulse Intestinal muscular weakness: anorexia, vomiting, distension, paralytic ileus

ETHACRYNIC ACID
(Edecrin)

AHFS 40:28
CATEGORY Diuretic

Action and use

Ethacrynic acid exerts its major effect by blocking the reabsorption of sodium along the ascending branch of the loop of Henle. Additional effects probably occur in the proximal and distal convoluted tubules where the drug may exert a direct effect on electrolyte transport.

Characteristics

Onset: 30 min. (PO). Peak activity: 2 hr. Duration: 6 to 8 hr. Excretion: 33% fecal, 22% unchanged in urine, 44% metabolites. Dialysis: unknown.

Administration and dosage
Adult

PO—50 to 100 mg initially, followed by 50 to 200 mg daily.

IV—50 mg or a calculated dose of 0.5 to 1 mg/kg. Add 50 ml of dextrose 5% or saline solution to 50 mg of ethacrynic acid. Occasionally the addition of a diluent may result in an opalescent solution. These solutions should not be used.

Pediatric

NOTE: Safe use in infants has not been established. Dosage recommendations are unavailable.

PO   1. Initial: 25 mg daily
   2. Maintenance: increase the dosage in increments of 25 mg to desired effect.

IV—1 mg/kg. Dilute with dextrose 5% and administer over 5 min.

Special remarks and cautions

If given in excessive dosage or in patients with massive fluid accumulation, treatment with ethacrynic acid may lead to excessive diuresis with water and electrolyte depletion.

Vertigo, deafness, and tinnitus with a sense of fullness in the ears have occurred, most frequently in patients with severe impairment of renal function.

The drug should be discontinued and should not be readministered if increasing azotemia and/or oliguria occur during treatment of severe progressive renal disease or if severe watery diarrhea occurs.

Gastrointestinal bleeding may result, especially in patients receiving IV therapy.

See General information on monitoring diuretics (p. 129).

Drug interactions

Ethacrynic acid can produce ototoxicity, which may add to or potentiate the ototoxicity of aminoglycoside antibiotics (kanamycin, gentamicin, neomycin, and streptomycin).

Potassium-losing diuretics produce a predisposition to digitalis toxicity.

Ethacrynic acid may displace warfarin from protein-binding sites, resulting in overanticoagulation and spontaneous bleeding.

FUROSEMIDE
(Lasix)

AHFS 40:28
CATEGORY Diuretic

Action and use

Furosemide exerts its major effect by blocking the reabsorption of sodium along the ascending branch of the loop of Henle. Additional effects probably occur in the proximal and distal convoluted tubules. After PO administration the diuretic effect usually begins within 1 hr, peaks in the first or second hour, and lasts 6 to 8 hr. After IV injection the diuretic effect begins within 15 min and lasts about 2 hr. Maximum diuresis occurs within 30 min.

Characteristics

Onset: 5 min (IV), 30 to 60 min (PO, IM). Peak activity: 15 to 30 min (IV), 1 to 2 hr (PO, IM). Duration: 2 hr (IV), 6 to 8 hr (PO, IM). Half-life: biphasic, $\frac{1}{5}$ to $\frac{2}{5}$ hr, and 2 hr. Metabolism: hepatic. Excretion: 33% in feces, 66% in urine unchanged and as metabolites. Dialysis: unknown.

Administration and dosage
Adult

PO—20 to 80 mg given as a single dose preferably in the morning; a second dose can be administered 6 to 8 hr later.

IV—20 to 40 mg given over 1 to 2 min. Much larger doses are frequently administered IV. The rate of administration should be proportional to the dose administered.

Pediatric

PO—Initially, 2 mg/kg. If response is not satisfactory, increase by 1 to 2 mg/kg every 6 hr.

IV—Initially, 1 mg/kg. If diuresis is not satisfactory, increase by 1 mg/kg every 2 hr to a maximum of 6 mg/kg.

Special remarks and cautions

Furosemide is a potent diuretic that if given in excessive amounts can lead to a profound diuresis with water and electrolyte depletion. Therefore careful medical supervision is required, and the dosage schedule has to be adjusted to the individual patient's need.

The most commonly reported side effects are related to the GI tract. Flushing, pruritus, postural hypotension, weakness, dizziness, blurred vision, and various forms of dermatitis may occur.

With long-term use, serum uric acid excretion is diminished, resulting in hyperuricemia.

Patients with known sulfonamide hypersensitivity may manifest an allergic reaction to furosemide.

See General information on monitoring diuretics (p. 129).

Drug interactions

Excessive loss of potassium in patients receiving digitalis may precipitate digitalis toxicity.

Furosemide may enhance the nephrotoxicity of cephaloridine (Loridine). If used together, renal function must be monitored closely and large doses of cephaloridine avoided.

HYDROCHLOROTHIAZIDE
(Hydro-Diuril, Esidrix)

AHFS 40:28
CATEGORY Thiazide diuretic

Action and use

Thiazide diuretics inhibit the reabsorption of sodium in the distal portion of the loop of Henle and the proximal portion of the distal tubule. Relaxation of peripheral vascular smooth muscle provides at least part of an explanation for the antihypertensive properties of thiazides.

Characteristics

Onset: 2 hr. Peak activity: 4 hr. Duration: 6 to 12 hr. Half-life: 3 hr. Dialysis: unknown.

Administration and dosage
Adult

PO—25 to 200 mg/day as a diuretic, 25 to 100 mg/day as an antihypertensive.

Pediatric
Under 6 months of age

PO—0.4 to 0.6 mg/kg/24 hr in 2 divided doses.

Over 6 months of age

PO—Usual dose: 0.4 mg/kg (1 mg/lb)/24 hr in 2 divided doses.

Special remarks and cautions

Thiazide diuretics cause a loss of potassium that may be of clinical significance; therefore electrolyte balance must be monitored and maintained.

Thiazides may cause hyperglycemia in susceptible individuals, requiring alterations in insulin or oral hypoglycemic doses. Glycosuria may also increase.

Long-term use of thiazides may block uric acid excretion, possibly resulting in an acute attack of gout in susceptible patients.

See General information on monitoring diuretics (p. 129).

Drug interactions

Excess loss of potassium may result in digitalis toxicity.

Thiazides may be additive or potentiate the action of other antihypertensive drugs.

Thiazides may antagonize the activity of oral anticoagulants.

Hypokalemia may develop with use of thiazides during concomitant use of corticosteroids.

Thiazides may inhibit excretion of lithium carbonate, resulting in toxicity. Lithium serum levels should be closely monitored.

Table 4-2. Comparison of thiazide diuretics

Thiazide	Brand name	Dosage range (mg)	Onset (PO, hr)	Peak (PO, hr)	Duration (PO, hr)
Bendroflumethiazide	Naturetin	2.5-15	1-2	6-12	18-24
Benzthiazide	Exna, Hydrex	50-150	2	4-6	12-18
Chlorothiazide	Diuril	1000-2000	2	4	6-12
Cyclothiazide	Anhydron	1-2	6	7-12	18-36
Hydrochlorothiazide	Esidrix, HydroDiuril	25-100	2	4	6-12
Hydroflumethiazide	Saluron, Diucardin	25-100	1-2	3-4	12-24
Methyclothiazide	Aquatensen, Enduron	2.5-5	2	6	24
Polythiazide	Renese	1-4	2	6	24-36
Trichlormethiazide	Metahydrin, Naqua	1-4	2	6	24

Table 4-3. Comparison of other diuretics

Diuretic	Brand name	Dosage range (mg)	Onset (PO, hr)	Peak (PO, hr)	Duration (PO, hr)
Chlorthalidone	Hygroton	50-200	2	—	24-72
Metolazone	Zaroxolyn	2.5-10	1	2	12-24
Quinethazone	Hydromox	50-100	2	6	18-24

MANNITOL
(*Osmitrol*)

AHFS 40:28
CATEGORY Osmotic diuretic

Action and use

Mannitol is a hypertonic solution that when injected, draws water from the cells and extracellular spaces into the intravasculature. Plasma volume is increased, potentially enhancing renal blood flow and diuresis by increasing the osmotic pressure of the glomerular filtrate so that tubular reabsorption of water is diminished. Potassium, chloride, calcium, phosphorus, lithium, magnesium, urea, and uric acid are excreted in addition to sodium and water.

Mannitol is used as a diuretic to help prevent and/or treat the oliguric phase of acute renal failure. It is also used to reduce the pressure of intraocular and cerebrospinal fluids.

Characteristics

Onset: 1 to 3 hr (IV). Half-life: 100 min. Metabolism: minimal, to glycogen in liver. Excretion: 80% unchanged in urine in 3 hr.

Administration and dosage

IV—Oliguria and acute renal failure:
1. Test dose: 12.5 g of mannitol in 50 to 60 ml over 3 to 5 min. A successful response is indicated by a urine output of 30 to 50 ml/hr over the next 2 to 3 hr. If unsuccessful, a second test dose may be given.
2. Prevention: 100 g of mannitol in 500 ml over 90 min to several hours.

IV—Reduction of pressure of intraocular and cerebrospinal fluids: 1 to 3 g/kg as a 15% to 25% solution over 30 to 60 min.

NOTE: As a result of high concentration the drug usually appears in the ampule in crystalline form. Heating to greater than 50 C will dissolve the crystals. After cooling to body temperature the solution may be infused. The use of an in-line filter is strongly recommended.

NOTE: Dosages for patients under 12 years of age have not been established.

Special remarks and cautions

Renal function, urine output, serum electrolytes, and central venous pressure must be monitored during mannitol administration.

Rapid infusion of large doses or accumulation of mannitol resulting from inadequate urine output may result in fluid overload and pulmonary edema. It is recommended that if the central venous pressure rises, but changes in urinary output remain minimal, the infusion should be slowed or stopped.

Mannitol may also promote tissue dehydration and hypovolemia as a result of sustained diuresis, enhancing sodium and water retention leading to oliguria.

Other side effects are acidosis, nausea, vomiting, thrombophlebitis, chills, dizziness, hypotension, hypertension, tachycardia, and angina-like chest pain. Hypersitivity reactions have also occurred.

Safe use in pregnancy has not been established.

See General information on monitoring diuretics (p. 129).

Drug interactions

Mannitol enhances the urinary excretion of lithium, potentially diminishing the response to lithium carbonate therapy.

SPIRONOLACTONE
(Aldactone)

AHFS 40:28
CATEGORY Diuretic

Action and use

Spironolactone is a competitive antagonist of aldosterone. It is structurally related to aldosterone and binds to the receptor sites normally occupied when the mineralocorticoid is secreted. Inhibition of aldosterone results in diminished exchange of sodium for potassium in the distal convoluted renal tubule. Potassium elimination is spared and sodium, chloride, and water are excreted, promoting a weak diuresis.

Spironolactone is a mild diuretic that may be used in the treatment of essential hypertension, the edema of congestive heart failure, and nephrotic syndrome. It is also effective in promoting the slow excretion of ascitic and edematous fluid in patients who retain sodium as a result of hyperaldosterone secondary to hepatic cirrhosis.

When administered in combination with thiazide diuretics, spironolactonie exerts a supplementary diuretic effect and offsets the usual potassium loss induced by other diuretics.

Characteristics

Onset: 48 to 72 hr. Metabolism: primarily to active canrenone, other inactive metabolites. Half-life: spironolactone, 10 min; canrenone, 13 to 24 hr. Excretion: metabolites in urine and feces. Dialysis: unknown.

Administration and dosage
Adult

PO—25 to 50 mg 4 times daily.

Pediatric

PO—3 mg/kg/day. Readjust dosage every 3 to 5 days.

Special remarks and cautions

Serum electrolytes should be monitored routinely. Spironolactone, because of its potassium-sparing effect, should be used with caution in patients with hyperkalemia and in patients with concomitant potassium supplementation and renal insufficiency. Dehydration and hyponatremia may also result from spironolactone therapy, especially when used in combination with other diuretics.

Hormonal irregularities such as gynecomastia and decreased libido in males and breast soreness and menstrual irregularities in females have resulted as a result of steroid-like structural similarities.

See General information on monitoring diuretics (p. 129).

Drug interactions

Spironolactone may promote the systemic acidosis produced by ammonium chloride.

Spironolactone spares potassium excretion. Potassium supplementation may result in hyperkalemia.

TRIAMTERENE
(Dyrenium)

AHFS 40:28
CATEGORY Diuretic

Action and use

The exact mechanism of action of triamterene is unknown, but its primary site of diuretic activity is in the distal renal tubule, where it blocks the exchange of sodium in the urine for potassium within the cells lining the distal nephron. It is a potassium-sparing agent used most effectively in conjunction with diuretics acting at other sites within the nephron.

Characteristics

Onset: 2 to 4 hr. Duration: 7 to 9 hr. Protein binding: approximately 66%. Excretion: renal. Dialysis: unknown.

Administration and dosage

PO—100 to 300 mg daily.

Special remarks and cautions

Triamterene should not be administered to patients with elevated serum potassium levels.

Side effects of triamterene are generally quite mild. Those reported include nausea, vomiting, diarrhea, headache, weakness, dry mouth, leg cramps, photosensitivity, and rash.

See General information on monitoring diuretics (p. 129).

Drug interactions

Potassium supplements must be used with caution in patients receiving triamterene.

CHAPTER FIVE

Anticoagulant agents

Heparin
Warfarin sodium

HEPARIN
(Heprinar, Liquaemin, Panheprin)

AHFS 20:12.04
CATEGORY Anticoagulant

Action and use

Heparin is a naturally-occurring, high molecular weight mucopolysaccharide. It acts directly on various plasma protein molecules (heparin co-factors) within the blood. Heparin does not affect the hepatic biosynthesis or the plasma levels of any coagulation factor.

In low concentrations, heparin inhibits the interactions of factors IX_a, VIII_a, and X_a. In higher concentrations heparin inhibits the actions of thrombin on fibrinogen, and in still higher concentrations it enhances fibrinolysis.

The action of heparin on platelets is variable and dose related. The aggregation and adhesiveness of platelets may be reduced, but other clinical factors make this activity difficult to predict.

Heparin anticoagulant therapy is indicated in the treatment of pulmonary embolism, deep venous thrombosis, cerebral embolism, heart valve prosthesis, and acute peripheral arterial embolism. It is also used prophylactically before and during cardiovascular surgery and hemodialysis procedures.

Characteristics

Heparin has no anticoagulant activity after PO administration, but is well absorbed after SC, IM, and IV injection. When administered IV in therapeutic doses, there is rapid clearance from circulation at a rate dependent on the dose. Onset of activity is immediate (IV). The half-lives of 100, 200, and 400 units/kg are 56, 96, and 152 min, respectively. Heparin is bound to plasma proteins at concentrations up to 2 units/ml of blood. Higher concentrations of heparin result in greater quantities of unbound heparin, which pass into other tissue spaces and appear in the lymphatic system. At concentrations above 7 units/ml, unchanged heparin is excreted in the urine (up to 50%). Heparin may have cumulative effects in patients with renal impairment. Heparin is metabolized in the liver and about 20% of a normal dose appears in the urine as uroheparin, which has about 50% of the anticoagulant activity of heparin. No dosage adjustment is required for hemodialysis.

Administration and dosage
Adult

SC 1. Prophylactic: 5000 units every 8 to 12 hr.
     2. Therapeutic: initial: 10,000 to 15,000 units; maintenance: 6000 to 10,000 units every 8 to 12 hr.
     Do not pinch the site or rub excessively.

IM—Not recommended because of the development of hematomas.

IV 1. Intermittent—initial, 10,000-unit bolus; maintenance, 5000 to 10,000 units every 4 to 6 hr. A "heparin-lock," consisting of a 20-gauge scalp vein needle attached to 3½-inch tubing ending in a resealing rubber diaphragm, may be used to administer intermittent IV doses of heparin. Advantages of a heparin-lock are the mobility that it provides the patient and the fewer venipunctures needed. After injecting the

bolus of heparin through the rubber diaphragm, flush the line with 1 ml of a solution containing 10 units of heparin/ml of saline solution. The heparin flush solution ensures that the patient will receive the entire heparin bolus and prevents the formation of a clot in the scalp vein needle.
2. Continuous infusion—initial, 5000-unit bolus; maintenance, 700 to 1200 units/hr. (Patient variation may require as little as 200 units/hr or as much as 2000 or more units/hr.) (See Table 5-1.)

Pediatric

IV—Intermittent—initial, 50 units/kg; maintenance, 50 to 100 units/kg every 4 hr.

Dosage is considered adequate when the partial thromboplastin time (PTT) is elevated 1½ to 2½ times the control value. (An exception is minidose heparin prophylactic therapy where changes in the PTT are minimal.) During intermittent IV therapy the PTT should be drawn 1 hr prior to the next dosage administration. During continuous IV therapy the PTT may be drawn at any time.

Special remarks and cautions

Firm, prolonged pressure must be applied following any venipuncture in a heparinized patient to avoid extravasation and the development of hematomas.

Factors that can influence the incidence of complications include age, weight, sex, and recent trauma. Spontaneous bleeding, such as hematomas, petechiae, hematuria, bleeding gums, and melena, after the administration of standard dosages is more frequent in women and occurs with increased incidence in those over 60 years of age. Hemorrhage is also more frequent in fully heparinized patients who have had recent trauma or who have undergone recent surgical procedures than in nontraumatized patients.

USP standards require that the potency is not less than 120 USP units in each milligram of heparin when derived from lungs and not less than 140 USP units in each milligram when derived from other tissues. Most commercial preparationis exceed these standards with a higher degree of purification (up to 170 units/mg). Consequently it is clinically safer

Table 5-1. Heparin infusion*

Units/500 ml	5000	10,000	15,000	20,000	25,000
Units/ml	10	20	30	40	50
ml/hr	Units/hr	Units/hr	Units/hr	Units/hr	Units/hr
5	50	100	150	200	250
10	100	200	300	400	500
15	150	300	450	600	750
20	200	400	600	800	1000
25	250	500	750	1000	1250
30	300	600	900	1200	1500
35	350	700	1050	1400	1750
40	400	800	1200	1600	2000
45	450	900	1350	1800	2250
50	500	1000	1500	2000	2500
55	550	1100	1650	2200	2750
60	600	1200	1800	2400	3000

*Using a microdrip administration set—60 gtts/ml.

and far more accurate to base the dose on units, rather than the old method of using milligrams.

Heparin therapy may be continued during menstruation unless bleeding becomes excessive.

Heparin must be used with caution during pregnancy and the immediate postpartum period.

Antidote

One mg of protamine sulfate will neutralize approximately 120 units of heparin. If protamine sulfate is given more than $\frac{1}{2}$ hr after the heparin was administered, then give only $\frac{1}{2}$ the dose of protamine sulfate.

Drug interactions

Aspirin, dipyridamole (Persantin) and glyceryl guiacolate should be used cautiously in patients receiving heparin. These agents inhibit platelet aggregation, thus predisposing a heparinized patient to hemorrhage.

WARFARIN SODIUM
(Coumadin, Panwarfin)

AHFS 20:12.04
CATEGORY Anticoagulant

Action and use

Warfarin inhibits the activity of vitamin K, which is required for the normal synthesis of blood coagulation factors II (prothrombin), VII (proconvertin), IX (Christmas factor), and X (Stuart-Prower factor). There is no direct effect on circulating coagulation factors.

Warfarin is indicated in the prophylaxis and treatment of venous thrombosis, atrial fibrillation with embolism, pulmonary embolism, and as an adjunct in the treatment of coronary occlusion.

Characteristics

Onset of anticoagulation: Dependent on the half-lives of the individual coagulation factors whose synthesis is suppressed. Peak prothrombin time effect: 24 to 96 hr. Duration: 1 to 5 days. Protein-binding: 97%. Half-life: 48 hr (15 to 55 hr). Metabolism: hepatic microsomal enzymes. Excretion: active and inactive metabolites in urine. Therapeutic level: 0.1 mg/100 ml to 1 mg/100 ml.

Administration and dosage

PO—10 to 15 mg daily for 3 days, then 2 to 15 mg daily maintenance.

IV—As for PO administration; onset of action is similar to that of PO administration because of dependence on individual coagulation factor synthesis.

NOTE: Dosage can be controlled only by determining the prothrombin time on a routine basis. Dosage is considered adequate when the prothrombin time is elevated 1½ to 2½ times the control value. For the patient's safety the prothrombin time should be drawn daily for the first week, weekly for the first 1 to 2 months, and monthly once the dosage has been safely established.

Special remarks and cautions

Hemorrhage is the principal adverse reaction to overdosage. Hemorrhagic tendency may be manifested by hematuria, petechiae in the skin, hemorrhage into or from a wound, or petechial and purpuric hemorrhages throughout the body. Patients receiving warfarin should be examined daily for evidence of these complications, and the urine should be tested routinely to detect hematuria. Patients should be counseled to report any excessive bleeding following shaving, oral hygiene, menstruation, or minor trauma.

Patients with impaired liver function may be more sensitive and require less warfarin for anticoagulation.

IM injections should be avoided in patients receiving anticoagulants.

Patients should be warned against self-medication with any over-the-counter product, especially those containing aspirin or other salicylates.

Warfarin crosses the placental barrier and is excreted in breast milk. Warfarin should be used in pregnant or nursing women only when the benefits outweigh the risk. The nursing infant should also be monitored with routine coagulation studies.

Antidote

The antidote to overdosage is vitamin K (Aquamephyton), 5 to 25 mg IM or IV. Following IV administration the effects of Aquamephyton appear within 15 min; bleeding is usually controlled within 6 hr, and normal prothrombin level may be obtained in 12 to 14 hr.

Drug interactions

Drugs reported to increase anticoagulant activity:

Aspirin	Disulfiram	Nortriptyline
Quinidine	Glucagon	Chloral hydrate
Phenylbutazone	Anabolic steroids	Mefenamic acid
Oxyphenbutazone	Tolbutamide	Diazoxide
Antibiotics	Phenothiazines	Nalidixic acid
Dextrothyroxine	Ethacrynic acid	Levothyroxine
Methylphenidate	Indomethacin	Cholestyramine
Vitamin E	Allopurinol	Clofibrate

Drugs reported to decrease anticoagulant activity:

Alcohol	Rifampin	Phenytoin
Ethchlorvynol	Barbiturates	Oral contraceptives
Glutethimide	Cholestyramine	Adrenocortical steroids
Meprobamate	Griseofulvin	

Respiratory agents

Acetylcysteine   *Isoproterenol*
Aminophylline U.S.P.   *Oxtriphylline*
Chromolyn sodium   *Pseudoephedrine hydrochloride*
Epinephrine   *Terbutaline*

ACETYLCYSTEINE
(*Mucomyst*)

AHFS 48:00
CATEGORY Mucolytic

Action and use

Acetylcysteine reduces the viscosity of purulent and nonpurulent pulmonary secretions by breaking disulfide bonds. This facilitates their removal by coughing, postural drainage, or mechanical means.

Acetylcysteine is used as an adjunct in the treatment of acute and chronic bronchopulmonary disorders such as pneumonia, bronchitis, emphysema, atelectasis caused by mucous obstruction, tuberculosis, and pulmonary complications of cystic fibrosis.

Characteristics

Liquifaction after inhalation is apparent within 1 min; maximal effects occur in 5 to 10 min.

Administration and dosage

Acetylcysteine may be administered by nebulization, direct application, or intratracheal instillation.

When nebulized into a face mask, mouthpiece, or tracheostomy, 1 to 10 ml of the 20% solution or 2 to 20 ml of the 10% solution may be given every 2 to 6 hr.

The recommended dosage for most patients is 3 to 5 ml of the 20% solution 3 to 4 times daily.

NOTE: After administration an increased volume of bronchial secretions may occur. Some patients with inadequate cough reflex may require mechanical suctioning to maintain an open airway.

Special remarks and cautions

Common side effects may include stomatitis, hemoptysis, nausea, severe rhinorrhea, and an unpleasant, transient odor.

Bronchospasm is most likely to occur in asthmatic patients. To prevent spasm and to maximize bronchodilatation, nebulize 0.5 ml 1:200 isoproterenol or 1% Bronkosol-2 in 5 ml of saline solution with or just prior to the use of acetylcysteine.

Adjunct measures to aid in the removal of any pulmonary secretions include increasing hydration and humidifying the environment.

Drug interactions

Acetylcysteine inactivates a number of antibiotics, including the penicillins, so it should not be mixed with them for aerosol administration.

AMINOPHYLLINE U.S.P.

AHFS 86:00
CATEGORY Bronchodilator, diuretic,
myocardial stimulant

Actions and use

Aminophylline is used in the treatment of pulmonary emphysema, congestive heart failure, bronchial or cardiac asthma, status asthmaticus, Cheyne-Stokes respiration, and bronchitis. It is a direct myocardial stimulant, bronchodilator, and weak diuretic. It increases the depth and rate of respiration, cardiac output, and renal blood flow and diminishes bronchospasm.

Administration and dosage
Adult

PO 1. Initial: 3 mg/kg every 6 hr.
    2. Maintenance: readjust dosage every few days up to 6 mg/kg every 6 hr as indicated by serum levels and clinical response.
IM—Painful, with erratic absorption. Not recommended.
IV—Infusion: the usual initial loading dose is 5.6 mg/kg administered no faster than 25 to 50 mg/min.* The maintenance dose is adjusted according to the following schedule:

Young patients	— 0.9 mg/kg/hr*
Middle-aged patients	— 0.7 mg/kg/hr*
Patients with congestive heart failure or liver disease	— 0.45 mg/kg/hr*

For maintenance infusion rate adjustment see Table 6-1.

RECTAL SUPPOSITORY—125 to 500 mg every 6 to 12 hr. This may be quite irritating to rectal tissues.
RETENTION ENEMA—500 to 700 mg in 20 to 30 ml of tap water 2 to 3 times daily.

Pediatric (greater than 1 year of age)

PO—Non–status asthmaticus: initially, 5 mg/kg every 6 hr. Readjust dosage every few days to 8 mg/kg every 6 hr as indicated by serum levels and clinical response.
IV 1. Infusion: the usual initial loading dose is 5.6 mg/kg administered at a rate no faster than 25 to 50 mg/min.
    2. Maintenance: 1.1 mg/kg/hr by continuous infusion or 5 mg/kg every 6 hr by intermittent bolus administered at a rate of 25 to 50 mg/min.

Aminophylline therapy is now quite easily monitored by serum levels. The normal therapeutic range is 7 to 20 µg/ml. Anorexia, nausea, and vomiting may occur at serum levels of 15 to 30 µg/ml.

Special remarks and cautions

Common side effects particularly associated with rapid IV injection of aminophylline may produce nausea, headache, flushing, palpitation, dizziness, arrhythmias, tachycardia, hypotension, or precordial pain. PO administration is also irritating to the stomach and may result in erratic absorption.

Since aminophylline is frequently administered via continuous infusion, a question arises as to what may be compatible with it. Consult a pharmacist, since the lists of compatibilities and incompatibilities are long and aminophylline is fairly unstable as a result of a high pH.

---

*Dosage must be calculated on an estimated lean body weight.

The bronchodilatory effects of aminophylline are usually not influenced by beta-blocking agents (propranolol); therefore this drug may be useful in patients who develop bronchospasm while taking beta-blocking agents.

Drug interactions

Aminophylline may increase the renal excretion of lithium carbonate. Patients may require increased dosages of lithium if they are on concomitant aminophylline and lithium carbonate therapy.

Aminophylline and propranolol may be mutually antagonistic in their actions. Patients must be observed for inhibition of either drug.

Table 6-1. Aminophylline infusion*

mg/500 ml	500		1000		1500		2000	
Final volume	520		540		560		580	
mg/ml	0.96		1.85		2.68		3.45	
50 kg μgtts/min	mg/kg/hr	mg/hr	mg/kg/hr	mg/hr	mg/kg/hr	mg/hr	mg/kg/hr	mg/hr
10	0.2	9.6	0.4	18.5	0.5	26.8	0.7	34.5
20	0.4	19.2	0.7	37	1.1	53.6	1.4	69
30	0.6	28.8	1.1	55.5	1.6	80.4	2	103.5
40	0.8	38.4	1.5	74	2.1	107.2	2.8	138
50	1.0	48	1.8	92.5	2.7	134	3.5	172.5
60	1.1	57.6	2.2	111	3.2	160.8	4.1	207
60 kg μgtts/min	mg/kg/hr	mg/hr	mg/kg/hr	mg/hr	mg/kg/hr	mg/hr	mg/kg/hr	mg/hr
10	0.2	9.6	0.3	18.5	0.5	26.8	0.6	34.5
20	0.3	19.2	0.6	37	0.9	53.6	1.2	69
30	0.5	28.8	0.9	55.5	1.3	80.4	1.7	103.5
40	0.6	38.4	1.3	74	1.8	107.2	2.3	138
50	0.8	48	1.5	92.5	2.2	134	2.9	172.5
60	1.0	57.6	1.9	111	2.7	160.8	3.5	207
70 kg μgtts/min	mg/kg/hr	mg/hr	mg/kg/hr	mg/hr	mg/kg/hr	mg/hr	mg/kg/hr	mg/hr
10	0.2	9.6	0.3	18.5	0.4	26.8	0.5	34.5
20	0.3	19.2	0.5	37	0.8	53.6	1.	69
30	0.4	28.8	0.8	55.5	1.1	80.4	1.5	103.5

	mg/kg/hr	mg/hr	mg/kg/hr	mg/hr	mg/kg/hr	mg/hr	mg/kg/hr	mg/hr
40	0.5	38.4	1.0	74	1.6	107.2	2.	138.5
50	0.7	48	1.3	92.5	1.9	134	2.5	172.5
60	0.8	57.6	1.6	111	2.3	160.8	3.	207

80 kg								
μgtts/min	mg/kg/hr	mg/hr	mg/kg/hr	mg/hr	mg/kg/hr	mg/hr	mg/kg/hr	mg/hr
10	0.1	9.6	0.2	18.5	0.3	26.8	0.4	34.5
20	0.2	19.2	0.5	37	0.7	53.6	0.9	69
30	0.4	28.8	0.7	55.5	1.0	80.4	1.3	103.5
40	0.5	38.4	0.9	74	1.3	107.2	1.7	138.5
50	0.6	48	1.2	92.5	1.7	134	2.2	172.5
60	0.7	57.6	1.4	111	2	160.8	2.6	207

90 kg								
μgtts/min	mg/kg/hr	mg/hr	mg/kg/hr	mg/hr	mg/kg/hr	mg/hr	mg/kg/hr	mg/hr
10	0.1	9.6	0.2	18.5	0.3	26.8	0.4	34.5
20	0.2	19.2	0.4	37	0.6	53.6	0.8	69
30	0.3	28.8	0.6	55.5	0.9	80.4	1.2	103.5
40	0.4	38.4	0.8	74	1.1	107.2	1.5	138
50	0.5	48	1.0	92.5	1.5	134	1.9	172.5
60	0.6	57.6	1.2	111	1.8	160.8	2.3	207

100 kg								
μgtts/min	mg/kg/hr	mg/hr	mg/kg/hr	mg/hr	mg/kg/hr	mg/hr	mg/kg/hr	mg/hr
10	0.1	9.6	0.2	18.5	0.3	26.8	0.3	34.5
20	0.2	19.2	0.4	37	0.5	53.6	0.7	69
30	0.3	28.8	0.5	55.5	0.8	80.4	1	103.5
40	0.4	38.4	0.7	74	1	107.2	1.4	138
50	0.5	48	0.9	92.5	1.3	134	1.7	172.5
60	0.6	57.6	1.1	111	1.6	160.8	2	207

*Using a microdrip administration set—60 gtts/ml.

CROMOLYN SODIUM
(Intal)

AHFS 92:00
CATEGORY Unclassified

Action and use

Cromolyn sodium blocks the release of histamine and slow-reacting substance of anaphylaxis (SRS-A) from sensitized mast cells after the formation of specific antigen-antibody complexes. Cromolyn has no direct bronchodilator, antihistaminic, anticholinergic, or anti-inflammatory activity. Cromolyn is recommended as an adjunct in the management of patients with severe perennial bronchial asthma. Cromolyn is effective only as a prophylactic agent and has no role in the treatment of an acute asthmatic attack.

Characteristics

Between 5% and 10% absorbed from inhaler. Peak blood levels: 15 min. Half-life: about 80 min. Metabolism: insignificant. Excretion: equal quantities in urine and feces unchanged.

Administration and dosage

NOTE: Not recommended in children under 5 years of age.

Adult and pediatric

PO—Patients must be advised that cromolyn sodium capsules are not absorbed when swallowed and that the drug is inactive when administered by this route.

INHALATION—20 mg (1 capsule) via inhaler 4 times daily. Patient education on proper use of the inhaler is particularly important to the therapeutic benefit of this agent.
1. Load the inhaler with a capsule and pierce (only once) the capsule immediately before use.
2. Holding the inhaler away from the mouth, exhale, emptying the air from lungs as much as possible.
3. With the head tilted backwards and teeth apart, close lips around the mouthpiece.
4. Inhale deeply and rapidly through the inhaler with a steady, even breath.
5. Remove the inhaler and hold the breath for a few seconds, then exhale. (Do not exhale through the inhaler because moisture from the breath will interfere with proper function of the inhaler.)
6. Repeat several times until the powder is inhaled. A light dusting of powder remaining in the capsule is normal.

A 2- to 4-week course of therapy is usually required to determine clinical response. Therapy should only be continued if there is a decrease in the severity of clinical symptoms of asthma and/or requirements for concomitant drug therapy.

Special remarks and cautions

The most common side effect of cromolyn therapy is irritation of the throat and trachea caused by inhalation of the dry powder, resulting in cough and/or bronchospasm.

If the patient is being treated with steroids and/or bronchodilators when cromolyn therapy is initiated, therapy should be continued. If the patient shows clinical signs of improvement, an attempt should be made to reduce the corticosteroid dosage. Reduction should be gradual and with close supervision to avoid an exacerbation of the asthma. Alternate-day steroid therapy may also be considered.

Caution should be used when decreasing the dosage of cromolyn because asthmatic symptoms may recur.

Use in pregnancy is not recommended as its safety has not been established.

EPINEPHRINE
(Adrenalin, Sus-Phrine)

AHFS 12:12
CATEGORY Bronchodilator

Action and use

Epinephrine is one of the primary catecholamines of the body, stimulating both alpha- and beta-receptor cells. It is a potent bronchodilatory agent, acting directly on the beta cells of the bronchi. It also increases the respiratory tidal volume by stimulating the alpha-receptor cells, relieving congestion within the bronchial mucosa, and constricting pulmonary vessels. Epinephrine may also block the antigen-induced release of histamine making it an effective agent in the treatment of asthma and anaphylactic reactions.

Administration and dosage

For anaphylaxis and asthmatic attacks:

Adult

sc—Epinephrine aqueous suspension 1:200 (Sus-Phrine): initial test dose: 0.1 ml (0.5 mg). Subsequent doses of 0.1 to 0.3 ml (0.5 to 1.5 mg) may be given only when necessary and not within 4 hr.

NOTE: Shake vial to disperse the suspension before drawing dose into syringe. A tuberculin syringe with a 26 gauge ½-inch needle is recommended. Do *NOT* administer the suspension IV. Refrigerate.

sc—Epinephrine 1:1000:0.3 to ml (0.3 to 1 mg) every 5 to 15 min as needed.

IV—Epinephrine 1:10,000: 3 to 10 ml (0.3 to 1 mg).

Pediatric

sc—Epinephrine aqueous suspension 1:200 (Sus-Phrine): initially, 0.005 ml/kg. The maximum single dose should not exceed 0.15 ml.

sc—Epinephrine 1:1000: 0.01 ml/kg (maximum dose: 0.5 ml). May repeat dose every 15 min for 2 doses, then every 4 hr as needed.

IV—Epinephrine 1:10,000: 0.05 to 0.1 ml/kg.

NOTE: Do not use if discolored (red or brown) or if sediment is present.

Special remarks and cautions

Be extremely cautious with dosage calculations and administration.

Isoproterenol and epinephrine should not be administered simultaneously, since both drugs are potent cardiac stimulants. They may be given alternately, however.

Palpitation, tachycardia, headache, tremor, weakness, and dizziness are common side effects. Serious arrhythmias, ventricular fibrillation, anginal pain, nausea, respiratory difficulty, and cerebral hemorrhage may also occur. Vital signs should be monitored during and after the administration of epinephrine.

Dosage should be adjusted carefully in elderly patients; in patients with coronary insufficiency, diabetes, hyperthyroidism, and hypertension; and in psychoneurotic individuals. All patients are particularly sensitive to sympathomimetic amines.

Drug interactions

Tricyclic antidepressants, such as doxepin (Sinequan), nortriptyline (Aventyl), amitriptyline hydrochloride (Elavil), protriptyline hydrochloride (Vivactil), imipramine (Tofranil), and desipramine (Norpramin), strongly potentiate the actions of epinephrine. If they must be used concurrently, start with significantly lower doses of epinephrine.

Use epinephrine with caution in patients receiving propranolol. Vagal reflex has resulted in marked bradycardia.

Epinephrine causes hyperglycemia. Diabetic persons may require increased doses of insulin or oral hypoglycemic agents.

Epinephrine may produce arrhythmias in patients anesthetized with cyclopropane.

ISOPROTERENOL

AHFS 12:12

(Isuprel)

CATEGORY Bronchodilator

Action and use

Isoproterenol is a beta-receptor stimulant that relaxes smooth muscle, particularly the bronchial and gastrointestinal musculature. It relieves bronchoconstriction in the smaller bronchi caused by drugs and bronchial asthma. Isoproterenol is used as a bronchodilator to treat bronchospasm associated with acute and chronic bronchial asthma, pulmonary emphysema, bronchitis, bronchiectasis, and laryngospasm caused by anesthesia. For its use as a cardiovascular agent, see Isoproterenol (Chapter 2, pp. 77 and 78).

Administration and dosage
Adult and pediatric

INHALATION   1. Mistometer: 15 r.:l of isoproterenol 1:4000 solution, 2.8 mg/ml, 300 single inhalations per vial, each measured dose containing 125 μg of isoproterenol.

Acute bronchial asthma: 5 to 6 inhalations daily as necessary.

Bronchospasm in chronic obstructive lung disease: 6 to 8 inhalations daily, no more often than every 3 hr.

Use of the Mistometer
1. Hold the mistometer in an inverted position.
2. Close teeth and lips around the open end of the mouthpiece.
3. Expel as much air from the lungs as possible.
4. Press down on the sprayer while inhaling deeply. Hold the breath for several seconds before exhaling.
5. Wait at least 1 min to determine the effect before starting a second treatment.

2. Hand-bulb nebulizer: 1:100 and 1:200 solutions. Do not use if there is a precipitate or brownish discoloration.

Acute bronchial asthma: 5 to 6 treatments daily consisting of 3 to 7 deep inhalations of the 1:100 isoproterenol solution or 5 to 15 deep inhalations of the 1:200 isoproterenol solution.

Bronchospasm in chronic obstructive lung disease: 6 to 8 treatments daily consisting of 3 to 7 deep inhalations of the 1:100 isoproterenol solution or 5 to 15 deep inhalations of the 1:200 isoproterenol solution. Repeat each treatment no more often than every 3 hr.

NOTE: 5 to 7 inhalations from a hand-bulb nebulizer using a 1:100 isoproterenol solution is equivalent to 1 inhalation of the Mistometer.

3. Intermittent positive pressure breathing (IPPB): 0.5 ml of isoproterenol 1:200 or 0.25 ml of isoproterenol 1:100 diluted with 2 to 2.5 ml of water or saline solution to provide concentrations of 1:800 and 1:1000, respectively. Administer usually over 15 to 20 min, up to 5 times daily as needed.

PO—Elixir contains 2.5 mg of isoproterenol/tbsp. (15 ml). The solution also contains 6 mg phenobarbital, 12 mg ephedrine sulfate, 45 mg of theophylline, 150 mg of potassium iodide, and 19% ethanol/tbsp (15 ml). Doses should be individualized for patients needs, but an initial dosage is 2 tbsp 3 to 4 times daily.

NOTE: Patients using both the PO and inhalation forms of therapy may develop a tolerance to isoproterenol if the recommended dosages are exceeded frequently. Prolonged abuse has resulted in severe paradoxic airway resistance. If this should occur, isoproterenol therapy should be withdrawn immediately. Isoproterenol may also cause sputum and saliva to turn pink.

Special remarks and cautions

Administration of isoproterenol is contraindicated in patients with tachycardia caused by digitalis intoxication.

Isoproterenol and epinephrine should not be administered simultaneously, since both drugs are direct cardiac stimulants. They may be given alternately, however.

Dosage should be adjusted carefully in patients with coronary insufficiency, diabetes, and hyperthyroidism and in patients sensitive to sympathomimetic amines.

If the cardiac rate increases sharply, patients with angina pectoris may experience anginal pain until the cardiac rate decreases.

Palpitation, tachycardia, headache, and flushing of the skin are common side effects. Serious arrhythmias, anginal pain, nausea, tremor, dizziness, weakness, and sweating occasionally occur.

Patients should be advised that with prolonged use, isoproterenol may cause a pink discoloration of the sputum and saliva. It is, however, of no clinical significance.

Although there have been no teratogenic effects reported, safe use in pregnant or lactating women has not been established.

Drug interactions

The beta-adrenergic stimulant effects of isoproterenol are blocked by propranolol, a beta-adrenergic blocker.

Isoproterenol may produce arrhythmias in patients anesthetized with cyclopropane.

OXTRIPHYLLINE
(Choledyl)

AHFS 86:00
CATEGORY Bronchodilator

Action and use

Oxtriphylline is a theophylline derivative about 65% as potent as theophylline. When compared with theophylline or aminophylline, it is less irritating to the gastric mucosa, and because it is more stable and soluble, it is more readily absorbed from the gastrointestinal tract. Oxtriphylline is used in long-term therapy to reduce bronchospasm in patients with acute bronchial asthma, chronic bronchitis, and emphysema.

Administration and dosage
Adult

TABLETS—200 mg 4 times daily. (Some patients may require 1200 mg daily for adequate therapy.)

ELIXIR—200 mg (10 ml) 4 times daily.

Pediatric (ages 2 to 12)

ELIXIR—100 mg (5 ml)/27 kg 4 times daily.

Special remarks and cautions

CNS stimulation manifested by nervousness, insomnia, irritability, nausea, and vomiting may occur, particularly with children and with larger doses.

Drug interactions

Administration of oxtriphylline in conjunction with other theophylline derivatives or with sympathomimetic agents may enhance cardiovascular and CNS adverse effects. Use with caution in drug combinations.

PSEUDOEPHEDRINE HYDROCHLORIDE
(Sudafed)

AHFS 12:12
CATEGORY Vasoconstrictor

Action and use

Pseudoephedrine is a sympathomimetic agent that stimulates the alpha-adrenergic receptors and releases catecholamines within the upper respiratory tract to cause vasoconstriction. The reduced blood flow to the area results in shrinkage of swollen nasal mucous membranes, allowing the airways to reopen and sinus secretions to drain. It also has some beta-adrenergic activity that may cause minor bronchodilatation. Pseudoephedrine may be used alone as a nasal decongestant, but it is also used in combination with antihistamine, analgesic, expectorant, and antitussive agents to provide symptomatic relief to patients with allergies or viral infections.

Characteristics

Onset: 30 min. Duration: 4 to 6 hr. Metabolism: liver to inactive metabolite. Excretion: 55% to 75% unchanged in urine. Dialysis: unknown.

Administration and dosage
Adult

PO—30 to 60 mg every 4 hr to a maximum dosage of 240 mg daily.

Pediatric
Ages 2 to 5

PO—15 mg every 4 hr to a maximum dosage of 60 mg daily.

Ages 6 to 12

PO—30 mg every 4 hr to a maximum dosage of 120 mg daily.

Special remarks and cautions

CNS stimulation manifested by nervousness, insomnia, irritability, dizziness, and headache may occur. Nausea and vomiting may result from large doses.

Patients known to have hypertension, hyperthyroidism, diabetes mellitus, prostatic hypertrophy, elevated intraocular pressure, or cardiac arrhythmias may be particularly sensitive to adverse reactions and must be monitored closely.

The effect of pseudoephedrine on the human fetus is unknown; therefore use in pregnant women must be determined on the basis of risk versus benefit. Infants are particularly susceptible to the pharmacologic actions of pseudoephedrine. The drug may enter breast milk and therefore should not be given to lactating women.

Drug interactions

Administration of pseudoephedrine in conjunction with other sympathomimetic agents may enhance cardiovascular and CNS side effects. Use with caution.

Use with extreme caution in patients receiving MAO inhibitors (pargyline [Eutonyl, Eutron] and tranylcypromine sulfate [Parnate]), because severe, prolonged hypertension may result.

TERBUTALINE
(Brethine, Bricanyl)

AHFS 12:12
CATEGORY Beta stimulant

Action and use

Terbutaline selectively stimulates $beta_2$ receptors, causing dilatation of bronchial, vascular, and uterine smooth muscle. In higher doses there is also stimulation of the $beta_1$ receptors of the heart. This selective activity makes terbutaline a useful agent in the treatment of symptoms of bronchial asthma and reversible bronchospasm that may occur in bronchitis and emphysema. Because of its ability to relax uterine musculature, it may also be used in cases of premature labor and threatened abortion.

Characteristics

Onset: 1 to 2 hr. Peak blood levels: 2 to 3 hr. Duration: 4 to 8 hr. Metabolism: liver. Excretion: 60% unchanged in urine, 3% in feces.

Administration and dosage
Adults

Guidelines for use in premature labor:
1. Initiate a control IV of dextrose 5%, Ringer's lactate, or saline solution and administer 400 to 500 ml in 15 to 20 min prior to initiation of the medication. Then decrease to 100 to 125 ml/hr.
2. Add 20 mg of terbutaline to 1000 ml of dextrose 5%.
3. Administer a loading dose of 250 μg IV over 1 to 2 min.
4. Start the infusion at a rate of 10 μg/min (30 ml/hr) (Table 6-2).
5. Increase the infusion rate by 3.5 μg/min (10 ml/hr) every 10 min until labor has stopped or a maximum dose of 26 μg/min (80 ml/hr) has been attained.
6. Maintain the effective dose for 1 hr or more, then begin decreasing the rate by 2 μg/min (6 ml/hr) every 30 min until the lowest effective dose is reached. Maintain the total IV fluid intake at 125 ml/hr.
7. When the lowest effective IV dose is reached, begin PO terbutaline, 2.5 mg every 4 hr.
8. If labor has stopped, discontinue the IV infusion 24 hr after PO administration was initiated if the uterus is not irritable.
9. Continue the PO regimen (2.5 mg every 4 hr or 5 mg every 8 hr) until 36 weeks' gestation.
10. If labor begins again, restart the IV infusion as above.

Guidelines for treatment of pulmonary disease:

PO—5 mg 3 times daily while the patient is awake. Total daily dosage should not exceed 15 ml.

SC—250 μg. The dose may be repeated if significant clinical improvement is not seen within 15 to 30 min. No more than 500 μg should be administered in a 4-hr period.

Table 6-2. Terbutaline administration in premature labor*

ml/hr	15	20	30	40	50	60	70	80	90
μg/min	5	6.6	10	13	16	20	23	26	30

*Administer 20 mg/1000 ml or 20 μg/ml.

Pediatric (12 to 15 years of age)

PO—2.5 mg 3 times daily.

NOTE: There are no dosage recommendations as yet for children under 12 years of age.

Special remarks and cautions

When terbutaline is used for premature labor a sometimes significant drop in blood pressure (due to vasodilatory effects) can be observed at the time of the loading dose and when the infusion is started. Blood pressure and pulse monitoring should be done prior to and every 5 min after the loading dose has been administered and the infusion started until the patient is stable. Use continuous fetal monitoring. If the maternal pulse exceeds 120 beats/min and does not decrease with an increase in fluids or when the patient is rolled on her left side, or if there is any evidence of a decrease in uterine perfusion, discontinue the infusion.

Most side effects are dose related. These include tachycardia, tremor, nervousness, palpitations, and dizziness. Headache, nausea, vomiting, restlessness, drowsiness, sweating, and tinnitus also have been reported.

Patients known to have hypertension, hyperthyroidism, diabetes mellitus, or cardiac disease with arrhythmias may be particularly sensitive to adverse reactions and must be observed closely.

Drug interactions

Propranolol (Inderal) may inhibit the pharmacologic effects of terbutaline.

Administration of terbutaline in conjunction with other sympathomimetic agents may enhance cardiovascular side effects. Therefore use terbutaline with caution.

Antihistaminic agents

Cyproheptadine hydrochloride
Diphenhydramine
Hydroxyzine
Meclizine hydrochloride

CYPROHEPTADINE HYDROCHLORIDE
(Periactin)

AHFS 4:00
CATEGORY Antihistamine, antipruritic

Action and use

Cyproheptadine has both anticholinergic and sedative effects. Its exact mechanism of action is unknown, but it is ia potent blocking agent against histamine and 5-hydroxytryptamine. Cyproheptadine is effective in various allergic diseases such as seasonal allergic rhinitis, conjunctivitis, pruritus, urticaria, and angioedema secondary to reactions to food, airborne allergens, and minor drug or serum reactions. It has also been used as an appetite stimulant in children.

Administration and dosage
Adult

PO—Up to 20 mg/day in divided doses. The initial dosage recommended is 4 mg 3 times daily. A few patients may require as much as 32 mg daily for symptomatic relief.

Pediatric
Ages 2 to 6

PO—2 mg 2 to 3 times daily. Do not exceed 12 mg/day.

Ages 7 to 14

PO—4 mg 2 to 3 times daily. Do not exceed 16 mg/day.

Special remarks and cautions

The most frequent adverse effects are sedation and sleepiness. This usually passes with continued use of the drug.

Less frequent effects include dry mouth, anorexia, nausea, dizziness, confusion, and ataxia.

Cyproheptadine is not recommended for use in pregnant women and is excreted in breast milk of nursing mothers.

Drug interactions

There are no specific drug interactions with cyproheptadine except for additive sedative and anticholinergic activity when used in combination with CNS depressants and anticholinergic agents.

DIPHENHYDRAMINE
(Benadryl)

AHFS 4:00, 48:00
CATEGORY Antihistamine

Action and use

Diphenhydramine blocks histamine activity by preventing the acess of histamine to its receptor sites. It is used prophylactically and therapeutically against milk, local allergic reactions such as insect bites, and mild drug and blood transfusion reactions characterized by angioedema, urticaria, and pruritus.

Diphenhydramine also has anticholinergic, antispasmodic, antitussive, antiemetic, and sedative effects. As an antiemetic, diphenhydramine may be effective in the treatment of motion sickness.

Diphenhydramine is also effective in treating extrapyramidal reactions induced by other drugs, such as phenothiazines, and as a bedtime sedative for relief of simple insomnia.

Characteristics

Peak blood levels: 1 hr (PO). Duration: 4 to 6 hr. Metabolism: liver. Excretion: as metabolites within 24 hr. Therapeutic level: 0.1 mg/100 ml to 0.5 mg/100 ml. Fatal level: 1 mg/100 ml. Dialysis: yes, H.

Administration and dosage
Adult

PO—25 to 50 mg 3 to 4 times daily.
IM—10 to 50 mg, not to exceed 400 mg daily.
IV—As for IM administration.

Pediatric
Infants and children under 10 kg

PO—½ to 1 tsp (6 to 12 mg) 3 to 4 times daily.

Children over 10 kg

PO—1 to 2 tsp (12 to 24 mg) 3 to 4 times daily, not to exceed 300 mg.
IM—5 mg/kg/24 hrs in 4 divided doses, not to exceed 300 mg.
IV—As for IM administration.
NOTE: Diphenhydramine must not be used in patients with narrow-angle glaucoma, asthmatic attacks, prostatic hypertrophy, or bladder-neck obstruction.

Special remarks and cautions

Patients may become drowsy and should be warned against engaging in activities requiring mental alertness.

Patients may complain of drowsiness, confusion, blurring of vision, difficulty in urination, dry mouth, nasal stuffiness, and constipation.

Antihistamines should be used with caution in patients with chronic pulmonary disease, since these agents may thicken bronchial secretions and cause tightness of the chest and wheezing.

The anticholinergic properties of diphenhydramine may inhibit lactation in nursing mothers.

Drug interactions

Diphenhydramine may have additive CNS depressant effects with alcohol, sedatives, hypnotics, tranquilizers, and narcotics.

HYDROXYZINE
(Atarax, Vistaril)

AHFS 28:16.08
CATEGORY Tranquilizer

Action and use

Hydroxyzine is a CNS depressant, anticholinergic, antiemetic, and antispasmodic as well as an antihistaminic agent. It is used as a mild tranquilizer in emotional and psychiatric states characterized by anxiety, tension, and agitation.

Hydroxyzine may also be effective as a preoperative or postoperative sedative to control emesis, diminish anxiety, and reduce the amount of narcotics needed for analgesia.

Administration and dosage
Adult

PO—Tranquilizer: 25 to 100 mg 3 to 4 times daily.
IM 1. Tranquilizer: 50 to 100 mg every 4 to 6 hr.
    2. Preoperative and postoperative: 25 to 100 mg.
    3. Antiemetic: 25 to 100 mg.

Pediatric
Under 6 years of age

PO—50 mg daily in divided doses.
IM 1. Preoperative and postoperative: 0.2 mg/kg.
    2. Antiemetic: 0.2 mg/kg.

Over 6 years of age

PO—50 to 100 mg daily in divided doses.
IM—As for children under 6 years of age.
NOTE: When hydroxyzine is used preoperatively, narcotic requirements may be reduced up to half the normal dosage.

Special remarks and cautions

Drowsiness may occur, especially during the first few days of therapy, and patients must be warned about performing hazardous tasks while taking hydroxyzine.

Dryness of the mouth and nasal stuffiness are common complaints.

Safe use of hydroxyzine in pregnancy has not been proved, and its use is not recommended in early pregnancy.

Drug interactions

Hydroxyzine may potentiate the action of other CNS depressants including narcotics, analgesics, barbiturates or other sedatives, anesthetics, tranquilizers, and alcohol.

MECLIZINE HYDROCHLORIDE

(Antivert, Bonine)

AHFS 56:20

CATEGORY Antihistamine, antinauseant

Action and use

Meclizine, a long-acting antihistaminic agent, is effective in controlling nausea, vomiting, and dizziness especially when associated with motion sickness or with diseases affecting the vestibular system. Its mechanism of action is unknown.

Characteristics

Duration: 12 to 24 hr.

Administration and dosage

PO 1. Motion sickness: initially, 25 to 50 mg 1 hr prior to embarkation. The dosage may be repeated every 24 hr for the duration of the journey.
2. Vertigo: 25 to 100 mg daily in divided doses, depending on clinical response.

NOTE: Meclizine is not recommended for the nausea and vomiting of pregnancy. Teratogenic effects have been observed in laboratory animals. Safe use has not been established in pediatric patients.

Special remarks and cautions

A common side effect of meclizine is drowsiness. Patients must be warned against performing hazardous tasks at this time.

Other side effects include blurred vision, dry mouth, constipation, and fatigue.

Drug interactions

Meclizine may display additive anticholinergic side effects (dry mouth, constipation, blurred vision) when administered with other antihistamines, phenothiazines, trihexyphenidyl (Artane), benztropine (Cogentin), and other agents with anticholinergic activity.

Analgesic agents

General information on analgesia
Acetaminophen
Alphaprodine hydrochloride
Aspirin
Butorphanol tartrate
Codeine
Ibuprofen

Indomethacin
Meperidine hydrochloride
Morphine sulfate
Pentazocine
Phenylbutazone
Propoxyphene hydrochloride

GENERAL INFORMATION ON ANALGESIA

Pain is an unpleasant subjective experience symptomatic of some underlying disorder. The "pain experience" includes, in addition to the sensation of pain, all the associated emotional sensations for a particular person under particular circumstances. Pain perception and response are influenced by such psychosocial factors as past experience, attention, and emotion. The intensity, duration, and location of harmful stimuli also influence pain perception and response. Whether it originates from physiologic or psychologic causes, it is still pain. Physiologically, it may serve as a key to pathology, that is, angina pectoris in coronary insufficiency, the pain of gout or rheumatoid arthritis. Pain also serves as a sign for other problems such as tense musculature, insomnia, stress, or high anxiety.

When the source of pain is not immediately obvious (that is, trauma), the diagnosis usually requires a detailed history and physical examination to determine the etiology. The region of pain can usually be localized (skin, skeletal muscle, or internal viscera), but the onset, course, and present status must also be identified. The patient should be asked what aggravates or relieves the pain, the effect of emotional disturbances, movement of the part, and other activities that may be associated with the intensity, quality, and distribution of pain.

If the diagnosis indicates that the source of pain has an emotional overlay without demonstrable physiologic changes, treatment of the psychologic dysfunction should be the primary approach to therapy.

When pain is related to a pathologic condition, factors to be considered when initiating therapy should include the cause, the site, the severity, and the probable duration of the pain. In selecting the type of analgesic to be used, the quality and intensity of pain are the most important factors. Mild analgesics (aspirin) are frequently and effectively used for pain originating in the integumental or musculoskeletal system. Those drugs that act centrally (morphine) are most effective for visceral pain.

Once an analgesic drug is selected, the optimal dose can be defined as the minimal dose repeated frequently enough to produce the desired therapeutic effect and yet be free of side effects that may further debilitate the patient or complicate therapy. Implicit in the selection of the optimal dose are the continued observation of the patient for proper evaluation of analgesia and the development of side effects. Analgesics must be administered on a regular basis for effective control of pain. It is essential, especially for patients with chronic and terminal pain, that the interval between doses is based on the half-life and duration of the analgesic, rather than on an arbitrary schedule. When a patient knows that he will not be expected to suffer until some appointed hour for the next dose, a cycle of anxiety, anticipation, and fear that may compound the pain will not develop. The evaluation of effective therapy may require the help of family members who may notice more subtle changes in patient behavior.

Tolerance to narcotic analgesics may develop relatively rapidly. Many patients and physicians fear that the use of pain-relieving drugs even for a short time must inevitably lead to a further problem of addiction. The number of people who become addicted after prolonged legitimate clinical use is small. When drugs are properly used in hospitals, few of the conditions predisposing to addiction exist. A critical factor predisposing to addiction is self-administration for immediate and continuing reward. A multifaceted approach frequently provides significant pain relief that is relatively uncomplicated by problems in drug dependence. Consequently, full and adequate doses of analgesic drugs should seldom be withheld simply because of fear of initiating drug dependence.

Considerations in the use of analgesics

Psychologic support and reassurance are quite important to a patient's sense of well-being. Patients are quick to sense an attitude of defeat or a lack of interest and may be easily demoralized by it. Feelings of isolation and anxiety may increase the patient's response to pain and decrease the effectiveness of analgesia. Therefore supportive, concerned communication is an effective tool in pain relief. Combine the analgesic with verbal assurance that it will be effective. Explain that the analgesic will help relieve pain and always indicate to the patient that you understand there is pain, that you have time to listen and to help.

Inform the patient of what may be expected—the quantity and duration of pain, how frequently the analgesic may be administered, by what routes, if and when it may be requested, and how long it will take for the effects to be noticeable.

Timing is of primary concern in planning analgesic care. Anticipate the need for pain medication, and don't force undue waiting as the therapeutic effects will then take longer; the patient's anxiety, fear, and anticipation will increase prior to the next encounter. While visiting with the patient, evaluate the effectiveness of the analgesic being administered.

Assess the need for the analgesic at the time of administration if the patient gives no indication of needing it. Be cautious of developing a judgmental attitude about personality characteristics associated with pain and the patient's pain threshold. Never assume that the pain is typically from one source. Encourage patients to describe pain in their own words and investigate all possible causes such as the development of infection of a wound or bandage tightness.

Nausea and vomiting are occasionally associated with the initial doses of morphine or meperidine. Maintaining a horizontal position for 15 to 20 min after administration and the use of antiemetics such as prochlorperazine or hydroxyzine will often control this adverse effect.

Constipation can result from the use of analgesics. Preventive treatment consists of bulk diet, adequate fluid intake, mobility, and the use of stool softeners.

Depression of the cough reflex by potent analgesics poses a serious threat to postoperative patients. It is essential that these patients deep-breathe, cough, and expectorate mucus secretions to prevent postoperative pulmonary complications.

Measures to increase the effectiveness of analgesics include repositioning, hygiene, and general comfort measures. Reduce unpleasant environmental stimuli and avoid painful activities such as deep breathing and ambulation until the effects of analgesics are apparent. Periodic rest and sleep are essential in assisting the patient to tolerate pain.

ACETAMINOPHEN
(Tylenol, Datril)

AHFS 28:08

CATEGORY Antipyretic analgesic

Action and use

Acetaminophen is a nonnarcotic, synthetic analgesic used in the treatment of mild to moderate pain. Its analgesic and antipyretic effectiveness is similar to that of aspirin in equal doses. Acetaminophen has no anti-inflammatory activity and is therefore ineffective (other than as an analgesic) in the symptomatic relief of rheumatoid arthritis.

Characteristics

Peak plasma levels: 10 to 60 min. Duration: 3 to 4 hr. Protein binding: 25%. Plasma half-life: 1½ to 3 hr. Metabolism: hepatic. Excretion: urine 3% active, more than 80% metabolites. Therapeutic serum levels: 3 mg/100 ml. Dialysis: yes, H; no, P.

Administration and dosage
Adult

PO—300 to 600 mg every 4 to 6 hr. Daily dosage should not exceed 2.6 g.

Pediatric
Under 1 year of age

PO—60 mg every 4 to 6 hr.

Ages 1 to 3

PO—60 to 120 mg every 4 to 6 hr.

Ages 3 to 6

PO—120 mg every 4 to 6 hr.

Ages 6 to 12

PO—240 mg every 4 to 6 hr.
RECTAL—As for PO.

Special remarks and cautions

During the past decade acetominophen has often been recommended as the drug of choice for the relief of mild pain and fever. Its acquisition does not require a prescription, and its use has climbed steadily. Unfortunately overdosage due to acute and chronic ingestion has risen dramatically in the last few years. Severe, life-threatening hepatotoxicity has been reported in patients who either ingest 5 to 8 g daily for several weeks or attempt suicide by consuming large quantities at one time.

Early indications of toxicity include anorexia, nausea, and vomiting—symptoms that are often attributed to other causes. A few days later the patient develops jaundice, and the SGOT and SGPT levels and prothrombin time rise dramatically. As more cases of toxicity are being recognized, the treatment modalities are becoming more refined. If acetaminophen toxicity is suspected, consult the manufacturer, a university drug information center, or a poison control center for the most current recommendations for therapy.

Blood dyscrasias, including thrombocytopenia, leukopenia, pancytopenia, and agranulocytosis are rare side effects that may result from prolonged administration of large doses.

Hemolytic anemia may be precipitated in those patients with a deficiency of glucose-6-phosphate dehydrogenase enzyme.

See General information on monitoring analgesics (pp. 160 and 161).

Drug interactions

There are no clinically significant drug interactions reported involving acetaminophen.

ALPHAPRODINE HYDROCHLORIDE
(*Nisentil*)

AHFS 28:08; C-II
CATEGORY Analgesic, narcotic

Action and use

Alphaprodine is a synthetically produced narcotic analgesic that is chemically related to meperidine. It is recommended for the relief of moderate to severe pain, but because of its short duration of action it is particularly well suited for use as an analgesic in minor surgical and obstetric procedures. For urgent situations IV injection will provide more prompt relief than any other analgesic.

Characteristics

Onset: 1 to 2 min (IV), 5 to 10 min (SC). Duration: ½ to 1 hr (IV), 2 hr (SC). Metabolism: liver. Excretion: primarily in urine as free drug and inactive metabolites.

Administration and dosage
Adult

SC—Usual range: 0.4 to 1.2 mg/kg. The initial dose should not exceed 60 mg.
IV—Usual range: 0.4 to 0.6 mg/kg. The initial dose should not exceed 30 mg.
NOTE: Doses of alphaprodine should be reduced 25% to 50% when phenothiazines or other tranquilizers are to be administered concomitantly.
NOTE: The total dose administered by any route should not exceed 240 mg/24 hr.

Pediatric

Use of alphaprodine is not recommended in children under 12 years of age.

Special remarks and cautions

Alphaprodine must be used with extreme caution in patients with chronic, severe respiratory disease. Normal therapeutic doses have occasionally produced respiratory depression (see Antidote).

If alphaprodine is used as a postoperative analgesic, the patient must be encouraged to cough and deep-breathe, to ambulate with caution or assistance, and to change positions every 2 hr to prevent respiratory pooling. Additional forms of comfort and support should be offered.

Repeated use may lead to tolerance, dependence, and addiction. Therefore evaluate the *patient's* response to the analgesic and suggest a change to milder analgesics if indicated.

See General information on monitoring analgesics (pp. 160 and 161).

Antidote

Administer Naloxone (Narcan) 0.4 mg (1 ml) IV, IM, or SC. If the desired degree of counteraction and improvement in respiratory function is not obtained immediately, the dose may be repeated at 2- to 3-min intervals (see Naloxone, p. 306).

Drug interactions

The depressant effects of alphaprodine are additive with those of general anesthetics, phenothiazines, tranquilizers, sedative-hypnotics, tricyclic antidepressants antihistamines, and other CNS depressants, including alcohol. Respiratory depression, hypotension, and profound sedation or coma may result from these interactions unless the dose of alphaprodine has been reduced appropriately (usually by one third to half the normal dose).

ASPIRIN
(A.S.A., Aspergum)

AHFS 28:08

CATEGORY Analgesic, antipyretic, anti-inflammatory agent

Action and use

The pharmacology of aspirin is rather extensive and quite dose dependent.

Analgesia: aspirin is the most popular and effective agent for relief of mild to moderate pain. Relief comes from a combination of peripheral and central nervous system effects. The analgesic potency of 325 mg of aspirin is approximately equivalent to 32 mg of codeine.

Antipyresis: aspirin lowers elevated body temperature by action within the hypothalamus and by producing vasodilatation peripherally to allow heat dissipation.

The mechanism of aspirin's anti-inflammatory effect is unknown, but is thought to involve inhibition of prostaglandin synthesis and other inflammatory and immunologic processes.

Diminished platelet adhesiveness may result from minimal doses of 300 to 600 mg/day. Aspirin blocks the adhesion of platelets to connective tissue and collagen fibers by several mechanisms, thus prolonging the bleeding time for several days. In doses greater than 6 g/day, aspirin reduces the plasma prothrombin level by decreasing blood clotting factor VII plasma levels.

Small doses (1 to 2 g daily) inhibit tubular secretion of uric acid and may elevate serum uric acid levels. Doses greater than 5 g daily promote urinary excretion of uric acid, resulting in lower serum uptake levels.

Characteristics

Onset: 15 to 30 min. Peak activity: 1 to 2 hr. Duration: 4 to 6 hr. Protein binding: 50% to 80%. Plasma half-life: 5 to 9 hr. Metabolism: liver, plasma, and erythrocytes. Excretion: urine—time-dose dependent. Therapeutic blood levels: 20 mg/100 ml to 30 mg/100 ml. Toxic blood levels: 40 mg/100 ml to 50 mg/100 ml. Fatal levels: 90 mg/100 ml to 120 mg/100 ml. Dialysis: yes, H, P.

Administration and dosage
Adult

PO
1. Analgesia and antipyresis: 300 mg to 1 g every 3 to 6 hr.
2. Rheumatoid disorders: 2.4 to 3.6 g (8 to 12 325-mg tablets) in 4 to 6 daily divided doses. Doses may be increased if needed. Gastrointestinal side effects can usually be reduced by administering the dose with food, milk, antacids, or large amounts of water.

RECTAL—Analgesia and antipyresis: as for PO administration.

Pediatric

PO
1. Analgesia and antipyresis: 65 mg/kg/day divided into 4 to 6 doses. Daily dosage should not exceed 3.6 g.
2. Rheumatoid disorders: as tolerated, to 3.6 g in 4 to 6 daily divided doses.

RECTAL—Analgesia and antipyresis: as for PO administration.

Special remarks and cautions

In normal therapeutic doses aspirin may produce gastrointestinal discomfort, nausea, vomiting, gastric hemorrhage, peptic ulcer, and occult blood loss. Extreme caution should be used with administration to those patients with a history of peptic ulcer, liver disease, or coagulation disorders.

In patients receiving higher dosages, salicylism (salicylate intoxication) may result. Symptomatology includes tinnitus, fever, sweating, dizziness, mental confusion, lethargy, dimness of vision, nausea, vomiting, and impaired hearing. This condition is reversible on reduction of dosage.

"Analgesic nephropathy," resulting in papillary necrosis, chronic interstitial nephritis, and possible pyelonephritis, occurs with increasing frequency in patients who ingest large doses of combination products containing aspirin, phenacetin, and caffeine.

Aspirin in various dosages will alter blood test results. Test results that may be elevated by aspirin either by interference with testing procedure or by pharmacologic effects include amylase, glucose, and red cell T_3 uptake. Tests results decreased by aspirin include cholesterol, glucose, potassium, PBI, and platelets.

Urine tests altered by aspirin include ketones, PSP, protein, steroids, and VMA. Ingestion of 8 to 18 325-mg tablets of aspirin daily may result in false-positive Clinitest and false-negative Tes-Tape urine glucose determinations.

Aspirin crosses the placental barrier and is excreted in breast milk. It may be used moderately during pregnancy, but is not recommended in the last month of pregnancy.

See General information on monitoring analgesics (pp. 160 and 161).

Drug interactions

Coagulation studies must be watched closely when anticoagulants (heparin, warfarin) are administered with aspirin. Aspirin inhibits platelet adhesiveness as well as potentially displacing oral anticoagulants from protein binding, especially in large doses. Aspirin has also been shown to reduce plasma prothrombin levels.

Aspirin displaces oral hypoglycemics (Diabinese, Orinase) from protein-binding sites, potentially producing hypoglycemia. This displacement has occurred at aspirin serum levels of less than 10 mg/100 ml.

Although often clinically indicated for concomitant use, aspirin and corticosteroids may produce gastrointestinal ulceration.

Salicylates may displace phenytoin (Dilantin) from protein-binding sites, increasing active serum levels and, potentially, the toxicity of phenytoin.

Aspirin may enhance the pharmacologic and adverse effects of methotrexate by displacement of methotrexate from protein-binding sites, as well as by blocking the renal tubular secretion of methotrexate.

Low doses of aspirin block the excretion of uric acid by sulfinpyrazone (Anturane) and probenecid (Benemid), while sulfinpyrazone and probenecid may inhibit the excretion of uric acid by large doses (5 g) of aspirin.

BUTORPHANOL TARTRATE
(*Stadol*)

AHFS 28:08
CATEGORY Analgesic

Action and use

Butorphanol tartrate is a new synthetic analgesic recommended for use in moderate to severe pain. Clinical trials indicate that it has the analgesic advantages of standard doses of morphine and meperidine, but has limited respiratory depressant effects and low physical dependence liability. Although the exact mechanism of action is unknown, it is believed that the drug acts in the subcortical and possibly the sublimbic portions of the CNS.

Characteristics

Onset: less than 30 min (IM), less than 15 min (IV). Duration: 2 to 4 hr. Metabolism: liver to glucuronides.

Administration and dosage
Adult

IM—Initially, 2 mg every 3 to 4 hr. Dosage range is 1 to 4 mg, depending on the severity of pain.

IV—Initially, 1 mg every 3 to 4 hr. Dosage range is 0.5 to 2 mg, depending on the severity of pain.

Pediatric

Butorphanol is currently not recommended for use in children under 18 years of age. NOTE: Butorphanol increases the work load of the heart and is therefore not recommended for patients with pain of cardiac origin unless a patient reacts adversely to morphine or meperidine.

Special remarks and cautions

The possibility that butorphanol may cause respiratory depression should be considered in the treatment of patients with bronchial asthma, obstructive respiratory diseases, cyanosis, or other respiratory depression from any cause.

The respiratory depressant effects of butorphanol and its potential for elevating cerebrospinal fluid pressure may be markedly exaggerated in the presence of head injury, other intracranial lesions, or a preexisting increase in intracranial pressure. The use of butorphanol can produce effects such as miosis that may obscure the clinical course of patients with head injuries.

The most commonly reported adverse reactions are sedation, nausea, a clammy and sweaty sensation, and dizziness.

Butorphanol has weak narcotic antagonist activity. It is not potent enough to antagonize the respiratory depression produced by morphine; however, when given to patients who have been receiving opiates on a regular basis, it may precipitate withdrawal symptoms.

Safety of butorphanol during pregnancy or lactation has not been established.

See General information on monitoring analgesics (pp. 160 and 161).

Antidote

Naloxone (Narcan) is a specific antidote for butorphanol. The usual adult dose is 0.4 mg (1 ml) administered IV, IM, or SC. If the desired degree of counteraction and improvement in respiratory function is not obtained immediately, the dose may be repeated at 2- to 3-min intervals (see Naloxone, p. 306).

Drug interactions

The depressant effects of butorphanol are additive with those of general anesthetics, phenothiazines, tranquilizers, sedative-hypnotics, tricyclic antidepressants, antihistamines, and other CNS depressants, including alcohol. Respiratory depression, hypotension, and profound sedation or coma may result from this interaction unless the dose of butorphanol has been reduced appropriately (usually by one third to half the normal dose).

CODEINE
(Codeine)

AHFS 28:08; C-II
CATEGORY Analgesic, narcotic

Action and use

Codeine has properties similar to morphine. Its analgesic and respiratory depressant effects are equivalent on an equianalgesic basis (120 mg codeine = 10 mg morphine parenterally). A particular advantage of codeine is its effectiveness on PO administration. It is approximately two thirds as effective orally as parenterally. Codeine is an effective antitussive agent as well as an analgesic in mild to moderate pain.

Characteristics

Onset: 15 to 30 min. Duration: 4 to 6 hr. Metabolism: liver, primarily inactive, 10% to morphine. Excretion: urine, primarily inactive, less than 16% active. Therapeutic level: 2.5 mg/100 ml. Fatal level: 0.2 mg/100 ml. Dialysis: unknown.

Administration and dosage
Adult

PO 1. Analgesia: 15 to 60 mg every 4 hr.
2. Antitussive: 8 to 20 mg every 4 hr as needed.
SC—Analgesia: 15 to 60 mg every 4 hr.
IM—Analgesia: as for SC administration. Do not inject IM to anticoagulated patients or those suspected of suffering a myocardial infarction. Use with caution in debilitated patients and those with chronic obstructive pulmonary disease.

Pediatric

PO 1. Analgesia: 3 mg/kg/24 hr in 6 divided doses.
2. Antitussive: 1 to 1.5 mg/kg/24 hr in 4 to 6 divided doses.
SC—Analgesia: as for PO administration.

Special remarks and cautions

Adverse reactions occur infrequently with codeine when it is used in normal doses. Reactions that may occur are listed in the morphine monograph.

Additional supportive antitussive actions include maintaining high humidity, avoiding smoking, limiting talking. Deep-breathing exercises should be encouraged.

Codeine appears in the milk of lactating women.

See General information on monitoring analgesics (pp. 160 and 161).

Antidote

Administer 0.4 mg (1 ml) of naloxone (Narcan) IV, IM, or SC to reverse respiratory depression. The dose may be repeated in 2 to 3 min (see Naloxone, p. 306).

Administer 5 mg of nalorphine (Nalline) IV every 3 to 5 min to 15 mg until the respiratory rate increases and the sensorium clears.

Drug interactions

See Drug interactions for morphine (p. 175).

IBUPROFEN
(*Motrin*)

AHFS 28:08
CATEGORY Antipyretic analgesic

Action and use

In higher doses ibuprofen has anti-inflammatory activity. Its mechanism of action is unknown, but thought to involve the inhibition of synthesis of prostaglandins. Ibuprofen is used in the chronic symptomatic treatment of rheumatoid arthritis and osteoarthritis. It may be considered an alternative to aspirin therapy in those patients who cannot tolerate the side effects of salicylates. The drug is contraindicated in those patients who are allergic to aspirin. Clinical studies indicate that the anti-inflammatory and analgesic effects are similar to those of salicylates and significantly less than indomethacin and phenylbutazone.

Characteristics

Protein binding: 90% to 99%. Plasma half-life: 2 to 4 hr. Excretion: less than 10% in urine unchanged, 50% to 60% as metabolites in 24 hr. Therapeutic level: unknown.

Administration and dosage
Adult

PO—Initially, 300 to 400 mg 3 to 4 times daily. The dosage may be increased to a maximum of 2.4 g daily.

Pediatric

For juvenile rheumatoid arthritis:

Under 20 kg

PO—Maximum daily dose: 400 mg.

Between 20 and 30 kg

PO—Maximum daily dose: 600 mg.

Between 30 and 40 kg

PO—Maximum daily dose: 800 mg.

Over 40 kg

PO—As for adult dosages.
Once control is achieved, the lowest effective dose must be maintained. Adequate dosages may need to be maintained for up to 2 weeks before a therapeutic response may be fully evaluated. Ibuprofen may be given with food or milk to minimize gastric irritation.
NOTE: Ibuprofen is contraindicated in patients who are allergic to aspirin.

Special remarks and cautions

Gastric irritation causing nausea, vomiting, heartburn, diarrhea, gas, and constipation are the most common side effects of ibuprofen. Gastrointestinal ulceration and perforation have been reported, and the drug should be used with caution in patients with a history of ulcer disease.

Other adverse effects that have been attributed to this agent include dizziness, headache, tinnitus, drowsiness, mental confusion, vision disturbances, and various rashes.

There are many other rare side effects that are caused by ibuprofen. These include blood dyscrasias such as anemia, thrombocytopenia, and agranulocytosis; various dermatoses such as urticaria, purpura, pruritus, and rashes; and hepatotoxicity and renal toxicity All these adverse effects warrant cessation of therapy.

Safe use during pregnancy has not been established, and the use of ibuprofen is not recommended in patients less than 14 years of age. In preliminary studies, ibuprofen has not been detected in the milk of lactating women.

See General information on monitoring analgesics (pp. 160 and 161).

Drug interactions

As a result of limited clinical studies, no drug interactions have been reported. Possible reactions that may occur include displacement of oral anticoagulants (warfarin) from protein-binding sites, enhancing the effects of the anticoagulant and potentiation of the ulcerogenic effects of salicylates, phenylbutazone, indomethacin, and corticosteroids when administered concomitantly with ibuprofen.

INDOMETHACIN
(*Indocin*)

AHFS 28:08
CATEGORY Antipyretic analgesic

Action and use

Indomethacin is a nonsteroidal, anti-inflammatory, and antipyretic analgesic. Although the exact mechanism of action is unknown, it is thought that indomethacin inhibits the biosynthesis of prostaglandins, which appear to contribute to inflammation. Indomethacin relieves pain and stiffness and reduces swelling and tenderness of joints. It may be effective in the treatment of active rheumatoid arthritis, rheumatoid (ankylosing) spondylitis, and degenerative joint disease of the hip. Because of its high incidence of side effects with chronic administration, its use is not recommended unless aspirin therapy is ineffective or not tolerated. About 25% of patients using this agent show significant improvement; however, if the patient does not show symptomatic improvement with 75 to 100 mg/day after 2 to 3 weeks, alternative therapy is recommended.

Characteristics

Onset: 1 to 2 hr. Duration: 4 to 6 hr. Protein binding: 90%. Plasma half-life: 2 hr. Metabolism: liver and kidneys. Excretion: metabolites, 35% in feces, 65% in urine. Therapeutic level: 10 to 18 mg/ml. Dialysis: unknown.

Administration and dosage
Adult

PO—Initially, 25 mg 3 to 4 times daily, increasing the dosage by increments of 25 mg daily to a maximum of 150 to 200 mg daily. After the acute phase of the disease subsides, the dosage should be reduced until discontinued. Indomethacin should be administered with food, immediately after meals, or with antacids to reduce gastric irritation.
NOTE: Do not use in the pediatric age group.

Special remarks and cautions

CNS effects are frequent. Headaches occurring 1 hr after administration and with increased severity in the morning are most common (25% to 50%). Patients also complain of dizziness, lightheadedness, and mental confusion. Patients should avoid activities requiring mental alertness, coordination, or judgment during the initiation of therapy.

Gastrointestinal complaints include anorexia, nausea, vomiting, abdominal pain, and diarrhea. Indomethacin may initiate or reactivate ulcers of the stomach, esophagus, duodenum, or small intestine. This ulcerogenic property appears to be unrelated to dosage. These complications may be minimized by administration with food or antacids.

There are many other rare side effects caused by indomethacin that suppress bone marrow function and produce ophthalmic disorders, various dermatoses, hepatotoxicity, and hypersensitivity and warrant cessation of the drug.

Use of indomethacin is not recommended in children under 14 years of age. Indomethacin crosses the placental barrier and is found in breast milk.

See General information on monitoring analgesics (pp. 160 and 161).

Drug interactions

Concurrent administration with salicylates, phenylbutazone, or corticosteroids may enhance the ulcerogenic properties of indomethacin.

Caution must be used in patients receiving anticoagulants because of possible indomethacin-induced bleeding and possible displacement of oral anticoagulants from protein-binding sites.

Probenecid blocks the renal tubular secretion of indomethacin, resulting in the accumulation and prolongation of the half-life of indomethacin.

MEPERIDINE HYDROCHLORIDE
(Demerol)

AHFS 28:08; C-II
CATEGORY Analgesic, narcotic

Action and use

Meperidine, like other narcotic analgesics, exerts its primary pharmacologic activity on the central nervous system. Therapeutic doses of meperidine produce analgesia, sedation, euphoria, and respiratory depression. Meperidine is recommended for the relief of moderate to severe pain and for preoperative analgesia (parenteral form only). Meperidine may also be indicated in patients with gallbladder disease or pancreatitis, since in equianalgesic doses it causes less spasm of Oddi's sphincter or the biliary tract.

Characteristics

Onset: 10 min (IM). Peak analgesia: 30 to 50 min (IV). Duration: 2 to 4 hr. Protein binding: 40%; half-life. 5½ hr. Excretion: 5% unchanged in urine. Therapeutic level: 60 μg/100 ml to 65 μg/100 ml. Toxic level: 200 μg/100 ml. Fatal level: 0.5 mg/100 to 3 mg/100 ml. Dialysis: unknown.

Administration and dosage
Adult

PO—50 to 150 mg every 3 to 4 hr.

IM—50 to 150 mg every 3 to 4 hr. Inject deeply since meperidine irritates subcutaneous tissue. Do not inject IM to anticoagulated patients or to those suspected of suffering a myocardial infarction.

IV—50 to 100 mg every 3 to 4 hr. Doses should be diluted and administered slowly. Severe tachycardia and hypotension may result. Side effects may also be diminished by having the patient in a recumbent position.

Pediatric

PO—1 to 2 mg/kg every 3 to 4 hr as needed. Do not exceed 100 mg/dose.

IM—As for PO administration.

SC—As for PO administration.

NOTE: Doses of meperidine should be reduced 25% to 50% when phenothiazines or other tranquilizers are to be administered concomitantly.

Special remarks and cautions

Adverse reactions are much the same as for morphine—dizziness, nausea, vomiting, and postural hypotension.

Meperidine must be used with extreme caution in patients with chronic severe respiratory disease. Normal therapeutic doses may decrease respiratory drive while increasing airway resistance.

Meperidine may precipitate or aggravate seizures in patients prone to convulsive activity.

If meperidine is used as a postoperative analgesic, the patient must be encouraged to cough and deep-breathe, to ambulate with caution or assistance, and to change positions every 2 hr to prevent respiratory pooling. Offer additional forms of comfort, support, and interest.

Repeated use may lead to tolerance, dependence, and addiction. Therefore evaluate the *patient's* response to the analgesic and suggest a change to milder analgesics when indicated.

Use meperidine with caution as an obstetric analgesic. Meperidine crosses the placental barrier and may produce respiratory depression in newborn infants. Meperidine is excreted in breast milk of lactating women.

See General information on monitoring analgesics (pp. 160 and 161).

Antidote

Nalorphine (Nalline) may be used to counteract the symptoms (particularly respiratory depression and hypotension) of excessive dosage of morphine, codeine, and meperidine. Dosage in the treatment of respiratory depression is 5 to 10 mg IV, repeated every 10 to 15 min if respirations remain depressed, but with a total dose not to exceed 40 mg.

Naloxone (Narcan), 0.4 mg (1 ml), may be administered IV, IM, or SC. If the desired degree of counteraction and improvement in respiratory function is not obtained immediately, the dose may be repeated at 2- to 3-min intervals (see Naloxone, p. 306).

Drug interactions

The depressant effects of meperidine are additive with those of general anesthetics, phenothiazines, tranquilizers, sedative-hypnotics, tricyclic antidepressants, antihistamines, and other CNS depressants, including alcohol. Respiratory depression, hypotension, and profound sedation or coma may result from this interaction unless the dose of meperidine has been reduced appropriately (usually by one third to half the normal dose).

MORPHINE SULFATE

AHFS 28:08; C-II
CATEGORY Analgesic, narcotic

Action and use

Morphine is recommended for the relief of severe pain as a preanesthetic medication, for acute vascular occlusion, and to produce sleep in selected cases. It may also be quite effective in low doses to reduce anxiety and diminish venous return in acute pulmonary edema. Morphine has a biphasic action on the CNS. It sedates the cerebrum and has a mixture of stimulation and sedation on the medulla. In the medulla it sedates the respiratory center, emetic center, and the cough reflex. It also stimulates the chemoreceptor trigger zone in the medulla, which is responsible for the nausea and emesis noted as a side effect. The stimulation of the chemoreceptor trigger zone occurs before the sedative action on the emetic center.

Characteristics

Onset: immediate. Peak analgesia: 50 to 90 min (SC), 30 to 60 min (IM), and 20 min (IV). Duration: 4 to 5 hr. Metabolism: primariy liver. Excretion: 90% in urine primarily as metabolites in 24 hr, 7% to 10% in feces. Therapeutic level: 0.01 mg/100 ml. Fatal level: 0.05 mg/100 ml to 0.4 mg/100 ml. Dialysis: unknown.

Administration and dosage
Adult

IM or SC—2 to 20 mg (10 mg average) every 4 hr. Do not inject IM to anticoagulated patients or to those suspected of suffering a myocardial infarction.

    IV—2.5 to 16 mg diluted in 5 ml of saline solution. Inject slowly, observing patient's response (hypotension, respiratory depression).

Pediatric

SC—0.1 to 0.2 mg/kg. Do not exceed 15 mg.

    IV—0.05 mg/kg. Inject slowly, observing patient's response (hypotension, respiratory depression).

Special remarks and cautions

The major hazards of narcotic analgesics are respiratory depression and, to a lesser degree, circulatory depression, respiratory arrest, shock, and cardiac arrest. Morphine renders the respiratory centers less responsive to increases in alveolar and serum P_{CO_2}. This may occur before either reduction in the respiratory rate or tidal volume is noticeable. Check the respiratory rate and depth frequently. Return to normal should occur within 3 to 4 hr.

The most frequently observed adverse reactions include lightheadedness, dizziness, sedation, nausea, vomiting, and sweating. These effects seem to be more prominent in ambulatory patients and in those who are not suffering severe pain.

Use extreme caution in administration to patients with head injuries, increased cerebrospinal pressure, or decreased respiratory reserve.

Morphine may also cause constipation and urinary retention.

Morphine is excreted in small amounts in human breast milk.

See General information on monitoring analgesics (pp. 160 and 161).

Antidote

Nalorphine (Nalline) is used to counteract the symptoms (particularly respiratory depression and hypotension) of excess dosage of morphine, codeine, and meperidine.

Dosage in the treatment of respiratory depression is 5 to 10 mg IV, repeated every 10 to 15 min if respirations remain depressed, but with a total dose not to exceed 40 mg.

Naloxone (Narcan), 0.4 mg (1 ml), can be administered IV, IM, or SC. If the desired degree of counteraction and improvement in respiratory function is not obtained immediately, the dose may be repeated at 2- to 3-min intervals (see Naloxone, p. 306).

Drug interactions

The depressant effects of morphine are additive with those of general anesthetics, phenothiazines, tranquilizers, sedative-hypnotics, tricyclic antidepressants, antihistamines, and other CNS depressants, including alcohol. Respiratory depression, hypotension, and profound sedation or coma may result from this interaction unless the dose of morphine has been reduced appropriately (usually by one third to half the normal dose).

PENTAZOCINE
(Talwin)

AHFS 28:08
CATEGORY Analgesic

Action and use

Pentazocine exerts CNS effects similar to morphine, including analgesia, sedation, and respiratory depression. The cardiovascular responses to pentazocine differ somewhat from those of morphine and codeine in that high doses cause an increase in blood pressure and heart rate. Pentazocine is indicated for the relief of moderate to severe pain.

Characteristics

Peak plasma levels: 15 to 60 min (IM), 1 to 3 hr (PO). Duration: 5 hr (PO). Half-life: 2 hr. Metabolism: extensive variation among individuals. Excretion: 60% in urine in 24 hr, primarily as metabolites. Therapeutic level: 0.05 mg/100 ml. Toxic level: 0.2 mg/100 ml to 0.5 mg/100 ml. Fatal level: 0.3 mg/100 ml to 2 mg/100 ml. Dialysis: unknown.

Administration and dosage
Adult

PO—50 to 100 mg every 3 to 4 hr.

IM—30 to 60 mg every 3 to 4 hr. Do not administer IM to anticoagulated patients or those suspected of having a myocardial infarction.

IV—30 to 60 mg every 3 to 4 hr.

NOTE: Pentazocine is not recommended in children under 12 years of age.

Special remarks and cautions

The possibility that pentazocine may cause respiratory depression should be considered in treatment of patients with bronchial asthma, obstructive respiratory conditions, cyanosis, or other respiratory depression from any cause.

The respiratory depressant effects of pentazocine and its potential for elevating cerebrospinal fluid pressure may be markedly exaggerated in the presence of head injury, other intracranial lesions, or a preexisting increase in intracranial pressure.

The most commonly reported adverse reactions are nausea, dizziness or lightheadedness, vomiting, and euphoria.

Pentazocine has weak narcotic antagonist activity. It does not antagonize the respiratory depression produced by morphine; however, when given to patients who have been receiving opiates on a regular basis, it may precipitate withdrawal symptoms.

Use extreme caution in administration to patients with head injuries, increased cerebrospinal pressure, or decreased respiratory reserve.

Pentazocine, when used in higher doses (50 mg IM), may elevate serum amylase levels, resulting from spasm of Oddi's sphincter.

Seizures have occurred in association with the use of pentazocine in patients prone to convulsions. No direct cause-and-effect relationship has been found, however.

Repeated use may lead to tolerance, dependence, and addiction. Abrupt discontinuance following extended use of pentazocine may result in withdrawal symptoms. Evaluate the *patient's* response to the analgesic and suggest a change to milder analgesics when indicated.

No teratogenic effects have been reported with pentazocine, but it does cross the placental barrier. It should be administered with caution during pregnancy and delivery because both elevation and depression in fetal heart rate have occurred.

See General information on monitoring analgesics (pp. 160 and 161).

Antidote

Nalorphine (Nalline) is not effective in antagonizing pentazocine-induced respiratory depression.

Naloxone (Narcan) is a specific antidote for pentazocine. The usual adult dose is 0.4 mg (1 ml) administered IV, IM, or SC. If the desired degree of counteraction and improvement in respiratory function is not obtained immediately, the dose may be repeated at 2- to 3-min intervals (see Naloxone, p. 306).

Drug interactions

The depressant effects of pentazocine are additive with those of general anesthetics, phenothiazines, tranquilizers, sedative-hypnotics, tricyclic antidepressants, antihistamines, and other CNS depressants, including alcohol.

PHENYLBUTAZONE
(Azolid, Butazolidin)

AHFS 28:08

CATEGORY Anti-inflammatory, antipyretic analgesic

Action and use

Phenylbutazone is a nonsteroidal, anti-inflammatory, antipyretic analgesic used for the symptomatic relief of gout, rheumatoid arthritis, osteoarthritis, and rheumatoid spondylitis. Phenylbutazone does not alter the course of the disease process. As a result of many serious adverse effects it should be used only after other drugs have failed. If significant improvement is not observed within 7 days, the drug should be discontinued.

Characteristics

Peak blood levels: 2 hr. Protein binding: 98%. Plasma half-life: 50 to 100 hr. Metabolized to oxyphenbutazone and other active products. Excretion: 15% as metabolites in urine. Therapeutic level: 5 mg/100 ml to 15 mg/100 ml. Dialysis: unknown.

Administration and dosage
Adult

PO—300 to 600 mg daily in divided doses. Gastrointestinal side effects may be diminished by administering the dose with food or milk.

NOTE: Use of phenylbutazone is not recommended in children under 14 years of age and in senile, elderly patients. With patients 60 years of age and over, every effort must be made to discontinue the drug as soon as possible, especially after 7 days, because of the exceedingly high risk of potentially fatal reactions in this group. With all patients the goal of therapy should be short-term relief of severe symptoms with the smallest possible dose for the shortest administration time and course possible.

Special remarks and cautions

Known factors that increase the incidence of adverse reactions are age (over 40), weight, dosage, duration of therapy, concurrent diseases, and concurrent administration of other drugs.

Serious and fatal blood dyscrasias, including agranulocytosis, aplastic anemia, and hemolytic anemia, have been reported. It is crucial that biweekly blood counts with differential are completed.

Many gastrointestinal side effects have been attributed to phenylbutazone. These include creation and reactivation of ulcers, occult bleeding, nausea, vomiting, and abdominal distention.

Phenylbutazone causes significant sodium and chloride retention that may result in congestive heart failure, edema, or hypertension in susceptible individuals. Check for signs of fluid retention in ankles, feet, and sacrum.

Other complications include hypersensitivity reactions, various dermatoses, potentially fatal hepatitis, renal impairment, and visual disturbances.

Phenylbutazone inhibits the thyroid uptake of iodine and may result in hypothyroidism.

Phenylbutazone is not recommended in pregnant or nursing mothers. Teratogenic effects have been noted in animals, and the drug is found in breast milk.

See General information on monitoring analgesics (pp. 160 and 161).

Drug interaction

Phenylbutazone displaces warfarin (Coumadin) from protein-binding sites, enhancing the anticoagulant activity of warfarin.

Phenylbutazone inhibits the metabolism of tolbutamide (Orinase) and acetohexamide

(Dymelor) and may also displace tolbutamide from protein-binding sites, thus enhancing the hypoglycemic effects of these agents.

Phenytoin (Dilantin) metabolism may be inhibited by phenylbutazone, leading to phenytoin toxicities.

Phenylbutazone inhibits excretion of uric acid by high (5 g daily) doses of salicylates.

PROPOXYPHENE HYDROCHLORIDE
(Darvon)

AHFS 28:08
CATEGORY Analgesic

Action and use

Propoxyphene is a synthetic analgesic that acts on the central nervous system for pain relief. Propoxyphene has no antipyretic or anti-inflammatory activity. It is used for the relief of mild to moderate pain. Clinical studies indicate that 65 mg of propoxyphene may have equivalent analgesic strength to 60 mg of codeine or 650 mg of aspirin. Greater pain relief may be attained when used in combination with aspirin, phenacetin, or acetaminophen.

Characteristics

Onset: 1 hr. Peak plasma levels: 2 hr. Biologic half-life: 3½ to 4 hr. Therapeutic serum levels: 0.05 to 0.2 µg/ml. Toxic serum levels: 1 to 10 µg/ml. Dialysis: minimally effective.

Administration and dosage

PO—65 mg every 4 to 6 hr.

NOTE: Propoxyphene is not recommended in children.

Special remarks and cautions

Side effects of propoxyphene include gastrointestinal disturbances, headache, dizziness, somnolence, and skin rashes.

Tolerance and psychologic and physical dependence have been reported.

Symptoms of acute overdose are similar to those of acute narcotic intoxication. These include coma, respiratory depression, pulmonary edema, circulatory collapse, and convulsions. Symptoms may be complicated by salicylism if combination products are consumed.

See General information on monitoring analgesics (pp. 160 and 161).

Antidote

Naloxone (Narcan), 0.4 mg (1 ml), may be administered IV, IM, or SC. If the desired degree of counteraction and improvement in respiratory function is not obtained immediately, the dose may be repeated at 2- to 3-min intervals (see Naloxone, p. 306).

For respiratory depression administer nalorphine (Nalline), 5 to 10 mg IV. Repeat the dose every 10 to 15 min if respirations remain depressed, but with a total dose not to exceed 40 mg.

Drug interactions

Orphenadrine (Norflex, Disipal) and propoxyphene may cause mental confusion, anxiety, and tremors if used together.

AHFS 28:08

Table 8-1. Other nonsteroidal anti-inflammatory agents

Drug	Peak levels	Duration (hr)	Protein binding (%)	Half-life (hr)	Excretion	Dialysis H	Dialysis P	Dosage Pediatric	Dosage Adult
Fenoprofen* (Nalfon)	30-180 min	—	99	3	Metabolized to inactive metabolites in liver, 3% excreted unchanged in urine	?	?	—	PO†: initially, 600 mg 4 times daily; increase dosage every few days according to patient's response and tolerance Do not exceed 3.2 g/day
Naproxen* (Naprosyn)	2-4 hr	—	99	13	Metabolized to inactive metabolites in liver, 10% excreted unchanged in urine	?	?	—	PO: initially, 250 mg 2 times daily; increase dose to a maximum of 750 mg Maximal improvement may take 4 weeks
Tolmetin‡ (Tolectin)	30-60 min	—	99	1	Metabolized to inactive metabolites in liver, 20% excreted unchanged in urine	?	?	—	PO§: initially, 400 mg 3 times daily; do not exceed 2 g daily Maximal improvement may take several weeks.

*See monograph on ibuprofen (pp. 169 and 170) for Special remarks and cautions and Drug interactions.
†Food may interfere with absorption. Administer 30 min before or 2 hr after meals.
‡See monograph on indomethacin (p. 171) for Special remarks and cautions and Drug interactions.
§If gastric irritation occurs, administer doses with food, milk, or antacids.

Sedative-hypnotic agents

General information on sedative-hypnotics
General information on barbiturates
Phenobarbital
Secobarbital
Chloral hydrate

Ethchlorvynol
Flurazepam
Glutethimide
Methaqualone
Paraldehyde

GENERAL INFORMATION ON SEDATIVE-HYPNOTICS

Sleep is a naturally occurring phenomenon that occupies about one third of an adult's life. What constitutes optimal or *sound* sleep has been frequently debated and is a highly individual matter, but *adequate* sleep is important. Natural sleep is a rhythmic progression through stages that provide physical rest and psychic equilibrium. Stages I and II are light sleep periods that allow easy arousal. Stage III is a transition from the lighter to the deeper state of sleep, stage IV. These first four stages of sleep are called nonrapid eye movement (NREM) sleep. Stage V is referred to as rapid eye movement (REM) sleep, during which rapid eye movements occur, muscle tension increases, and most dreaming occurs. All stages of sleep are irregularly interrupted by REM sleep, which is thought to provide a psychic release of anxiety and tension.

Unfortunately many of the details of what constitutes *normal* sleep are unknown. Normal sleep patterns may be altered by anxiety, pain, environmental conditions, physical exhaustion, forced awakenings, and drugs.

The ideal sedative-hypnotic agent should induce and maintain sleep as naturally as possible, that is, rapid induction of stages I, II, and III without significantly diminishing the time of stages IV or V. Frequently the most commonly used sedative-hypnotics increase total sleeping time, especially in stages III and IV (NREM) sleep; however, they also decrease the number of REM periods and the total time in REM sleep. When REM sleep is decreased, there is a strong tendency to "make it up." Compensatory REM sleep seems to occur even when hypnotics are used for only 3 or 4 days.

After chronic administration of sedative-hypnotic agents, REM rebound may be severe, accompanied by restlessness and vivid nightmares. Depending on the frequency of hypnotic administration, normal sleep patterns may not be restored for weeks. It is suspected that the effects of REM rebound may enhance chronic use and dependence of these agents by the patient to avoid the unpleasant consequences of rebound.

A primary responsibility of patient care is to provide a resting and relaxing environment, and sleep is a major part of hospital therapy. Hypnotic agents should not be forced on patients ("a good patient is a quiet patient"), but patients should be aware that sleeping medication is available. Treatment should be continued only on an intermittent basis and the smallest dose suitable for obtaining the desired effects should be used.

Special remarks on monitoring sedative-hypnotics

Individual responses vary with these medications. Discuss with the patient the quality and quantity of sleep to assess whether adjustments in dosage and/or medication are indicated.

Irritation to the gastric mucosa and aftertaste may be minimized by administration with fruit juice, milk, or a bedtime snack if dietary requirements allow this.

Safety measures, such as siderails and assistance with ambulation, should be implemented shortly after ingestion. Hypnotic doses often have a rapid onset of action, resulting in transient dizziness and excitation. This occurs most frequently when administered on an empty stomach or to an ambulating patient.

Patients may complain of "morning hangover," drowsiness, blurred vision, and transient hypotension on arising. Explain to the patient the need for arising first to a sitting position, equilibrating, and then standing. Again, assistance with ambulation may be required. If "hangover" becomes troublesome, there should be a reduction in dosage and/or change in medication.

These drugs are psychologically and/or physiologically habit-forming. Withdrawal after long-term use may produce symptoms of anxiety, insomnia, tremors, vivid dreams, agitation, and confusion. Use as many natural aids as possible (for example, a relaxing backrub, a warm cup of milk, a quiet and soothing environment, a clean body and bed) to help produce relaxation and sleep.

Therapeutic, toxic, and fatal blood levels listed in the characteristics section of each monograph are much lower when more than one CNS depressant (for example, alcohol, tranquilizers, antihistamines, anesthetics, narcotics) have been ingested.

GENERAL INFORMATION ON BARBITURATES

The barbiturates are a class of structurally related chemicals that may reversibly depress the activity of all excitable tissues. The central nervous system is particularly sensitive, but the degrees of depression (ranging from mild sedation to deep coma and death) depend on the dosage, route of administration, tolerance from previous use, degree of excitability of the central nervous system at the time of administration, and condition of the patient. Usual hypnotic doses produce mild respiratory depression similar to that of natural sleep; with larger doses, the rate, depth, and volume of respiration are markedly diminished.

Barbiturate-induced sleep varies from normal sleep by decreased REM time. With chronic administration of hypnotic doses, the amount of REM sleep gradually returns to normal as tolerance develops to the REM suppressant effect. When barbiturate therapy is discontinued, a rebound increase in REM sleep occurs in spite of the tolerance. Irregularities in REM sleep cycles may take weeks to fully dissipate.

Barbiturates are recommended primarily for their sedative and hypnotic effects. Some of the intermediate (secobarbital, pentobarbital) and long-acting (phenobarbital) barbiturates are also used for their anticonvulsant activity. The ultrashort-acting (methohexital, thiopental) agents may be administered IV as general anesthetics.

Special remarks and cautions

General adverse effects of barbiturates include drowsiness, lethargy, headache, muscle or joint pain, and mental depression. Barbiturate "hangover" frequently occurs after administration of hypnotic doses or with long-term anticonvulsant therapy. Patients may display dulled affect, subtle distortion of mood, and impaired coordination.

Elderly patients and those in severe pain may respond paradoxically to barbiturates with excitement, euphoria, restlessness, and confusion.

Hypersensitivity reactions to barbiturates are infrequent, but the sequelae are quite serious and potentially fatal. Barbiturate therapy should be discontinued immediately if the patient develops symptoms of hypersensitivity, including high fever, inflammation of mucous membranes, or any type of dermatitis.

Blood dyscrasias have been attributed to barbiturate administration. Blood counts should be repeated periodically during long-term therapy. The patient should be reminded to report symptoms, including sore throat, easy bruisability, fever, or petechiae.

Barbiturates readily cross the placental barrier, appearing in fetal circulation. They are also present in breast milk. Neonates and nursing infants whose mothers receive barbiturates must be observed for signs of toxicity.

See General information on monitoring sedative-hypnotics (pp. 181 and 182).

Treatment of overdosage

General management should consist of symptomatic and supportive therapy, including gastric lavage, administration of IV fluids, and maintenance of blood pressure, body temperature, and adequate respiratory exchange.

Forced diuresis enhances excretion of all barbiturates, and alkalinization of the urine (pH = 7.5) further enhances the excretion of phenobarbital.

Barbiturate abuse

The habitual use of barbiturates may result in physical dependence. Rapid discontinuance of barbiturates after long-term use of high dosages may result in symptoms similar to alcohol withdrawal. They may vary from weakness and anxiety to delirium and grand mal seizures. Treatment consists of cautious and gradual withdrawal of barbiturates over a 2- to 4-week period.

Drug interactions

The CNS depressant effects of antihistamines, analgesics, anesthetics, tranquilizers, and sedative-hypnotics may be potentiated by the barbiturates.

Barbiturates, especially phenobarbital, may induce hepatic microsomal enzymes enhancing the metabolism of warfarin (Coumadin), digitoxin, corticosteroids (prednisone), doxycycline (Vibramycin), phenytoin (Dilantin), and chlorpromazine (Thorazine). If the barbiturate is discontinued, the patient must be observed closely for signs of secondary drug toxicity requiring reduction of dosage.

Disulfiram (Antabuse) inhibits metabolism of barbiturates, leading to potential barbiturate toxicity.

MAO inhibitors (isocarboxazid [Marplan], pargyline hydrochloride [Eutonyl], tranylcypromine sulfate [Parnate]) may inhibit the metabolism of barbiturates, resulting in prolonged barbiturate effects. Barbiturate dosage reduction may be required.

PHENOBARBITAL
(Luminal, Eskabarb)

AHFS 28:12, 28:24; C-IV
CATEGORY Sedative-hypnotic, anticonvulsant

Action and use

Phenobarbital is a long-acting barbiturate used as a daytime sedative and as an adjunct in the prophylactic management of epilepsy.

Characteristics

Onset: 2 to 3 hr (PO). Peak blood levels: 8 to 12 hr. Protein binding: 40% to 60%. Half-life: 2 to 6 days. Metabolism: hydroxylation in liver to inactive forms. Excretion: 10% to 25% unchanged in urine, 75% as inactive metabolites. Therapeutic level: 1 mg/100 ml to 2.5 mg/100 ml. Toxic level: 4 mg/100 ml to 6 mg/100 ml. Fatal levels: 8 mg/100 ml to 11 mg/100 ml. Dialysis: yes, H, P (only 25% as effective as hemodialysis).

Administration and dosage
Adult

PO 1. Sedation: 30 to 120 mg daily in 3 to 4 divided doses.
　　2. Hypnosis: 100 to 320 mg.
　　3. Anticonvulsant: 100 to 200 mg usually given at bedtime.
IM—As for PO administration.
IV—As for PO administration. Administer at a rate no greater than 60 mg/min. Monitor the respiratory rate and blood pressure closely and administer with extreme caution to patients with respiratory disease.

Pediatric

PO 1. Sedation: 2 to 3 mg/kg every 8 hr.
　　2. Hypnosis: 6 to 10 mg/kg.
　　3. Anticonvulsant—status epilepticus: initially, 5 to 8 mg/kg, then 3 to 4 mg/kg every 5 min until seizures stop.
　　4. Maintenance: 5 to 10 mg/kg/day divided into 4 doses.
IM—As for PO administration
IV—As for PO administration. Administer at a rate no greater than 60 mg/min. Monitor the respiratory rate and blood pressure closely.

Special remarks and cautions

See General information on barbiturates (pp. 183 and 184).
Phenobarbital may produce paradoxic excitement and hyperactivity in children.
Alkalinization of the urine and forced diuresis significantly increase the excretion of phenobarbital.

Drug interactions

See General information on barbiturates (pp. 183 and 184).

SECOBARBITAL
(Seconal)

AHFS 28:24; C-III
CATEGORY Sedative-hypnotic

Action and use

Secobarbital is a short-acting barbiturate used as a sedative-hypnotic and as an anesthetic in the control of acute convulsive conditions such as status epilepticus, tetanus, and toxic reactions to strychnine.

Characteristics

Onset: 10 to 30 min (PO). Duration: 6 to 8 hr. Half-life: 20 to 28 hr. Metabolism: liver. Therapeutic level: 0.1 mg/100 ml to 0.5 mg/100 ml. Toxic level: 1 mg/100 ml to 3 mg/100 ml. Fatal level: 3 mg/100 ml to 5 mg/100 ml. Dialysis; no, H, P; however, dialyzable as a poison.

Administration and dosage
Adult

PO—Hypnosis: 100 mg at bedtime.
Preoperatively: 200 to 300 mg 1 to 2 hr before surgery.
NOTE: When secobarbital sodium is being prepared for parenteral administration, use sterile water for injection as a diluent. Do not use if the solution is not absolutely clear within 5 min of reconstitution. As a result of instability, use within 30 min of opening the ampule.

IM—Doses exceeding 250 mg are not recommended. After deep IM injection the patient should be watched closely for 20 to 30 min to ensure that respiratory depression does not develop.

IV—Injections should not exceed 50 mg/15-sec intervals. Rapid administration may cause respiratory depression, apnea, laryngospasm, vasodilatation, and hypotension.

RECTAL—120 to 200 mg.

Pediatric

PO 1. Sedation: 2 mg/kg/day in 4 divided doses.
2. Hypnosis: 6 mg/kg.
3. Preoperatively: 50 to 100 mg 1 to 2 hr before surgery.

To 6 months of age

RECTAL—15 to 60 mg.

Ages 6 months to 3 years

RECTAL—60 mg.

Over 3 years of age

RECTAL—60 to 120 mg.

Special remarks and cautions

See General information on barbiturates (pp. 183 and 184).

Drug interactions

See General information on barbiturates (pp. 183 and 184).

CHLORAL HYDRATE
(Noctec, Somnos)

AHFS 28:24; C-IV
CATEGORY Sedative-hypnotic

Action and use

Chloral hydrate is rapidly metabolized to trichlorethanol, which is believed to cause the CNS depression seen with this product. Chloral hydrate is used as a nocturnal sedative and does not have any specific restrictions as to the type of patient, other than those who should not receive any CNS depressant. Suppression of REM sleep may occur at doses greater than 800 to 1000 mg.

Characteristics

Onset: 15 to 30 min. Duration: 5 to 8 hr. Half-life (trichloroethanol): 8 hr. Metabolism: chloral hydrate is rapidly metabolized by alcohol dehydrogenase to trichloroethanol, which is subsequently conjugated and excreted in the feces and urine. Therapeutic level: 1 mg/100 ml. Toxic level: 10 mg/100 ml. Fatal level: 10 mg/100 ml to 25 mg/100 ml. Dialysis: yes, H.

Administration and dosage
Adult

PO—500 mg to a maximum of 2 g.

Pediatric

PO   1. Sedative: 8 mg/kg 3 times daily (maximum dose: 1500 mg daily).
     2. Hypnosis: 50 mg/kg to a single maximum dose of 1 g.
NOTE: Chloral hydrate should be administered well diluted with milk, water, or fruit juices to minimize irritation and mask an aftertaste.

Special remarks and cautions

The habitual use of chloral hydrate may result in physical dependence and addiction similar to that of alcohol. Sudden withdrawal may result in delirium.

Allergic reactions, although rare, include erythema, urticaria, and dermatitis. The eruption usually begins on the face or back and spreads to the neck, chest, and arms. The dermatitis may occur soon after administration or as long as 10 days after administration.

Large doses may produce false-positive results with Clinitest tablets.

Chloral hydrate passes the placental barrier and is excreted in breast milk.

See General information on monitoring sedative-hypnotics (pp. 181 and 182).

Drug interactions

Trichloroacetic acid, a major metabolite of chloral hydrate, displaces warfarin from protein-binding sites, thereby increasing anticoagulant activity and lengthening the prothrombin time. This reaction is potentially more significant in patients stabilized on warfarin therapy when chloral hydrate therapy is being initiated.

Ethanol may significantly potentiate the sedative action of chloral hydrate.

Chloral hydrate may be potentiated by other CNS depressants such as phenothiazines, narcotics, barbiturates, antihistamines, and antidepressants.

ETHCHLORVYNOL
(*Placidyl*)

AHFS 28:24; C-IV
CATEGORY Sedative-hypnotic

Action and use

Ethchlorvynol is a nonbarbiturate CNS depressant with a rapid onset and short duration of action. It is used as a hypnotic agent in the short-term management of insomnia.

Characteristics

Onset: 15 to 30 min. Peak plasma levels: 1 to 1½ hr. Duration: 5 hr. Protein binding: minimal. Half-life: biphasic-distribution phase—5 to 6 hr, elimination phase—70 hr. Metabolism: liver, possibly kidneys, activity of metabolites unknown. Excretion: negligible amounts in urine unchanged. Therapeutic level: 0.2 mg/100 ml to 1.5 mg/100 ml. Toxic level: 2 mg/100 ml. Fatal level: 10 mg/100 ml to 15 mg/100 ml. Dialysis: yes, H,P.

Administration and dosage
Adult

PO—500 mg to 1 g at bedtime. Ethchlorvynol should be administered with food or milk to
    help prevent aftertaste, transient giddiness, dizziness, and ataxia.
NOTE: Ethchlorvynol is not recommended in children.

Special remarks and cautions

Chronic use of ethchlorvynol may result in physical and psychologic dependence. Sudden discontinuance may result in withdrawal symptoms similar to delirium tremens.
Mild "hangover" effects from the drug are relatively common.
As a result of rapid onset of action (15 to 20 min), side effects (dizziness, giddiness, ataxia) are likely to occur before the induction of sleep. Safety measures such as maintenance of bedrest, siderails, and observation should be implemented during this period.
Ethchlorvynol administration is not recommended during the first and second trimesters of pregnancy.
See General information on monitoring sedative-hypnotics (pp. 181 and 182).

Drug interactions

Ethchlorvynol may enhance the metabolism of oral anticoagulants, such as warfarin (Coumadin), resulting in a decreased prothrombin time. Use particular caution when discontinuing ethchlorvynol with patients receiving oral anticoagulants.
Transient delirium has been reported with the combination of amitriptyline (Elavil) and ethchlorvynol.
Ethchlorvynol may be potentiated by other CNS depressants such as alcohol, phenothiazines, narcotics, barbiturates, and antihistamines.

FLURAZEPAM
(Dalmane)

AHFS 28:24; C-IV
CATEGORY Hypnotic

Action and use

Flurazepam is a benzodiazepine derivative used specifically for inducing and maintaining sleep. It may be effective in those patients who have difficulty falling asleep, those patients with frequent awakenings and/or early morning awakenings, and in those patients with acute or chronic medical situations where restful sleep is essential. Laboratory data indicates that doses of 30 mg or less generally do not alter REM sleep, or cause rebound on withdrawal of the drug. Doses of 60 mg do inhibit REM sleep, but again, there appears to be no rebound on discontinuance of therapy.

Characteristics

Onset: 20 to 45 min. Duration: 6 to 8 hr. Half-life: active metabolites—50 to 100 hr. Metabolism: liver. Excretion: renal. Dialysis: unknown.

Administration and dosage
Adult

PO—15 to 30 mg at bedtime. It is recommended that elderly and debilitated patients start with 15 mg at bedtime to determine response.

NOTE: The use of flurazepam is not recommended in patients under 15 years of age.

Special remarks and cautions

See General information on benzodiazepines (p. 215).

Overdosage may be manifested by somnolence, confusion, coma, and respiratory depression. Treatment consists of general physiologic and supportive measures including maintenance of an airway and administration of oxygen. Methylphenidate (Ritalin) or caffeine may be used for severe CNS or respiratory depression. Do not use barbiturates in patients who develop excitation after ingestion of flurazepam.

See General information on monitoring sedative-hypnotics (pp. 181 and 182).

Drug interactions

See General information on benzodiazepines (p. 215).

GLUTETHIMIDE
(Doriden)

AHFS 28:24; C-III
CATEGORY Sedative-hypnotic

Action and use

Glutethimide is a nonbarbiturate hypnotic used for insomnia of short-term duration. Its mechanism of CNS depression is unknown, but is thought to be similar to that of the barbiturates. It, too, suppresses REM sleep but will not diminish the number of nocturnal awakenings or prolong the total sleeping time. It also appears to lose its effectiveness after a few weeks of continual administration.

Characteristics

Onset: 30 min. Duration: 4 to 8 hr. Protein binding: 50%. Half-life: 10 hr. Metabolism: almost complete. Excretion: urine and feces, inactive. Dialysis: no, H, P.

Administration and dosage

PO   1. Daytime sedation: 125 to 250 mg 3 times daily after meals.
      2. Hypnosis: 500 mg at bedtime.
NOTE: Total daily dosages above 1 g are not recommended. Glutethimide is not recommended in children under 12 years of age.

Special remarks and cautions

Chronic use of glutethimide may result in physical and psychologic dependence. Sudden discontinuance may result in withdrawal symptoms that include, nausea, abdominal discomfort, tremors, and delirium.

General adverse effects include nausea, vomiting, headache, dizziness, confusion, and generalized skin rash. Anticholinergic effects of blurred vision, constipation, dry mouth, and tenacious secretions are also occasionally seen.

Glutethimide must be used with caution in pregnancy. Newborn infants of mothers dependent on glutethimide may also exhibit withdrawal symptoms.

See General information on monitoring sedative-hypnotics (pp. 181 and 182).

Drug interactions

Glutethimide enhances the metabolism of warfarin (Coumadin) by induction of hepatic microsomal enzymes. Use particular caution when discontinuing glutethimide in patients stabilized on oral anticoagulants.

Patients receiving tricyclic antidepressants and glutethimide concurrently may display additive anticholinergic effects.

Glutethimide may be potentiated by other CNS depressants such as alcohol, phenothiazines, narcotics, barbiturates, and antihistamines.

METHAQUALONE
(Quaalude, Sopor)

AHFS 28:24; C-II
CATEGORY Sedative-hypnotic

Action and use

Methaqualone is a CNS depressant that acts on the cortex, mid-brain, and spinal cord. In addition to its sedative-hypnotic activity, methaqualone has mild antitussive and anticonvulsant activity. The primary use of methaqualone is to produce sleep in simple insomnia. There is disagreement in the literature as to whether or not methaqualone suppresses REM sleep. In low doses it may be used as a daytime sedative.

Characteristics

Onset: 15 to 30 min. Duration: 6 to 8 hr. Half-life: 2½ hr. Metabolism: liver microsomal enzymes to 9 metabolites. Excretion: primary urine, inactive. Therapeutic level: 0.5 mg/100 ml. Toxic level: 1 mg/100 ml to 3 mg/100 ml. Fatal levels: 2 mg/100 ml. to 3 mg/100 ml. Dialysis: yes, H, P.

Administration and dosage
Adult

PO—150 to 300 mg at bedtime for insomnia; 75 mg 3 to 4 times daily as a sedative.
NOTE: Methaqualone is not recommended for continuous use for periods exceeding 3 months. It is also not recommended for use in pediatric patients.

Special remarks and cautions

Psychologic and physiologic dependence have been observed with methaqualone. It has also been a popular agent of abuse with the drug culture. Severe grand mal seizures may occur after withdrawal from high doses. Use of succinylcholine accompanied by assisted respiration has been proposed for prolonged convulsions.

Patients frequently complain of "hangover," fatigue, dizziness, and headache after ingestion of hypnotic doses.

Patients may occasionally experience transient numbness and tingling in extremities, restlessness, and anxiety before falling asleep after ingestion of hypnotic doses.

Methaqualone administration is not recommended in pregnant women or those who may become pregnant. Teratogenic effects have been noted in offspring of laboratory animals.

See General information on monitoring sedative-hypnotics (pp. 181 and 182).

Drug interactions

One case has been reported of a patient who developed apnea after receiving diazepam (Valium), 10 mg IV, to treat an overdose of diphenhydramine and methaqualone combination (Mandrax).

The CNS depressant activity of methaqualone is enhanced by barbiturates, reserpine, phenothiazines, narcotics, antihistamines, and alcohol.

PARALDEHYDE
(Paral)

AHFS 28:24; C-IV
CATEGORY Sedative-hypnotic

Action and use

The mechanism of action of paraldehyde is unknown although it does depress many levels of the central nervous system. Its sedative-hypnotic properties may be effective in suppressing the withdrawal symptoms of alcohol, narcotics, and barbiturates. It may also be used to control seizures arising from tetanus, poisons, and status epilepticus.

Characteristics

Onset: 10 to 15 min (PO). Peak activity: 30 to 60 min. Duration: 8 hr. Half-life: 7½ hr. Metabolism: 70% to 80 % metabolized in liver. Excretion: 11% to 28% exhaled, up to 2.5% in urine. Therapeutic level: 5 mg/100 ml to 8 mg/100 ml. Toxic level: 20 mg/100 ml to 40 mg/100 ml. Fatal level: 50 mg/100 ml. Dialysis: unknown.

Administration and dosage
Adult

PO— 10 to 30 ml well diluted in milk or iced fruit juice to disguise the odor and taste and to minimize gastrointestinal irritation.

IM—5 to 10 ml undiluted deep into the buttocks with no more than 5 ml/injection site. Use caution; permanent sciatic nerve injury, sterile abscesses, and skin sloughing have been reported.

IV—5 to 10 ml diluted with several volumes of 0.9% sodium chloride and injected slowly with caution.

RECTAL—5 to 10 ml diluted in 200 ml of 0.9% sodium chloride or 120 ml of olive oil to minimize mucosal irritation.

Pediatric

PO—0.15 ml/kg well diluted in milk or iced fruit juice to disguise the odor and taste and to minimize gastrointestinal irritation.

IM—0.15 ml/kg undiluted. Use caution; permanent sciatic nerve injury, sterile abscesses, and skin sloughing have been reported.

IV—0.15 ml/kg mixed with several volumes of 0.9% sodium chloride and injected slowly with caution.

RECTAL—0.3 ml/kg diluted with at least 2 volumes of olive or cottonseed oil to prevent rectal irritation.

NOTE: Paraldehyde should not be stored or administered in plastic containers such as syringes and cups, because of the instability with various plastics.

Preparations with a brownish color or a sharp odor of acetic acid (vinegar) should not be used. The unused contents of any container should be discarded within 24 hours after being opened.

Special remarks and cautions

Paraldehyde must be used with caution in patients with hepatic disease. The drug is metabolized more slowly, and the hypnotic effects may be prolonged.

Paraldehyde by-products are excreted through the lungs, giving the breath a characteristic odor.

The most frequent adverse effects associated with normal doses are gastric irritation and erythematous skin rash.

Acetaldehyde, a metabolic by-product, may produce false-positive serum and urine ketone values when Acetest tablets are used.

Paraldehyde readily diffuses across the placenta and appears in fetal circulation in quantities sufficient to induce respiratory depression in newborn infants.

See General information on monitoring sedative-hypnotics (pp. 181 and 182).

Drug interactions

Disulfiram may slow the metabolism of paraldehyde, resulting in more prolonged blood levels of paraldehyde and acetaldehyde.

Paraldehyde may be potentiated by other CNS depressants such as alcohol, phenothiazines, narcotics, barbiturates, and antihistamines.

Tranquilizing agents

Chlordiazepoxide
Diazepam
Haloperidol
Meprobamate
Molindone hydrochloride
General information on phenothiazines
   Chlorpromazine

Prochlorperazine
Promethazine hydrochloride
Thioridazine
Thiothixene
Trifluoperazine
General information on tricyclic
   antidepressants

CHLORDIAZEPOXIDE
(Librium)

AHFS 28:16.08; C-IV
CATEGORY Tranquilizer

Action and use

Chlordiazepoxide is a benzodiazepine derivative used in mild to moderate states of anxiety and tension. It is also frequently used as a tranquilizer for acute alcohol withdrawal syndrome.

Characteristics

Onset: 30 to 60 min (PO), 15 to 30 min (IM), 3 to 15 min (IV). Peak blood level: 2 to 4 hr (PO). Half-life: 24 to 30 hr. Metabolism: liver, to two active metabolites. Excretion: urine and feces. Therapeutic level: 0.1 mg/100 ml to 0.3 mg/100 ml. Toxic level: 0.5 mg/100 ml. Fatal level: 2 mg/100 ml to 3 mg/100 ml. Dialysis: no, H, P.

Administration and dosage
Adult

PO   1. Mild to moderate anxiety and tension: 5 to 10 mg 3 to 4 times daily.
      2. Severe anxiety and tension: 20 to 25 mg 3 to 4 times daily.
      3. Alcohol withdrawal syndrome: 50 to 100 mg initially, then 25 to 50 mg 3 to 4 times daily as needed.

IM—As for PO administration. IM administration appears to provide longer onset of activity and lower blood levels than PO administration. It may be more beneficial to administer dosage PO if the patient's clinical status will allow it. Add 2 ml of Special Intramuscular Diluent to the contents of the 5 ml dry-filled amber ampule to make 100 mg of IM chlordiazepoxide. Agitate gently to prevent formation of bubbles and inject deeply and slowly into a large skeletal muscle.

IV—As for PO administration. Add 5 ml of sterile water for injection or saline solution to the contents of the 5 ml dry-filled amber ampule to make 100 mg of the chlordiazepoxide for IV use. Administer at a rate no faster than 100 mg/min. Solutions prepared for IV administration are not recommended for IM use because of pain on injection.

NOTE: Total doses of greater than 300 mg/24 hr are not recommended.

Pediatric

NOTE: Not recommended in children under 6 years of age.
PO—Initially, 5 mg 2 to 4 times daily.
IM—0.5 mg/kg/24 hr in 3 or 4 divided doses. See IM administration instructions for adult dosages.

Special remarks and cautions

Acute overdosage or cumulative effects from chronic ingestion may be manifested by somnolence, confusion, coma, and respiratory depression. Treatment consists of general physiologic supportive measures including maintenance of an airway and administration of oxygen. Methylphenidate (Ritalin) or caffeine may be effective against severe respiratory depression. Do not use barbiturates in patients who develop excitation after ingestion of chlordiazepoxide.

Hypotension and tachycardia may occur, particularly on parenteral administration. Severe hypotensive effects may be reversed with levarterenol (Levophed), dopamine (Intropin), or metaraminol (Aramine).

Use with caution in pregnant women. Fetal blood levels are similar to that of maternal circulation. Safe use in pregnancy has not been established.

See General information on benzodiazepines (p. 215).

Drug interactions

See General information on benzodiazepines (p. 215).

Rare cases have been reported where chlordiazepoxide has inhibited the metabolism of phenytoin (Dilantin), resulting in increased serum levels of phenytoin.

DIAZEPAM
(Valium)

AHFS 28:16.08; C-IV
CATEGORY Tranquilizer, anticonvulsant

Action and use

Diazepam is a benzodiazepine derivative used in mild to moderate states of anxiety and tension. It may also be used as a tranquilizer for acute alcohol withdrawal syndrome.

Diazepam has beneficial tranquilizing and amnesic effects when administered parenterally for the relief of anxiety and tension prior to endoscopy, surgical procedures, and cardioversion of atrial fibrillation. Diazepam displays some mild muscle relaxant properties, as do other CNS depressants.

Diazepam is often effective in controlling grand mal, psychomotor, petit mal, and Jacksonian seizures and in controlling status epilepticus.

Characteristics

Onset: immediate (IV), 15 to 30 min (IM), 30 to 60 min (PO). Peak plasma levels: 1 to 3 hr (PO). Protein binding: highly bound. Half-life: 1 to 2 days (parent compound and active metabolites). Metabolism: liver, active. Excretion: metabolites in urine and feces. Therapeutic level: 0.1 mg/100 ml to 0.25 mg/100 ml. Toxic level: 0.5 mg/100 ml to 2 mg/100 ml. Fatal level: 2 mg/100 ml. Dialysis: no, H.

Administration and dosage
Adult

PO—2 to 10 mg 2 to 4 times daily.

IM—Should be discouraged; it is painful, with erratic absorption.

IV—2 to 40 mg depending on use and should be added in small increments. Inject slowly, monitoring the patient's response. Take at least 1 min for each 5 mg (1 ml) given. A fine, white precipitate will develop when diazepam is added to other solutions, including dextrose 5% and saline solution. Administer as close to the venipuncture site as possible.

Pediatric

PO—0.12 to 0.8 mg/kg/24 hr divided into 3 or 4 doses.

IV—0.1 to 0.3 mg/kg repeated in 2 to 4 hr as needed.

NOTE: Diazepam is not recommended in infants less than 30 days of age. However, if seizure activity cannot be arrested with maximum doses of phenobarbital, 0.1 to 0.8 mg/kg/24 hr may be used. Sodium benzoate, a preservative in parenteral solutions of diazepam, has been associated with clinically significant displacement of bilirubin from protein-binding sites.

Special remarks and cautions

See General information on benzodiazepines (p. 215).

Overdosage may be manifested by somnolescence, confusion, coma, and respiratory depression. Treatment consists of general physiologic supportive measures including maintenance of an airway and administration of oxygen. Methylphenidate (Ritalin) or caffeine may be effective against severe CNS or respiratory depression. Do not use barbiturates in patients who develop excitation after ingestion of diazepam.

Hypotension may occur, particularly with parenteral administration. Severe hypotensive effects may be reversed with levarterenol (Levophed) or metaraminol (Aramine).

Use with caution in pregnant women. Fetal blood levels are similar to those in maternal circulation. Small amounts are found in breast milk.

Drug interactions

When diazepam is used with a narcotic analgesic, the dosage of the narcotic should be reduced by at least one third and administered in small increments.

Rare cases have been reported where diazepam has inhibited the metabolism of phenytoin (Dilantin), resulting in increased serum levels of phenytoin and potential toxicity.

See General information on benzodiazepines (p. 215).

HALOPERIDOL
(Haldol)

AHFS 28:16.08
CATEGORY Tranquilizer

Action and use

Haloperidol is a butyrophenone derivative structurally unrelated but with pharmacologic properties similar to the piperazine group of phenothiazine tranquilizers. Haloperidol may be effective in the control of agitated states associated with psychotic behavior such as schizophrenia and manic phases of manic-depressive psychoses. The exact mechanism of action is unknown.

Characteristics

Peak plasma levels: 10 to 15 min (IM), 2 to 6 hr (PO). Duration: up to 72 hr. Metabolism: concentration in liver. Excretion: urine and feces.

Administration and dosage

NOTE: Dosage must be carefully adjusted according to individual requirements and tolerance. Geriatric or debilitated patients frequently require lower initial doses to achieve the same therapeutic effect. Haloperidol is not approved for use in children.

PO   1. Initial: moderate symptoms, 0.5 to 2 mg 2 to 3 times daily; severe symptoms, 3 to 5 mg 2 to 3 times daily. Dosages up to 100 mg daily may be required in severely disturbed individuals.

   2. Maintenance: after achieving a desired therapeutic response, dosage should be gradually reduced to the lowest effective maintenance level.

IM—2 to 5 mg for immediate control of the acutely agitated patient. Depending on the patient's response, doses may be repeated every hour, but may need to be repeated only every 4 to 8 hr.

Special remarks and cautions

Extrapyramidal symptoms (akathisia or parkinsonian manifestations of marked drowsiness and lethargy, drooling and hypersalivation, fixed stare, and muscular rigidity) are the most common side effects of haloperidol. These symptoms often occur during the first few days of therapy and may require reduction in dosage, initiation of antiparkinsonian drug therapy (benztropine, [Cogentin] 2 to 4 mg) or complete discontinuance of haloperidol therapy. Antiparkinsonian drugs should be continued after haloperidol has been discontinued because the slow elimination of haloperidol may cause a recurrence of the extrapyramidal symptoms.

Tardive dyskinesia, manifested by recurrent protrusion of the tongue, puffing of the cheeks, puckering of the mouth, and chewing movements, may develop with long-term treatment with haloperidol. There appears to be a higher incidence in elderly female patients on high-dose therapy. This syndrome is irreversible in some patients, but may be prevented if the drug is discontinued at the first sign of fine tremor-like movements of the tongue.

Haloperidol should be administered with caution in patients prone to seizures since haloperidol may lower the convulsive threshold. Dosages of anticonvulsant therapy may require readjustment.

Hypotension occurs infrequently but may be observed on IM injection or overdosage. It may be treated with IV fluids, plasma, albumin, or vasopressors such as norepinephrine or phenylephrine. Do not use epinephrine, since haloperidol blocks its vasopressor effects, resulting in further lowering of blood pressure.

Other general adverse effects of haloperidol include mild and transient leukopenia and leukocytosis, impaired liver function and/or jaundice, skin rashes and alopecia, anorexia, dry mouth, constipation, nausea and vomiting, blurred vision, urinary retention, bronchospasm, drowsiness, euphoria, and agitation.

Haloperidol therapy is not recommended in pregnant women. Teratogenic effects have been reported; however, a causal relationship has not been established. Haloperidol also appears in the milk of lactating mothers.

Drug interactions

Haloperidol may reverse the hypotensive effects of guanethidine.

Haloperidol may have additive CNS depressant effects with ethanol, barbiturates, sedatives, antihistamines, anesthetics, analgesics, and tranquilizers.

MEPROBAMATE
(Equanil, Miltown)

AHFS 28:16.08; C-IV
CATEGORY Tranquilizer

Action and use

Meprobamate is a minor tranquilizer used effectively as an antianxiety agent and mild skeletal muscle relaxant. It acts on multiple sites within the central nervous system, producing mild sedation and relaxation. Meprobamate is indicated for the relief of anxiety and tension and for the promotion of sleep in anxious, tense patients. Meprobamate is of little value in the treatment of psychoses.

Characteristics

Onset: 30 min. Peak activity: 2 to 3 hr. Plasma half-life: 10 hr. Metabolism: microsomal enzymes in the liver; may produce enzyme induction. Excretion: 10% unchanged in urine. Therapeutic level: 0.5 mg/100 ml to 2 mg/100 ml. Toxic level: 5 mg/100 ml to 20 mg/100 ml (lower with ethanol). Lethal dose: 12 to 40 g. Dialysis: yes, H, P.

Administration and dosage
Adult

PO—400 mg 3 to 4 times daily. Smaller doses may suffice for elderly and debilitated patients. Maximum daily doses should not exceed 2400 mg.

Pediatric

PO—The usual dosage in children 6 to 12 years of age is 100 to 200 mg 2 or 3 times daily. Meprobamate is not recommended in children under 6 years of age.

Special remarks and cautions

Psychologic and physiologic dependence and abuse have occurred. Symptoms of the chronic use of high doses include ataxia, slurred speech, and dizziness. Withdrawal reactions such as vomiting, tremors, confusion, hallucinosis, and grand mal seizures may develop within 12 to 48 hr after abrupt discontinuance. Symptoms usually abate within the next 12 to 48 hr. Withdrawal from high and prolonged dosage should gradually be completed over 1 to 2 weeks. Alternatively, a patient may be stabilized on short-acting barbiturates and then gradually tapered from the barbiturate.

Meprobamate may precipitate seizures in patients prone to convulsive episodes.

Adverse reactions to meprobamate are generally mild and include dizziness, slurred speech, headache, paradoxic excitement, various arrhythmias, hypotension, dermatologic and allergic reactions, blood dyscrasias, and exacerbation of intermittent porphyria.

Meprobamate may interfere with urinary steroid determinations as a result of interference with the testing procedure.

Meprobamate readily crosses the placental barrier and is found in breast milk in concentrations 2 to 4 times that of the mother's blood level. Neonates and nursing infants whose mothers receive meprobamate must be observed for signs of toxicity.

Drug interactions

The CNS depressant effects of antihistamines, analgesics, anesthetics, other tranquilizers, and sedative-hypnotics may be potentiated by meprobamate.

Meprobamate may induce hepatic microsomal enzymes, enhancing the metabolism of warfarin (Coumadin), digitoxin, corticosteroids (for example, prednisone), doxycycline (Vibramycin), phenytoin (Dilantin), and chlorpromazine (Thorazine). If meprobamate is discontinued, the patient must be observed closely for signs of secondary drug toxicity requiring reduction of dosage.

MOLINDONE HYDROCHLORIDE
(Moban hydrochloride)

AHFS 28:16.08
CATEGORY Tranquilizer

Action and use

Although not structurally related to the butyrophenones, thioxanthenes, or phenothiazines, molindone has pharmacologic properties similar to these agents. Molindone is used to control the symptoms of schizophrenia such as grandiosity, tension, disorientation, perceptual distortion, and withdrawal. The exact mechanism of activity is unknown.

Characteristics

Peak plasma levels: 1 hr. Duration: 36 hr. Plasma half-life: $1\frac{1}{2}$ hr. Metabolism: liver. Excretion: 3% unchanged in urine, small amount via lungs as CO_2, remainder in urine and feces as inactive metabolites. Therapeutic level: unknown. Dialysis: no, H, P.

Administration and dosage

NOTE: Dosage must be carefully adjusted to individual requirements and tolerance. Geriatric or debilitated patients frequently require lower initial doses to achieve the same therapeutic effect. Molindone is not recommended for use in children under 12 years of age.

PO 1. Initial: mild, 5 to 15 mg 3 to 4 times daily; moderate, 10 to 25 mg 3 to 4 times daily; severe, daily dosages as high as 225 mg may be required.
     2. Maintenance: once the patient is stabilized, a single daily dose is adequate.

Weeks or months of therapy with molindone may be necessary to produce maximun clinical improvement.

Special remarks and cautions

Transient initial drowsiness is the most frequently reported side effect.

Extrapyramidal symptoms (akathisia or parkinsonian reactions characterized by muscle rigidity, recurring drowsiness and lethargy, drooling and hypersalivation, fixed stare, reduction of voluntary movement, and tremor) are frequently noted, particularly with increasing doses. These extrapyramidal symptoms may require control by antiparkinsonian drugs (benztropine or trihexyphenidyl).

Other adverse effects noted with molindone include restlessness, depression, dizziness, blurred vision, hyperactivity, nausea, vomiting, euphroia, dry mouth, and tachycardia.

Although molindone differs structurally and to some degree pharmacologically from the phenothiazines, similar adverse reactions should be anticipated. Grouping these potential adverse reactions into classes, they include liver dysfunction and jaundice, hematologic dyscrasias, hypotensive effects, allergic reactions, endocrine disorders, skin pigmentation, and ocular changes. Many of these reactions have not yet been reported, but as molindone gains more widespread use, the possibility of the development of these effects increases.

Molindone is not recommended for use in pregnant or nursing women. No teratogenetic abnormalities in animals have yet been observed. Data are not available on the content of molindone in breast milk.

Drug interactions

No drug interactions have as yet been reported; however, molindone may be expected to have additive CNS depressant effects with ethanol, sedatives, antihistamines, anesthetics, analgesics, and tranquilizers.

GENERAL INFORMATION ON PHENOTHIAZINES

The phenothiazine derivatives are among the oldest and most popular antipsychotic agents used in medicine today. There are several classes of phenothiazine derivatives, all based on different structural substituents attached to the basic phenothiazine molecule. These subgroups (with examples) are: (1) ethylamino derivatives (promethazine—Phenergan), (2) propylamino derivatives (chlorpromazine—Thorazine, promazine—Sparine), (3) piperazine derivatives (trifluroperazine—Stelazine, fluphenazine—Prolixin), and (4) piperidine derivatives (thioridazine—Mellaril). See the individual monographs on these agents for particular advantages and disadvantages of these classes of phenothiazines.

Phenothiazines are major tranquilizers believed to act by blocking receptors in the brain to dopamine and norepinephrine. The exact mechanisms of action are unknown. Their actions on the central and autonomic nervous systems affect many different sites within the body, thus giving rise to the many varied actions and side effects of phenothiazines.

Administration and dosage

Dosages must be individualized according to the degree of mental and emotional disturbance. It will often take several weeks for a patient to show optimal improvement and to become stabilized on an adequate maintenance dosage. As a result of the cumulative effects of phenothiazines, patients must be periodically reevaluated to determine the lowest effective dosage necessary to control psychiatric symptoms.

After patients have become stabilized on the lowest effective maintenance dosage, phenothiazines can often be given in a single daily dose. Single daily dosages at bedtime offer the advantages of improved sleep, which masks minor side effects. Other patients, however, may experience fewer side effects when the doses are spread out. Consequently patients must be placed on an individualized dosage regimen that will provide optimal symptomatic improvement and compliance with the fewest adverse effects.

Special remarks and cautions

Some of the most troublesome side effects noted with antipsychotic agents are "extrapyramidal" effects. These include the parkinsonian symptoms of tremor, muscular rigidity, masklike facies, shuffling gait, and loss or weakness of motor function; dystonias and dyskinesias, which are spasmodic movements of the body and limbs (dystonias) and coordinated, involuntary rhythmic movements (dyskinesias); and akathisias, which consist of involuntary motor restlessness, constant pacing, inability to sit still, and are often accompanied by fidgeting, with lip and limb movements.

Tardive dyskinesia is a drug-induced neurologic disorder manifested by facial grimaces and involuntary movement of the lips, tongue, and jaw, producing smacking and frequent, recurrent protrusions of the tongue. This adverse drug effect is usually irreversible and appears after several years of antipsychotic therapy. The incidence appears to be higher in patients taking both antiparkinsonian and antipsychotic agents concomitantly. It has been reported that fine movements of the tongue may be an early sign of tardive dyskinesia. If the medication is stopped, the syndrome may not develop.

Dry mouth and constipation are other frequent side effects that may caused decreased compliance. Sugarless hard candy or gum may help the dry mouth. The use of stool softeners such as dioctyl sodium sulfosuccinate (Colace) and occasionally a potent laxative such as bisacodyl (Dulcolax) may be required for constipation.

Chronic drowsiness and fatigue may occur during initiation or adjustment in therapy. Tolerance will usually develop, but a single daily dose at bedtime may also be effective.

Phenothiazines lower the seizure threshold. Seizures may occur in those with and without a history of seizure activity. Adjustment of anticonvulsant therapy may be required, especially in those seizure-prone patients.

Hypersensitivity reactions include cholestatic jaundice (upper abdominal pain, yellow skin, rash, fever, eosinophilia, elevated liver function tests), blood dyscrasias, dermatoses, and photosensitivity. Most hypersensitivity reactions occur within the first few months of therapy.

Adverse effects, listed according to organ systems involved, include:

1. Hematologic: blood dyscrasias are rare, but the mortality rate can be high. Agranulocytosis occurs most frequently in women and after 4 to 10 weeks of therapy. Leukopenia frequently occurs after prolonged therapy with high dosages of phenothiazines and is usually an indication to stop therapy. Other blood dyscarasias include eosinophilia, hemolytic anemia, thrombocytopenia, and aplastic anemia. If signs of blood dyscrasias (sore throat, fever, weakness) occur, phenothiazine therapy should be discontinued until a complete blood count has eliminated the possibility of a blood dyscrasia.

2. Hepatic: a cholestatic jaundice may appear in 0.5% to 4% of those patients ingesting phenothiazines. It usually appears within 2 to 4 weeks after initiating therapy. Patients may complain of upper abdominal pain, yellow skin, rash, and fever, and display elevated levels in liver function tests (SCOT, SGPT, bilirubin, alkaline phosphatase).

3. Skin: photosensitivity may develop while a patient is on phenothiazine therapy. Patients should be warned to wear protective clothing and avoid direct sunlight. A contact dermatitis may develop in those patients who have contact with solutions of phenothiazine derivatives. These patients should avoid physical contact with these solutions. Skin pigmentation, usually yellowish brown but possibly changing to greyish-purple, may result from long-term (3 years or more) administration of large doses of phenothiazines. The pigmentation is more frequent in women, is usually restricted to exposed areas of the body, and may fade on discontinuance of therapy.

4. Ophthalmic: long-term administration may lead to deposition of fine particulate matter in the lens and cornea. These eye lesions appear to be reversible on discontinuance of phenothiazine therapy.

5. Cardiovascular: hypotension, tachycardia, fainting, and dizziness may occur, especially after parenteral administration. ECG changes similar to those caused by hypokalemia or quinidine may also occur.

6. Endocrine: menstrual irregularities, delayed ovulation, galactorrhea, alterations in libido, hyperglycemia, glycosuria, hypoglycemia, weight gain, and high or prolonged glucose tolerance curves may occur.

7. Other: phenothiazines may produce a myriad of side effects other than those already listed. These include gastrointestinal effects, alterations in body temperature regulation, particularly hypothermia, and respiratory depression, especially in those with impaired pulmonary function.

Phenothiazines cross the placental barrier and may appear in the milk of nursing mothers. The effects of phenothiazine therapy on the human fetus is unknown. Therefore these derivatives should be used on a risk versus benefit basis in pregnant women or those women planning to become pregnant while on phenothiazine therapy.

Overdosage

Treatment of phenothiazine overdosage is essentially symptomatic. Establish and maintain an airway. Early gastric lavage may be helpful. Extrapyramidal effects may be treated with diphenhydramine (Benadryl) 2.5 to 5 mg/kg with a maximum single IV dose of 50 mg over 2 min. Hypotension may be treated with an infusion of levarterenol (Levophed) or phenylephrine (Neo-Synephrine). Epinephrine is not recommended. As a result of the alpha-adrenergic blocking activity of phenothiazines, a paradoxic hypotension may result after the use of epinephrine.

Drug interactions

Phenothiazines display enhanced CNS depressant activity with ethanol, barbiturates, narcotics, tranquilizers, antihistamines, sedative-hypnotics, and anesthetics. Because of enhanced activity the phenothiazines may allow a dosage reduction to about half the usual dosage of these other agents.

The absorption of orally administered phenothiazines may be diminished by antacids. Spacing the time intervals between administration of the two products will minimize the gastrointestinal mixing that leads to diminished absorption.

Barbiturates may increase the rate of metabolism by enzyme induction, potentially leading to decreased phenothiazine activity.

Although the mechanism is unknown, phenothiazines may produce hyperglycemia. Diabetic patients controlled on insulin or oral hypoglycemic agents may require readjustment of dosages to control the diabetes mellitus.

Although the cases are rare, there are reports of phenytoin (Dilantin) metabolism being inhibited by prochlorperazine and chlorpromazine. Caution is recommended, and the dosage of phenytoin may require adjustment to maintain antiarrhythmic or anticonvulsant control.

Phenothiazines may inhibit the antihypertensive effect of guanethidine by diminishing the uptake of guanethidine into the adrenergic neurons. Patients must be observed for loss of antihypertensive control. Remember that phenothiazines also cause hypotension and may enhance the drop in blood pressure.

Propranolol may enhance the hypotensive effect of phenothiazines. Patients should be observed for hypotensive effects, especially during adjustment to either propranolol or phenothiazine therapy.

Phenothiazine effects on the heart are in some respects similar to those of quinidine. Phenothiazine-induced ventricular tachycardia should not be treated with quinidine, but should be treated similar to quinidine toxicity.

CHLORPROMAZINE
(Thorazine)

AHFS 28:16.08
CATEGORY Tranquilizer

Action and use

Chlorpromazine is a representative of the propylamino phenothiazine derivatives. It may be used in the treatment of psychomotor agitation associated with various types of acute and chronic psychoses, control of the manic phase of manic-depressive illness, moderate to severe agitation, hyperactivity or aggressiveness in disturbed children, and control of nausea and vomiting. Sedative effects are predominant (although tolerance soon develops) while the frequency of extrapyramidal symptoms are moderate.

Characteristics

Absorption: dependent on formulation of the product, decreased significantly by the presence of food and anticholinergic drugs, as well as great intersubject variation. Peak plasma levels: 2 to 3 hr. Protein binding: 90%. Half-life (plasma): less than 6 hr. Metabolism: liver to greater than 100 metabolites. Excretion: about 10% unchanged in urine, metabolites about equal in urine and feces. Some metabolites are detectable in the urine 6 months after discontinuance of therapy. Therapeutic level: plasma concentrations of free chlorpromazine do not correlate with the therapeutic responses. Dialysis: no, H, P.

Administration and dosage

For anxiety, tension, and agitation:

Adult

PO—Initially 10 to 50 mg 4 times daily. Increase daily dosages by 25 to 50 mg semiweekly until the patient becomes calm and cooperative.

IM—25 to 50 mg for prompt control of severe symptoms. This dosage may be repeated in 1 hr. Observe patient closely for hypotensive effects, especially on initial dosages. Gradually increase dosages over several days. As a result of irritation, inject deeply into the upper outer quadrant slowly. Rotate injection sites.

IV—Not recommended because of potential cardiovascular effects.

Pediatric

PO—2 mg/kg/24 hr divided into 4 to 6 doses.

NOTE: Maximum improvement may not be seen for several weeks. Daily dosages of 1 to 2 g may be required in some patients with severe symptomatology. After symptoms have been controlled for a few weeks, dosages should be slowly reduced to the lowest effective level.

For nausea and vomiting:

Adult

PO—10 to 25 mg every 4 to 6 hr as needed.

IM—25 mg. Observe closely for hypotension. If hypotension is not evident, subsequent dosages may be increased to 50 mg every 3 to 4 hr as needed.

IV—If symptoms persist, inject 25 to 50 mg in 500 ml of saline slowly. The patient should remain flat in bed, and the blood pressure be monitored closely.

RECTAL—50 to 100 mg suppository every 6 to 8 hr as needed.

Pediatric

PO—0.1 mg/kg every 4 to 6 hr.

IM—0.1 mg/kg every 6 to 8 hr.

RECTAL—0.2 mg/kg every 6 to 8 hr as needed.

NOTE: Not recommended in children under 6 months of age unless potentially lifesaving.

NOTE: Pain on IM injection may be minimized by diluting with 2% procaine or saline. Abrupt withdrawal after long-term use of high dosages of chlorpromazine may result in symptoms of physical dependence (gastritis, nausea, vomiting, dizziness, and tremulousness). Gradual dosage reduction or continuation of antiparkinsonian agents for several weeks may avoid these complications.

Special remarks and cautions

See General information on phenothiazines (pp. 202 to 204).

Overdosage

See General information on phenothiazines (pp. 202 to 204).

Drug interactions

See General information on phenothiazines (pp. 202 to 204).

PROCHLORPERAZINE
(Compazine)

AHFS 56:20 and 28:16.08
CATEGORY Antiemetic, tranquilizer

Action and use

Prochlorperazine is a piperazine phenothiazine derivative. It is an antipsychotic agent effective in controlling the psychomotor agitation of schizophrenia; the manic phase of manic-depressive psychosis; and the anxiety, tension, and confusion associated with various neuroses. Its most frequent use however, is in the prevention and control of severe nausea and vomiting.

Administration and dosage

For severe nausea and vomiting:

Adult

PO—5 to 10 mg 3 to 4 times daily or 15 mg (in sustained release form) on arising or 10 mg (in sustained release form) every 12 hr.

IM—Initially, 5 to 10 mg injected deeply into the upper outer quadrant of the buttock. Repeat every 3 to 4 hr as needed. Total IM dosage should not exceed 40 mg/day.

IV—Initially, 5 to 10 mg. Observe for hypotension. An infusion of 20 mg of prochlorperazine/L of solution may be used to control nausea during surgery.

RECTAL—25 mg 2 times daily.

Pediatric

NOTE: Prochlorperazine should be used with caution when administered to children. There has been some suspicion that centrally acting antiemetics may contribute, in combination with viral illnesses, to the development of Reye's syndrome, a potentially fatal acute childhood disease. Administration of antiemetics is not recommended until the cause of vomiting can be determined.

Under 10 kg or 2 years of age

PO or RECTAL—Not recommended.

Between 10 and 14 kg

PO or RECTAL—2.5 mg 1 or 2 times daily, not to exceed 7.5 mg/day.

IM—One half the PO or rectal dosage. More than 1 dose is seldom necessary.

Between 15 and 18 kg

PO or RECTAL—2.5 mg 2 or 3 times daily, not to exceed 10 mg/day.

IM—As for children between 10 and 14 kg.

Between 19 and 40 kg

PO or RECTAL—2.5 to 5 mg 2 or 3 times daily, not to exceed 15 mg/day.

IM—As for children between 10 and 14 kg.

NOTE: Prochlorperazine is not recommended for use in pediatric surgery. Children seem more prone to develop extrapyramidal reactions, even with moderate doses.

Special remarks and cautions

See General information on phenothiazines (pp. 202 to 204).

Other measures that enhance antiemetic activity include frequent small feedings or dry carbohydrates when allowed by dietary restrictions and avoidance of high fat foods and antacids. Decrease noxious stimuli in the environment such as odors, smoke, unpleasant sounds, drainage, and waste products. Good oral hygiene for improved patient comfort is frequently overlooked after emesis.

One must be aware of excessive vomiting and must observe patient for deficiencies in fluids, electrolytes, and nutrients. See Indications of fluid and electrolyte imbalance (p. 130).

Safe use during pregnancy has not been established.

Drug interactions

See General information on phenothiazines (pp. 202 to 204).

PROMETHAZINE HYDROCHLORIDE
(Phenergan)

AHFS 4:00 and 28:24
CATEGORY Antihistaminic and tranquilizer

Action and use

Promethazine hydrochloride is a representative of the ethylamino phenothiazine derivatives. Although promethazine is a phenothiazine and has the potential for many of the side effects of phenothiazines, it has no use as an antipsychotic agent. Ethylamino derivatives are used for their antihistaminic and sedative properties. Antihistaminic activity makes promethazine useful in the symptomatic treatment of seasonal allergies, mild hypersensitivity reactions of urticaria and angioedema, and for the prevention of allergic reactions to blood or plasma transfusions. The sedative effects may be useful for mild preoperative and postoperative apprehension. Antiemetic activity may be effective in preventing or treating motion sickness and postoperative nausea.

Administration and dosage

For allergy:

Adult

PO—12.5 to 25 mg 2 or 3 times daily.
RECTAL—25 mg suppositories. May be repeated within 2 hr if necessary.

Pediatric

PO—0.1 mg/kg every 6 hr and 0.5 mg/kg at bedtime as needed or 6.25 to 12.5 mg 3 times daily and 25 mg at bedtime as needed.

For motion sickness, prophylaxis:

Adult

PO—25 mg twice daily. The initial dose should be administered 30 to 60 min prior to departure.

Pediatric

PO—0.5 mg/kg every 12 hr as needed or 12.5 to 25 mg every 12 hr as needed.

For nausea and vomiting:

Adult

PO—25 mg every 4 to 6 hr as needed.
RECTAL—12.5 to 25 mg suppository every 4 to 6 hr as needed.

Pediatric

PO—12.5 to 25 mg every 4 to 6 hr as needed.
RECTAL—As for adult dosages or 0.25 to 0.5 mg/kg every 4 to 6 hr as needed.
IM—0.25 to 0.5 mg/kg every 4 to 6 hr as needed.

To relieve apprehension and induce sleep:

Adult

PO—25 to 50 mg.

Pediatric

    PO—12.5 to 25 mg.
RECTAL—12.5 to 25 mg.
    IM—0.5 to 1 mg/kg.

Special remarks and cautions

See General information on phenothiazines (pp. 202 to 204).

A paradoxic reaction manifested by hyperexcitability and nightmares has been reported in children receiving single PO doses of 75 to 125 mg.

Drug interactions

See General information on phenothiazines (pp. 202 to 204).

THIORIDAZINE
(Mellaril)

AHFS 28:16.08
CATEGORY Tranquilizer

Action and use

Thioridazine is a representative of the piperidine phenothiazine derivatives. It may be effective in reducing psychomotor excitement, agitation, and tension associated with various types of acute and chronic psychoses and neuroses. The piperidine group of phenothiazines display minimal antiemetic activity, prominent sedative effects, and have the lowest incidence of extrapyramidal side effects of any of the classes of phenothiazines.

Administration and dosage
Adult

For neurotic depressive reaction, psychoneuroses, senility:
PO—10 to 50 mg 3 to 4 times daily.

For psychotic manifestations:
PO—50 to 100 mg 3 times daily, with gradual increments to a maximum of 800 mg if required.

NOTE: Once effective control of symptoms is achieved, the dosage should be reduced gradually to determine the minimum maintenance dose.

Pediatric (2 to 12 years of age)

NOTE: Thioridazine is not intended for children under 2 years of age. Dosage range for children age 2 to 12 years: 0.5 to 3.0 mg/kg.

Children with moderate disorders

PO—10 mg 2 or 3 times daily is the usual starting dose

Children with severe disorders

PO—25 mg 2 to 3 times daily is the usual starting dose.

Dosage may be increased gradually until optimal therapeutic effect or maximal dosage has been attained.

Special remarks and cautions

See General information on phenothiazines (pp. 202 to 204).

Drug interactions

See General information on phenothiazines (pp. 202 to 204).

THIOTHIXENE
(Navane)

AHFS 28:16.08
CATEGORY Tranquilizer

Action and use

Thiothixene is an antipsychotic agent used in the treatment of acute and chronic psychoses. Its mechanism of action is not known, but it produces pharmacologic responses similar to those of the piperazine phenothiazines (trifluoperazine [Stelazine]) and butyrophenones (haloperidol [Haldol]). Thiothixene also displays some mild cholinergic and alpha-adrenergic blocking activity. Thiothixene may be used successfully in patients who are withdrawn, apathetic schizophrenics, and suffering from delusions and hallucinations. It is less effective in those patients displaying severe psychomotor excitement.

Characteristics

Onset: 1 to 6 hr (IM), a few days to several weeks (PO). Metabolism: liver. Excretion: primarily in bile and feces as unchanged drug and metabolites. Therapeutic level: unknown. Dialysis: no, H, P.

Administration and dosage
Adult

For mild to moderate psychotic states:

PO—Initially, 2 mg 3 times daily, gradually increased up to 15 mg daily. Dosage in elderly patients should be one third to half the normal adult dosage.

For severe psychotic states:

PO—Initially, 5 mg 2 times daily, with subsequent increases as needed. The usual optimal dose is 15 to 30 mg daily, although 60 mg daily may be required in some patients with severe symptomatology. A single daily dosage is usually adequate for maintenance therapy.

IM—In acutely agitated states, 4 mg 2 to 4 times daily may be effective. Subsequent doses may require adjustment. The usual optimal daily IM dose is 16 to 20 mg, with a total daily IM dosage not to exceed 30 mg. PO therapy should replace parenteral administration as soon as possible.

NOTE: Use in children under 12 years of age is not recommended.

Special remarks and cautions

See General information on phenothiazines (pp. 202 to 204).
Safe use in pregnancy has not been established.

Drug interactions

See General information on phenothiazines (pp. 202 to 204).

TRIFLUOPERAZINE
(Stelazine)

AHFS 28:16.08
CATEGORY Tranquilizer

Action and use

Trifluoperazine is a piperazine phenothiazine derivative used to treat anxiety, tension, and agitation associated with various neurotic and psychotic disorders. There appear to be fewer symptoms of sedation, blurred vision, and hypotension than with other classes of phenothiazine derivatives, but the extrapyramidal symptoms occur more frequently than with other classes of phenothiazines.

Administration and dosage
Adult

PO—1 to 5 mg 2 times daily. Optimal therapeutic dosage levels should be reached within 2 to 3 weeks. Most patients respond well at 15 to 20 mg/day, but an occasional patient will require 40 mg or more daily.

IM—1 to 2 mg by deep injection every 4 to 6 hr as needed. The injection should be protected from light. Slight yellow discoloration should not alter potency, but if markedly discolored, the solution should be discarded.

NOTE: As a result of the cumulative effects of trifluoperazine, patients should be periodically reevaluated to determine whether a lower maintenance dose may be adequate, or whether drug therapy may be discontinued.

Pediatric (hospitalized patients 6 to 12 years of age)

PO—1 mg 1 to 2 times daily. Most patients respond to less than 15 mg/day. Gradually increase dosages until symptoms are controlled or until side effects become unacceptable.

IM—1 mg 1 or 2 times daily. The injection should be protected from light. Slight yellow discoloration should not alter potency, but if markedly discolored, the solution should be discarded.

Special remarks and cautions

See General information on phenothiazines (pp. 202 to 204).

Overdosage

See General information on phenothiazines (pp. 202 to 204).

Drug interactions

See General information on phenothiazines (pp. 202 to 204).

GENERAL INFORMATION ON TRICYCLIC ANTIDEPRESSANTS

Tricyclic antidepressants are a class of compounds believed to act by inhibiting the pump mechanism responsible for the reuptake of norepinephrine and 5-hydroxytryptamine into adrenergic neurons. Investigators have proposed that this may potentiate or prolong sympathetic activity by accumulation of these amines at extracellular sites.

Tricyclic antidepressants have been found to be more specifically effective in treating patients with endogenous (psychotic) depression. Combination therapy with phenothiazine derivatives may be beneficial in treating the depression of schizophrenia or moderate to severe anxiety and depression associated with psychosis or psychoneurosis. Tricyclic antidepressants may also be used in conjunction with electroconvulsive therapy in treating depression. Although data is conflicting, the use of antidepressants may reduce the amount of electroconvulsive therapy required.

Administration and dosage

Dosage should be initiated at a low level and increased gradually, particularly in elderly or debilitated patients. Increases in dosage should be made in the evening, since increased sedation is often present.

Manifestations of depression may improve within a few days (that is, increase in appetite, sleep, and psychomotor activity). However, the depression still exists and it usually takes several weeks of therapeutic doses of antidepressants and psychotherapy before improvement is noted. Suicidal precautions should be maintained during this time.

After an optimal response has been obtained, dosage should be reduced to the minimum necessary to maintain relief of depression.

When tricyclic antidepressant therapy is abruptly discontinued after several months of therapy, withdrawal symptoms (abdominal cramping, nausea, vomiting, chills, insomnia, and irritability) often occur. Tapering should be done over a 1- or 2-month period.

See Table 10-1 for generic and brand names and recommended dosages.

Special remarks and cautions

Frequent side effects include dry mouth, blurred vision, tachycardia, constipation, and urinary retention. A fine rapid tremor of the hands may occur in about 10% of the patients on tricyclic therapy. Occasionally, patients have reported numbness and tingling of arms and

Table 10-1. Tricyclic antidepressants   AHFS 28:16.04

Generic	Brand	Initial dosage		Maintenance dosage (daily)	Maximum dosage (daily)
		PO	IM		
Amitriptyline hydrochloride	Elavil	25 mg 3 times a day	20 to 30 mg 4 times a day	150 to 250 mg	300 mg
Desipramine hydrochloride	Norpramin, Pertofrane	25 to 30 mg 3 times a day	—	75 to 100 mg	200 mg
Doxepin hydrochloride	Sinequan	25 mg 3 times a day	—	No less than 150 mg	300 mg
Imipramine hydrochloride	Presamine, Tofranil	30 to 75 mg daily	Up to 100 mg	150 to 250 mg	300 mg
Nortriptyline hydrochloride	Aventyl	25 mg 3 to 4 times a day	—	50 to 75 mg	100 mg
Protriptyline hydrochloride	Vivactil	5 to 10 mg 3 to 4 times a day	—	20 to 40 mg	60 mg

legs, peculiar taste, and temporary confusion. Sedation is a common side effect, particularly with amitriptyline. Desipramine, nortriptyline, and protriptyline are the least sedating of the tricyclic antidepressants.

Patients with cardiovascular disorders must be observed for development or aggravation of existing arrhythmias, sinus tachycardia, and hypotension. Orthostatic hypotension is commonly seen with therapeutic dosages. Tricyclic antidepressants may cause flattening or inversion of the T wave of an electrocardiogram in about 20% of patients without previous history of cardiovascular disease. Deaths from coronary occlusion, cardiac arrest, and ventricular fibrillation have been reported, as well as cases of severe arrhythmias.

High doses may produce grand mal seizure activity even in patients without a history of convulsions.

Safe use in pregnancy has not been established.

Overdosage

Toxicity caused by acute overdosage is characterized by hyperpyrexia, hypertension, hypotension, arrhythmias, seizures, and coma. Gastric lavage may be of value in acute overdosage. Vital signs and ECG should be monitored continuously. Sudden fatal arrhythmias have been reported late in the course.

Physostigmine salicylate (Antilirium) may reverse the anticholinergic manifestations of delirium, convulsions, coma, and arrhythmias. (See Physostigmine salicylate, p. 309, for use.)

Hypotensive activity may be reversed with fluids. If a pressor agent is required, levarterenol or dopamine may be titrated as needed. Initiate therapy with very low doses as tricyclics increase the pressor response to levarterenol.

Convulsions may be treated with IV diazepam (Valium). Arrhythmias refractory to physostigmine may be treated with phenytoin (Dilantin). Propranolol (Inderal) may be effective in arrhythmias caused by adrenergic hyperactivity resulting from blockade of the reuptake of catecholamines. In patients with conduction defects the doses of physostigmine, propranolol, and phenytoin should be reduced to prevent complete heart block.

Drug interactions

Severe reactions (convulsions, hyperpyrexia, and fatalities) have been observed with the concomitant administration of a MAO inhibitor (isocarboxazid [Marplan], pargyline hydrochloride [Eutonyl], tranylcypromine sulfate [Parnate]). It is recommended that 2 weeks lapse between discontinuing an MAO inhibitor and starting tricyclic antidepressants.

The antihypertensive effect of guanethidine (Ismelin) is blocked by tricyclic antidepressants because of the inhibition of uptake of guanethidine into the adrenergic neuron.

Tricyclic antidepressants may display additive anticholinergic effects (dry mouth, constipation, urinary retention, acute glaucoma, blurred vision) when administered with antihistamines (Benadryl), phenothiazines, trihexiphenidyl (Artane), benzotropine (Cogentin), meperidine (Demerol), and other agents with anticholinergic activity. Usually, however, the side effects are not serious enough to require discontinuance of therapy.

Methylphenidate (Ritalin) and thyroid hormones may increase serum levels of tricyclic antidepressants. This reaction has been advantageous in attempts to gain a faster onset of antidepressant activity.

Barbiturates may stimulate the metabolism of tricyclic antidepressants and may decrease their blood levels. Barbiturates may also potentiate the adverse effects (respiratory depression) of toxic doses of tricyclic antidepressants.

Tricyclic antidepression may enhance meperidine-induced respiratory depression. This reaction may be particularly significant in those patients with lung disease.

Tricyclic antidepressants may cause a synergistic response in patients receiving infusions of pressor amines—levarterenol (Levophed), epinephrine, phenylephrine (Neo-Synephrine).

CHAPTER ELEVEN

Anticonvulsant agents

General information on benzodiazepines
Clonazepam
Diazepam
Carbamazepine
Phenytoin
Primidone
Valproic acid

GENERAL INFORMATION ON BENZODIAZEPINES

The benzodiazepines are a group of structurally related chemicals that cause CNS depression. This class of compounds is believed to act on the limbic and subcortical levels of the central nervous system, producing varying degrees of sedation, skeletal muscle relaxation, and anticonvulsant activity. See specific agents for therapeutic use.

Special remarks and cautions

The more common side effects of benzodiazepines are extensions of their pharmacologic properties. Drowsiness, fatigue, lethargy, and ataxia are relatively common, dose-related, adverse effects of this class of agents.

Paradoxic reactions occasionally occur within the first few weeks of therapy. These reactions are manifested by increased anxiety, hyperexcitation, hallucinations, acute rage, and insomnia.

Physical and psychologic dependence is relatively rare, but may occur on discontinuance after prolonged therapy with high dosages. Abrupt withdrawal may result in seizure activity and symptoms similar to barbiturate withdrawal. The symptoms may not appear for more than a week after discontinuance as a result of the long half-lives and conversion to active metabolites.

Benzodiazepines should be administered with caution to patients with a history of blood dyscrasias or hepatic or renal damage. Cases of agranulocytosis, jaundice, and elevated SGOT, SGPT, bilirubin, and alkaline phosphatase levels have been reported.

Drug interactions

Benzodiazepines may be potentiated by other CNS depressants such as phenothiazines, narcotics, barbiturates, antihistamines, and antidepressants.

CLONAZEPAM
(Clonopin)

AHFS 28:12; C-IV
CATEGORY Anticonvulsant

Action and use

Clonazepam is a benzodiazepine derivative used in the prophylactic treatment of myoclonic, akinetic, and petit mal variant (Lennox-Gastaut syndrome) seizures. It is the first PO benzodiazepine derivative available for anticonvulsant use in the United States. Its mechanism of action is unknown. Clonazepam may also be effective in the management of petit mal (absence) seizures refractory to succinimide therapy. Investigationally, clonazepam has shown variable degrees of success in psychomotor, focal, and grand mal seizures when other first-line therapy has failed. IV clonazepam has been effective in various types of status epilepticus.

Characteristics

Onset: 20 to 60 min. Peak levels: 1 to 2 hr. Duration: 6 to 8 hr in infants and children, 12 hr in adults. Half-life: 19 to 50 hr. Metabolism: liver to 5 inactive metabolites. Excretion: 50% to 70% in urine, 13% to 30% in feces, as metabolites.

Administration and dosage
Adult

PO   1. Initial—up to 1.5 mg/day divided into 3 doses. Increase the dosage in increments of 0.5 to 1 mg every 3 days until seizures are controlled or side effects prevail.
   2. Maintenance: individualized for each patient. The maximum recommended daily dosage is 20 mg.

Pediatric (to 10 years of age or 30 kg)

PO   1. Initial: 0.01 to 0.03 mg/kg/day, not to exceed 0.05 mg/kg/day. Administer in 2 or 3 divided doses.
   2. Maintenance: increase dosage by no more than 0.25 to 0.5 mg every third day until the daily maintenance dose of 0.1 to 0.2 mg/kg is achieved, seizures are controlled, or side effects are unacceptable. Divide the dosage into 3 equal doses if possible. If not, administer the largest dose at bedtime.

NOTE: Dosage should be reduced slowly, especially after long-term, high-dose therapy, to avoid precipitating seizures or status epilepticus.

Special remarks and cautions

Addition of clonazepam to a therapeutic regimen of other anticonvulsants may allow reduction in dosage of the other anticonvulsants; however, paradoxic increases in seizure activity have also been reported.

Patients may become refractory to clonazepam after months or years of therapy. In some cases, increased doses may be effective, if tolerated. Addition of other antiepileptic agents may also be required.

The most commonly occurring side effects are related to CNS depression. Drowsiness and ataxia are frequently seen, especially on initiation of therapy. They do dissipate to some extent with time. They may be enhanced by the concurrent use of other anticonvulsants with CNS depressant effects.

Behavioral disturbances such as aggressiveness, agitation, and hyperkinesis have been reported, especially in patients with preexisting brain damage, mental retardation, or psychiatric disturbances.

Respiratory hypersecretion, chest congestion, shortness of breath, increased salivation, and rhinorrhea may occur.

Numerous other neurologic side effects have been reported, including nystagmus, double vision, slurred speech, headache, tremor, and vertigo.

Various dermatologic and hematologic effects have also been reported. Periodic blood counts and liver function tests should be performed on patients receiving long-term clonazepam therapy.

Clonazepam therapy is not recommended for pregnant or nursing women. It crosses the placental barrier, and its relationship to birth defects is not fully known.

See General information on benzodiazepines (p. 215).

Drug interactions

Ethanol, narcotics, barbiturates, anticonvulsants, sedative-hypnotics, tranquilizers, phenothiazines, and tricyclic antidepressants may potentiate the CNS depressant effects of clonazepam.

DIAZEPAM
(Valium)

AHFS 28:16.08; C-IV
CATEGORY Tranquilizer, anticonvulsant

Action and use

Diazepam is a benzodiazepine derivative used in mild to moderate states of anxiety and tension. It may also be used as a tranquilizer for acute alcohol withdrawal syndrome.

Diazepam has beneficial tranquilizing and amnesic effects when administered parenterally for the relief of anxiety and tension prior to endoscopy, minor surgical procedures, and cardioversion of atrial fibrillation.

Diazepam is often effective in controlling grand mal, psychomotor, petit mal, and jacksonian seizures and in controlling status epilepticus.

Characteristics

Onset: immediate (IV), 15 to 30 min (IM), 30 to 60 min (PO). Peak plasma levels: 1 to 3 hr (PO). Protein binding: highly bound. Half-life: 1 to 2 days (parent compound and active metabolites). Metabolism: liver, active; Excretion: metabolites in urine and feces. Therapeutic level: 0.1 mg/100 ml to 0.25 mg/100 ml. Toxic level: 0.5 mg/100 ml to 2 mg/100 ml. Fatal level: 2 mg/100 ml. Dialysis: no, H.

Administration and dosage
Adult

PO—2 to 10 mg 2 to 4 times daily.

IM—Should be discouraged: it is painful, with erratic absorption.

IV—2 to 40 mg depending on use; added in small increments. Inject slowly, monitoring the patient's response. Take at least 1 min for each 5 mg (1 ml) given. A fine, white precipitate will develop when diazepam is added to other solutions, including dextrose 5% and saline solution. Administer as close to the venipuncture site as possible.

Pediatric

PO—0.12 to 0.8 mg/kg/24 hr divided into 3 or 4 doses.

IM—0.1 to 0.3 mg/kg repeated in 2 to 4 hr as needed.

NOTE: Diazepam is not recommended in infants less than 30 days of age. However, if seizure activity cannot be arrested with maximum dosages of phenobarbital, 0.1 to 0.8 mg/kg/24 hr may be used. Sodium benzoate, a preservative used in parenteral solutions of diazepam, has been associated with clinically significant displacement of bilirubin from protein-binding sites.

Special remarks and cautions

See General information on benzodiazepines (p. 215).

Overdosage may be manifested by somnolence, confusion, coma, and respiratory depression. Treatment consists of general physiologic supportive measures including maintenance of an airway and administration of oxygen. Methylphenidate (Ritalin) or caffeine may be effective against severe CNS or respiratory depression. Do not use barbiturates in patients who develop excitation after ingestion of diazepam.

Hypotension may occur, particularly on parenteral administration. Severe hypotensive effects may be reversed with levarterenol (Levophed) or metaraminol (Aramine).

Use with caution in pregnant women. Fetal blood levels are similar to those in maternal circulation. Small amounts are found in breast milk.

Drug interactions

When diazepam is used with a narcotic analgesic, the dosage of the narcotic should be reduced by at least one third and administered in small increments.

Rare cases have been reported where diazepam has inhibited the metabolism of phenytoin (Dilantin), resulting in increased serum levels of phenytoin and potential toxicity.

See General information on benzodiazepines (p. 215).

CARBAMAZEPINE
(Tegretol)

AHFS 28:12
CATEGORY Anticonvulsant

Action and use

Carbamazepine is an anticonvulsant structurally related to the tricyclic antidepressants. Its mechanism for antiepileptic activity appears to be similar to that of the hydantoin derivatives (Dilantin); it elevates the convulsive threshold and limits the spread of the seizure discharge from its focus. Carbamazepine has been found to be effective in the prophylactic treatment of psychomotor, grand mal, and mixed seizure patterns. It is not effective in the control of petit mal seizures. Carbamazepine has also been used to successfully treat the pain associated with trigeminal neuralgia (tic douloureaux).

Characteristics

Peak plasma levels: 2 to 4 hr. Protein binding: 75% to 90%; Half-life: 14 to 36 hr. Metabolism: liver to several metabolites, activity unknown. Excretion: less than 1% unchanged in the urine. Therapeutic plasma level: 0.3 mg/100 ml. Toxic plasma level: 0.8 mg/100 ml to 1 mg/100 ml. Dialysis: unknown.

Administration and dosage
Adult

PO 1. Initial: 200 mg 2 times daily. Add up to 200 mg daily as tolerated until the best response is attained. Daily dosages above 1200 mg are not recommended; however, 1600 mg daily may be required in certain instances.
2. Maintenance: adjust dosage to the minimum effective level, usually 800 to 1200 mg daily.

Pediatric
Ages 12 to 15

PO—As for adults; dosage should generally not exceed 1000 mg daily.

Ages 15 and older

PO—As for adults; dosage should generally not exceed 1200 mg daily.

NOTE: Serious and sometimes fatal blood dyscrasias have been reported following treatment with carbamazepine. Use of this drug is not recommended unless other antiepileptic agents have been found to be ineffective or produce unacceptable side effects.

Patients sensitive to the tricyclic antidepressants must not receive carbamazepine. If serious side effects should require abrupt discontinuance of carbamazepine therapy, patients must be observed closely for increased seizure activity.

Special remarks and cautions

Side effects often observed on initiation of therapy include dizziness, drowsiness, nausea, and vomiting. Reduction in dosage or gradual increases in dosage will help minimize these adverse effects.

As a result of serious adverse reactions the manufacturer recommends that the following baseline studies be repeated at regular intervals:
1. Complete blood count with differential, platelet, and reticulocyte counts; serum iron determinations
2. Liver function tests
3. Urinalysis, BUN, and serum creatinine
4. Ophthalmologic examination

Congestive heart failure, hypertension, hypotension, edema, and aggravation of coronary artery disease have been reported. Although not reported specifically with carbamazepine, arrhythmias and myocardial infarction have been reported with other tricyclic compounds.

Neurologic side effects include incoordination, nystagmus, visual hallucinations, and oculomotor and speech disturbances.

Dermatologic manifestations of alopecia, pruritus, rashes, skin pigmentation, urticaria, and aggravation of systemic lupus erythematosus have been reported.

Carbamazepine anticonvulsant therapy should only be used in pregnant women on a risk-versus-benefit basis. Carbamazepine crosses the placental barrier, and teratogenic abnormalities have been reported in laboratory animals. It is recommended that lactating women *not* nurse their infants. Carbamazepine does appear in breast milk.

Drug interactions

Carbamazepine causes hepatic microsomal enzyme induction. It may enhance the metabolism of other anticonvulsants (phenytoin [Dilantin], phenobarbital, and primidone [Mysoline]) used concurrently with carbamazepine. Monitoring changes in serum levels should help warn of possible increased seizure activity.

Warfarin (Coumadin) metabolism may be increased by enzyme induction from carbamazepine. Monitor the prothrombin time more closely while carbamazepine therapy is being started or stopped.

The clinical effectiveness of doxycycline (Vibramycin) may be reduced by enhanced metabolism caused by carbamazepine.

MAO therapy should be discontinued at least 1 week before initiating carbamazepine therapy.

PHENYTOIN
(Dilantin)

AHFS 28:12
CATEGORY Anticonvulsant

Action and use

Phenytoin may be effective in the treatment of epilepsy. It appears to stabilize the normal seizure threshold and prevent the spread of seizure activity. It does not abolish the primary focus of seizure discharges. It is indicated for the control of grand mal and psychomotor seizures.

Characteristics

Onset: 1 to 2 hr following an IV loading dose of 1 to 1.5 g, 2 to 24 hr following a PO loading dose of 1 g. Protein binding: 95%. Half-life: 18 to 24 hr. Metabolism: liver to inactive metabolits. Excretion: 1% unchanged in urine, 75% in urine as metabolites. Therapeutic levels: 7.5 to 20 µg/ml. Toxic level: 10 to 50 µg/ml. Dialysis: yes, H.

Administration and dosage
Adult

PO—Initial: 100 mg 3 times daily. For most adults the daily maintenance dosage is 100 to 400 mg.

IM—Avoid if at all possible: the dosage is painful and quite erratically absorbed.

IV—Status epilepticus: 750 to 100 mg at *a rate no faster than 50 mg/min,* with monitoring of the ECG and pulse rate.

Pediatric

PO—Initial: 5 to 7 mg/kg/24 hr in 1 or 2 doses.

IM—Avoid if at all possible; the dosage is painful and quite erratically absorbed.

IV—Status epilepticus: 15 to 20 mg/kg at *a rate no faster than 50 mg/min,* with monitoring of the ECG and pulse rate. Maintain response with 5 to 8 mg/kg/day in 1 or 2 divided doses.

NOTE: If given too rapidly by the IV route, bradycardia and severe hypotension may result. The diluent, propylene glycol, will also potentiate the hypotensive effect of phenytoin and cause ECG changes. Cardiac and respiratory arrest may occur with excessive dosage and rate of administration. Blood pressure and the ECG should be monitored carefully, especially during administration.

Phenytoin should not be mixed with any drugs or added to any IV infusion solutions. The solubility is very pH dependent, and use with other medications or solutions will result in a white precipitate.

Each IV injection should be followed by an injection of sterile saline solution through the same needle or IV catheter to avoid local venous irritation.

Special remarks and cautions

Frequent side effects include nystagmus, ataxia, slurred speech, and mental confusion. Dizziness, insomnia, and transient nervousness may also occur. These side effects are usually dose related and disappear at reduced dosage levels.

Phenytoin may elevate blood glucose levels, especially if larger doses are used. Patients with diabetes mellitus or renal insufficiency may be more susceptible to hyperglycemia.

Fatal dermatologic manifestatons sometimes accompanied by fever, blood dyscrasias, toxic hepatitis, and liver damage have been attributed to phenytoin.

Gingival hyperplasia occurs frequently, but the incidence may be reduced by good oral hygiene including gum massage, frequent brushing, and proper dental care.

There have been reports suggesting a correlation between birth defects and the administration of anticonvulsant drugs. Use of phenytoin must on a risk-versus-benefit basis.

Drug interactions

Barbiturates may enhance the rate of metabolism of phenytoin.

Warfarin (Coumadin), disulfiram (Antabuse), phenylbutazone (Butazolidin), chloramphenicol (Chloromycetin), and isoniazid (INH) inhibit the metabolism of phenytoin, resulting in signs of phenytoin toxicity (nystagmus, ataxia, lethargy, and confusion).

Complex relationships exist between folic acid, phenytoin, and anticonvulsant activity. Phenytoin may induce folic acid defieiency, while folic acid replacement may result in partial loss of seizure control.

Phenytoin stimulates microsomal enzyme activity that enhances the metabolism of corticosteroids.

PRIMIDONE
(Mysoline)

Action and use

Primidone is an anticonvulsant structurally related to phenobarbital. It has anticonvulsant properties of its own, but is also metabolized to phenobarbital and phenyethylmalonamied (PEMA), both of which are also active anticonvulsants. Primidone is a useful adjunct to the treatment of several types of seizures; some clinicians consider it the drug of choice for psychomotor seizures. It is also effective in the prophylactic control of grand mal and focal epileptic seizures, and is often used in combination with phenytoin (Dilantin) therapy.

Characteristics

Peak serum levels: 3 to 4 hr (PO). Protein binding: insignificant. Metabolism: to phenobarbital, PEMA (active). Half-life: primidone, 3 to 24 hr; PEMA, 24 to 48 hr; phenobarbital, 48 to 120 hr. With chronic administration, patients may accumulate high serum levels of phenobarbital. Excretion of primidone: 15% to 25% unchanged in urine, 15% to 25% metabolized to phenobarbital, 50% to 70% excreted in urine as PEMA. Therapeutic serum level: of primidone, 1 mg/100 ml to 2 mg/100 ml; of phenobarbital, 1 mg/100 ml to 2.5 mg/100 ml. Toxic level of primidone: 5 mg/100 ml to 8 mg/100 ml. Dialysis of primidone: yes, H, P.

Administration and dosage
Adult

PO—Initial: 250 mg daily, with incremental increases of 250 mg at weekly intervals to tolerance or therapeutic effectiveness. The average adult dose is 0.75 to 1.5 g/day. Maximum daily doses should not exceed 2 g.

Pediatric
Under 8 years of age

PO—Initial: 125 mg daily, with incremental increases of 125 mg at weekly intervals to tolerance or therapeutic effectiveness. The average pediatric dosage is 500 to 750 mg/day.

Over 8 years of age

PO—As for adult dosages.

Special remarks and cautions

Common adverse effects include sedation, drowsiness, dizziness, ataxia, diplopia, and nystagmus. These symptoms tend to disappear with continued therapy and possible readjustment of dosage.

Primidone has been reported to produce paradoxic hyperexcitability in children (as does phenobarbital).

Severe adverse effects such as maculopapular and morbilliform rash, leukopenia, thrombocytopenia, megaloblastic anemia, and systemic lupus erythermatosus are rare occurrences, but have been reported. A complete blood count is recommended every 6 months during prolonged therapy.

Neonatal hemorrhage has been reported in newborns whose mothers were taking primidone. It is recommended that pregnant women under anticonvulsant therapy should receive prophylactic phytonadione (Mephyton) therapy for 1 month prior to and during delivery. Primidone also appears in breast milk in substantial quantities and may result in somnolence and drowsiness in nursing newborns.

Drug interactions

Phenytoin (Dilantin) appears to increase the phenobarbital serum levels when taken concurrently with primidone. This may be beneficial in the control of epilepsy, but patients must also be observed for increased signs of sedation and lethargy caused by high phenobarbital levels.

VALPROIC ACID
(Depakene)

AHFS 28:12
CATEGORY Anticonvulsant

Action and use

Valproic acid is an anticonvulsant chemically unrelated to other agents used to treat seizure disorders. Its mechanism of action is unknown. Valproic acid is most effective, either alone or in combination with other anticonvulsants, in the management of simple and complex absence (petit mal) seizures.

Characteristics

Peak serum levels: 1 to 4 hr (PO). Protein binding: 90%. Half-life: 8 to 12 hr. Metabolism: liver to inactive metabolites. Excretion: primarily in urine, small amounts in feces and via lungs; Therapeutic levels: 50 to 100 μg/ml (estimated). Dialysis: unknown.

Administration and dosage
Adult and pediatric

PO—Initial: 5 mg/kg every 8 hr. The dosage may be increased by 5 to 10 mg/kg/day at weekly intervals, depending on patient response. The maximum recommended daily dosage is 30 mg/kg/day. Between 2 and 4 weeks are required to fully assess the effectiveness of therapy.

NOTE: Valproic acid may be given with food or milk to minimize gastric irritation.

Special remarks and cautions

Gastric irritation resulting in nausea, vomiting, and indigestion is a common side effect on initiation of valproic acid therapy. Gradual increases in therapy or dosage reduction usually controls gastrointestinal discomfort.

Sedative effects have been reported, particularly when valproic acid is used in conjunction with other anticonvulsant therapy. Atoxia, dizziness, diplopia, nystagmus, "spots before eyes," and headache have occasionally been reported. These side effects are usually dose related and disappear when the dosage of valproic acid or other anticonvulsant therapy is reduced. Patients should also be warned against engaging in activities requiring mental alertness.

As a result of rare reports of impaired platelet aggregation, thrombocytopenia, and elevated liver enzymes, the manufacturer recommends that the following baseline studies be completed before therapy is initiated and at regular intervals thereafter:

1. Liver function tests
2. Bleeding time determination
3. Platelet count

One of the metabolites of valproic acid is a ketone-containing derivative. It is excreted in the urine and may produce a false-positive test (Ketostix, Acetest) for urine ketones.

Valproic acid anticonvulsant therapy should only be used in pregnant women on a risk-versus-benefit basis. Valproic acid crosses the placental barrier, and teratogenic abnormalities have been reported in laboratory animals. It is recommended that lactating women *not* nurse their infants. Valproic acid does appear in breast milk.

Drug interactions

Ethanol, narcotics, barbiturates, anticonvulsants, sedative-hypnotics, tranquilizers, phenothiazines, and tricyclic antidepressants may enhance the CNS depressant effects of valproic acid.

Valproic acid may increase serum phenobarbital levels and may increase or decrease phenytoin (Dilantin) serum levels. Serum phenobarbital and phenytoin levels should be determined periodically, and dosages should be adjusted if necessary.

Absence status (continuous absence seizure activity) has been induced when the benzodiazepine-derivative anticonvulsant clonazepam was used concomitantly with valproic acid.

Coagulation studies should be monitored closely when valproic acid is prescribed for concurrent use with medications such as warfarin (Coumadin), sulfinpyrazone (Anturane), and aspirin.

Antiemetic agents

Benzquinamide
Cyclizine
Trimethobenzamide

BENZQUINAMIDE
(Emete-Con)

AHFS 56:20
CATEGORY Antiemetic

Action and use

Benzquinamide is structurally unrelated to other phenothiazine or antihistaminic antiemetics. Its mechanism of action in humans is unknown, but is believed to involve suppression of the chemoreceptor trigger zone in the medulla oblongata.

Characteristics

Onset: antiemetic 15 min (IM or IV). Peak blood levels: 30 min (IM). Duration of action: 3 to 4 hr. Protein binding: 55% to 60%. Half-life: 30 to 40 min. Metabolism: liver. Excretion: 3% to 10% unchanged in urine, metabolites in feces and urine. Dialysis: no, H, P.

Administration and dosage

Reconstitute benzquinamide 50 mg/vial with 2.2 ml of sterile water or bacteriostatic water for injection to yield a solution containing 25 mg benzquinamide/ml. Do not reconstitute with 0.9% sodium chloride injection because precipitation may result. Potency is maintained for 14 days at room temperature. *Do not refrigerate.*

IM—50 mg or 0.5 to 1 mg/kg by deep IM injection in a large muscle mass. May repeat in 1 hr, with subsequent doses every 3 to 4 hr.

IV—25 mg or 0.2 to 0.4 mg/kg. Subsequent doses should be given IM.

NOTE: Sudden increase in blood pressure and transient cardiac arrhythmias (premature atrial and ventricular contractions) have been reported following IV use. Use with extreme caution in patients with heart disease or those patients receiving preanesthetic or cardiovascular agents.

NOTE: Safe use in children has not been established.

Special remarks and cautions

Drowsiness and sedation appear to be the most commonly observed side effects of benzquinamide. Others include dry mouth, blurred vision, hypertension, hypotension, dizziness, and arrhythmias. Hypersensitivity reactions, nausea, vomiting, tremor, weakness, and abdominal cramps have also been reported.

Antiemetics may obscure signs of overdosage of other drugs or of symptoms of such conditions as appendicitis, intestinal obstruction, or brain tumor.

Other measures to enhance the antiemetic effect include frequent small amounts of dry carbohydrate feedings when allowed by the patient's diet, avoidance of high-fat foods, and antacids. Decrease noxious stimuli in the environment such as odors, smoke, unpleasant sounds, drainage, and waste products. Good oral hygiene is frequently overlooked after emesis.

Be aware of excessive vomiting, and observe for deficiencies in fluids, electrolytes, and nutrients. See Indications of fluid and electrolyte imbalance (p. 130).

No teratogenic effects have yet been reported, but use in pregnancy is not recommended. It is not known whether benzquinamide crosses the placental barrier or appears in breast milk.

Drug interactions

None have been specifically reported; however, additive anticholinergic, antihistaminic, and sedative effects may be expected with other drugs with similar properties.

CYCLIZINE
(Marezine)

AHFS 56:20
CATEGORY Antihistamine, antinauseant

Action and use

Cyclizine is a short-acting antihistaminic agent with CNS depressant, anticholinergic, and antiemetic properties. It is used in the prophylaxis and treatment of the nausea, vomiting, and dizziness of motion sickness and vestibular disease.

Characteristics

Duration of action: 4 to 6 hr. Dialysis: unknown.

Administration and dosage
Adult

PO 1. Motion sickness: 50 mg 30 min before departure; may be repeated every 4 to 6 hr as needed. Do not exceed 4 tablets daily.
2. Vertigo: 50 mg 3 to 4 times daily.
IM—As for PO administration.
RECTAL—100 mg suppository every 4 to 6 hr.
NOTE: Cyclizine is not recommended for the nausea and vomiting of pregnancy. Teratogenic effects have been observed in laboratory animals.

Pediatric
Under 6 years of age

PO AND RECTAL—One fourth the adult dosages.

Between 6 and 12 years of age

PO AND RECTAL—Half the adult dosages.

Special remarks and cautions

A common side effect of cyclizine is drowsiness. Patients must be warned about performing tasks requiring mental alertness and coordination.

Other side effects may include blurred vision, dry mouth, constipation, and fatigue.

Drug interactions

Cyclizine may display additive anticholinergic side effects (dry mouth, constipation, and blurred vision) when administered with other antihistamines, phenothiazines, trihexyphenidyl (Artane), benztropine (Cogentin), and other agents with anticholinergic activity.

TRIMETHOBENZAMIDE
(Tigan)

AHFS 56:20
CATEGORY Antiemetic

Action and use

Trimethobenzamide is a nonphenothiazine antiemetic structurally related to diphenhydramine-like antihistamines. It is believed to control nausea and vomiting by suppression of the chemoreceptor trigger zone in the medulla oblongata through which impulses pass to the vomiting center.

Characteristics

Onset: 10 to 40 min (PO), 15 to 30 min (IM). Duration: 2 to 3 hr (IM), 4 to 6 hr (PO). Metabolism: liver. Excretion: 30% to 50% unchanged in urine within 48 to 72 hr, metabolites in urine and feces. Therapeutic level: 0.1 to 0.2 mg/100 ml.

Administration and dosage
Adult

PO—250 mg 2 to 4 times daily.
IM—200 mg 3 to 4 times daily.
IV—Not recommended.
RECTAL—200 mg 3 to 4 times daily.
NOTE: The suppository form contains benzocaine. It should not be administered to patients known to be sensitive to local anesthetics.

Pediatric

NOTE: Trimethobenzamide should be used with caution when administered to children. There has been some suspicion that centrally acting antiemetics, in combination with viral illnesses, may contribute to the development of Reye's syndrome, a potentially fatal acute childhood disease. Administration of antiemetics is not recommended until the cause of vomiting can be determined.

Under 13.5 kg

RECTAL—½ suppository (100 mg) 3 or 4 times daily.

Between 13.5 and 40.5 kg

PO—100 to 200 mg 3 or 4 times daily.
RECTAL—½ to 1 suppository (100 to 200 mg) 3 or 4 times daily.
NOTE: Do not administer suppositories to premature or newborn infants.
NOTE: IM administration is not recommended for use in children.

Special remarks and cautions

CNS reactions (opisthotonos, convulsions, coma, and extrapyramidal symptoms) may occur with and without the use of antiemetics during the course of acute febrile illness, encephalopathies, gastroenteritis, dehydration, and electrolyte imbalance. Trimethobenzamide should be used with caution especially in patients who have recently received other CNS-acting agents such as phenothiazines, barbiturates, and belladonna derivatives.

Drowsiness, dizziness, and hypotension may occur. Patients should be warned about performing hazardous tasks requiring mental alertness or physical coordination.

Antiemetics may obscure signs of overdosage of other drugs or of symptoms of such conditions as appendicitis, intestinal obstruction, or brain tumor.

Blood dyscrasias, blurring of vision, coma, convulsions, depression of mood, diarrhea, disorientation, jaundice, msucle cramps, and exacerbation of preexisting nausea have also been reported.

Safety in pregnancy and in nursing mothers has not been established. Teratogenic effects have been noted in animal studies.

Drug interactions

None have been specifically reported; however, additive anticholinergic, antihistaminic, and sedative effects may be expected with other drugs with similar properties.

Antidiabetic agents

General information on diabetes mellitus
General information on insulins
General information on sulfonylureas

GENERAL INFORMATION ON DIABETES MELLITUS

Diabetes mellitus is a chronic, progressive disease manifested by abnormalities in carbohydrate, protein, and fat metabolism resulting from a relative or absolute lack of insulin. As the altered states of metabolism progress, complications of the disease become evident. Premature vascular degeneration with coronary and peripheral atherosclerosis, retinopathies, and nephropathies develop. These patients have a much higher incidence of nerve degeneration (neuropathies), and the incidence of infections is markedly enhanced.

Diabetes is a common disease, appearing with increasing frequency as the population ages. In the United States approximately 4 million persons have diabetes. Of those 4 million, about 50% are unidentified. Undiagnosed diabetic adults with few or no symptoms present a major challenge to the health profession. Because early diabetic symptoms are minimal, the patient does not seek medical advice and indications of the disease are discovered only at the time of routine physical examination. Those persons with a predisposition to developing diabetes include (1) persons who have relatives with diabetes (2½ times greater incidence of developing the disease), (2) obese persons (85% of diabetic patients are overweight), and (3) older persons (4 out of 5 diabetics are over 45 years of age).

The American Diabetes Association has developed a classification based on the degree of abnormality in carbohydrate metabolism. The first stage is prediabetes. The patient has neither signs nor symptoms and may only be suspected as diabetic because of a strong familial history of the disease. Patients who usually have a normal glucose tolerance test curve but who, during pregnancy, infection, stress, or obesity develop an abnormal curve, are known as latent or stress diabetics. Chemical or asymptomatic diabetics have normal fasting blood sugars, but postprandial levels are usually elevated and the glucose tolerance curve is abnormal. Patients may have no frank symptoms of diabetes for years, or symptomatology may progress rapidly to the next stage of overt or clinical diabetes. At the clinical stage the patient displays hyperglycemia, glycosuria, and, possibly, ketoacidosis.

The overt diabetic stage is usually subclassified into two categories: juvenile onset and adult onset. The juvenile or growth onset form of the disease usually has a rapid progression of symptomatology characterized by polydipsia (increased thirst), polyphagia (increased appetite), and polyuria (increased urination), loss of weight and strength, irritability, and often ketoacidosis. These patients may be known as brittle diabetics, since the disease is often difficult to control. There is no insulin secretion from the pancreas, and obese patients are quite sensitive to the administration of exogenous insulin. Insulin dosage adjustment is easily influenced by inconsistent patterns of physical activity and dietary irregularities.

Adult onset or maturity diabetes usually has a much more insidious onset. The pancreas still maintains some capability to produce and secrete insulin. Consequently, symptoms are minimal or absent for quite some time. The patient may seek medical attention several years later only after symptoms of the complications of the disease have become apparent. Patients may complain of weight gain or loss. Blurred vision may be an indication of diabetic retinopathy. Neuropathies may be first observed as numbness or tingling of the extremities (paresthesia), loss of sensation, orthostatic hypotension, impotence, and difficulty in controlling urination (neurogenic bladder). An indication of chronic vascular disease may be nonhealing ulcers of the lower extremities.

Since a cure for diabetes mellitus is unknown at present, the minimal purpose of treatment is to prevent ketoacidosis and symptoms resulting from hyperglycemia. The lifelong objectives of control must involve mechanisms to stem the progression of the complications of the disease. Major determinants involve a balanced diet, insulin or oral hypoglycemic therapy, routine exercise, and good hygiene. Patient education and reinforcement are tantamount to successful therapy. The intelligence and motivation of the diabetic patient and an awareness of the potential complications contribute significantly to the ultimate outcome of the disease and the quality of life the patient may lead.

Control

Patients with diabetes can lead a full and satisfying life. However, free diets and unrestricted activities are not possible. Dietary treatment of diabetes constitutes the basis for management of most patients, especially those with the adult onset form of disease. With adequate weight reduction and dietary control, patients may not require the use of exogenous insulin or oral hypoglycemic drug therapy. Juvenile onset diabetics will always require exogenous insulin as well as dietary control because the pancreas has lost the capacity to produce and secrete insulin. The aims of dietary control are (1) the prevention of excessive postprandial hyperglycemia, (2) the prevention of hypoglycemia in those patients being treated with hypoglycemic agents or insulin, and (3) the achievement and maintenance of an ideal body weight. A return to normal weight is often accompanied by a reduction in hyperglycemia. The diet should also be adjusted to reduce elevated cholesterol and triglyceride levels in an attempt to retard the progression of atherosclerosis.

To help maintain adherence to dietary restrictions, the diet should be planned in relation to the patient's food preferences, economic status, occupation, and physical activity. Emphasis should be placed on what food the patient may have and what exchanges are acceptable. Food should be measured for balanced portions, and the patient should be cautioned not to omit meals or between-meal and bedtime snacks.

All diabetic patients must receive adequate instruction on personal hygiene, especially regarding care of the feet, skin, and teeth. Development of infection is a common precipitating cause of ketosis and acidosis and must be treated promptly.

Insulin is required in the control of juvenile onset diabetes and in those patients whose diabetes cannot be controlled by diet, weight reduction, or oral hypoglycemic agents. Patients normally controlled with oral hypoglycemic agents will require insulin during situations of increased physiologic and psychologic stress such as pregnancy, surgery, and infections. The dosage of insulin is usually adjusted according to the blood glucose levels and the degree of glucosuria. The patient should test the urine before each meal and at bedtime while the insulin is being regulated. See General information on insulins (pp. 233 to 239) for types and dosages of insulin, monitoring guidelines, and other medications that may cause hyperglycemia or hypoglycemia.

Another adjunct in the therapy of maturity onset diabetes is the use of oral hypoglycemic agents. They are recommended only in those patients who cannot be controlled by diet alone and who are not prone to develop ketosis, acidosis, and/or infections. Patients most likely to benefit from treatment are those who have developed diabetes after 40 years of age and who require less than 40 units of insulin/day. See General information on sulfonylureas (pp. 240 and 241).

GENERAL INFORMATION ON INSULINS   AHFS 68:20.08

Insulin is a hormone produced in the beta cells of the pancreas and is a key regulator of metabolism. The protein molecule is composed of 51 amino acids divided into two chains. Insulins of various animal species have similar biologic activity and differ only in the sequence of one to three amino acids on one of the chains. Factors that promote the secretion of insulin are increased blood levels of glucose, various amino acids, ketone bodies, glucagon, sulfonylureas, gastrin, secretin, beta-receptor stimulants such as isoproterenol (Isuprel) and alpha-receptor blockers such as phentolamine (Regitine). Alpha-receptor stimulants—norepinephrine (Levophed), epinephrine (Adrenalin), and diazoxide (Hyperstat)—may inhibit the release of insulin.

Insulin promotes the entry of glucose into skeletal and heart muscle and fat and plays a significant role in protein and lipid metabolism. It is not required for glucose transport into brain or liver tissue. A deficiency of insulin, known as diabetes mellitus, results in cellular deprivation of essential nutrients.

Several preparations of insulin isolated from beef and pork pancreas are commercially available. Various extracton procedures, as well as the addition of various proteins, modify the onset, peak, and duration of activity. In 1972 the American Diabetes Association recommended the elimination of production of the U-40 and U-80 insulins. The replacement with the U-100 dosage form for all types of insulin will help reduce the chance of patient error in using multiple dosage forms and dually calibrated syringes. U-500 regular insulin (pork) is also available for those patients developing resistance to insulin.

Regular insulin

Insulin precipitated from solution in the amorphous (noncrystalline) form (Insulin Injection, USP) or insulin prepared by precipitation with zinc chloride in the crystalline form (Insulin Injection, USP. "Insulin made from zinc-insulin crystals") may have either an acidic or neutral pH. As a result of improved manufacturing technology, regular insulin is now being produced at a neutral pH by most manufacturers. This allows a more stable product, both in terms of shelf-life without refrigeration and in mixing with other insulins, although there is no clinical difference between neutral and acid regular insulins. Neutral regular insulin (NRI) retains its potency at room temperature for at least 1 year and may be premixed with NPH or Lente up to 2 to 3 months before use. In contrast, acid (pH = 2.8 to 3.5) regular insulin (ARI) must be refrigerated and has mixing restrictions (Table 13-2). See Table 13-1 for the activity of the regular insulins.

Protamine zinc insulin (PZI)

Insulin precipitated with zinc in the presence of a protein, protamine, produces protamine zinc insulin. PZI is poorly soluble and absorbed slowly when injected in subcutaneous tissue. See Table 13-1 for the activity of protamine zinc insulin.

Globin zinc insulin

Insulin precipitated with zinc and another protein, globin, produces globin zinc insulin.

Neutral-protamine-hagedorn (NPH) insulin

NPH insulin is an intermediate-acting insulin containing specific amounts of insulin and protamine so that the crystals formed leave behind no protamine or insulin. The activity of NPH is similar to that of a mixture of regular insulin and protamine zinc insulin (Tables 13-1 and 13-2).

Table 13-1. Commercially available forms of insulin

Type of insulin	Onset* (hours)	Peak* (hours)	Duration* (hours)	Protein	pH†	Appearance	Shape of bottle	Glycosuria‡	Hypoglycemia‡
Fast-acting									
Insulin injection USP (regular insulin)	½-1	3-6	5-8	None	A or N	Clear	Round	Early AM[1]	Before lunch[3]
Prompt insulin zinc suspension USP (Semilente)	½-1	4-6	12-16	None	A or N	Opaque	Hexagonal	Early AM[1]	Before lunch[3]
Intermediate-acting									
Globin zinc insulin injection USP	1-4	6-8	16-18	Globin	A	Clear	Round	Before breakfast and lunch[2]	3 PM to supper[3]
Insulin zinc suspension USP (Lente)	1-2	8-12	24-28	None	N	Opaque	Hexagonal	Before lunch[2]	3 PM to supper[3]
Isophane insulin suspension USP (NPH)	1-2	8-12	24-28	Protamine	N	Opaque	Square	Before lunch[2]	3 PM to supper[3]
Long-acting									
Extended insulin zinc suspension USP (Ultralente)	4-8	16-18	36+	None	N	Opaque	Hexagonal	Before lunch and bedtime[2]	2 AM to breakfast[3]
Protamine zinc insulin (PZI) suspension USP	1-8	16-24	36+	Protamine	N	Opaque	Round	—	2 AM to breakfast[3]

*The times listed are averages based on a newly diagnosed diabetic patient. Factors modifying these times include patient variation, site and route of administration, and dosage.

†N, neutral; A, acid.

‡Most frequently occurs when insulin is administered at (1) bedtime the previous night, (2) before breakfast the previous day, (3) before breakfast the same day.

Table 13-2. Compatibility of insulin combinations

Combination	Ratio	Mix prior to administration
NRI* + NPH	Any combination	2 to 3 months
NRI + Lente	Any combination	2 to 3 months
ARI† + NPH	Any combination	Immediately
ARI + Lente	No greater than 1:1§	Immediately
ARI or NRI + PZI‡	1:1 = action like PZI alone	Immediately
	2:1 = action like NPH	Immediately
	3:1 = action like NPH + ARI or NRI	Immediately
Lentes	Any combination	Stable indefinitely

*NRI = Neutral regular insulin
†ARI = Acid regular insulin
‡PZI contains excess protamine that binds with regular insulin prolonging the activity of the regular insulin.
§If the amount of ARI exceeds that of Lente, incompatibilities result in an unpredictable duration of action.

Lente insulins

Another manufacturing process using much higher concentrations of zinc and an acetate buffer (phosphate buffers are used with insulins containing protamine) produces two physical forms, one crystalline and the other amorphous, at a neutral pH. The long-acting crystalline form is marketed as Ultralente and the amorphous fast-acting compound is available as Semilente. The intermediate-acting Lente insulin is a mixture containing approximately 30% Semilente and 70% crystalline Ultralente insulin.

See Table 13-1 for a comparison of the properties of available forms of insulin and Table 13-2 for the compatibility of insulin mixtures.

Characteristics

Onset, peak activity, duration: see Table 13-1. Plasma half-life: less than 9 min. Metabolism: 40% liver, 40% kidney. Excretion: less than 10% unchanged in urine. Dialysis: unknown.

Administration and dosage
Adult

For ketoacidosis:

SC AND IV—Initially, 50 to 100 units of regular insulin SC and 50 to 100 units IV. Follow with doses of 50 to 100 units every 2 to 4 hr until the blood glucose level falls to 250 mg/100 mg. The total dose of insulin required generally ranges between 200 and 400 units. Maintain the patient on regular insulin every 4 to 6 hr as needed, then start intermediate-acting insulin the next morning if the patient is doing well.*

IM—Initially, 10 to 20 units of regular insulin, followed by 5 to 10 units hourly until the blood glucose is 150 to 300 mg/100 ml.†

IV—2 to 12 units of regular insulin/hr. (Addition of 50 units regular insulin to 500 ml one-half saline solution administered at a rate of 1 ml/min provides an insulin dose of 6 units/hr.) Various studies indicate a 20% to 33% loss of insulin po-

*N. Eng. J. Med. **290:**1360, 1974.
†Lancet **2:**515, 1973.

tency caused by adsorption of insulin to the bottle and tubing. The addition of 3.5 mg of human serum albumin/ml of solution (7 ml of 25% albumin/500 ml of solution) has been found to prevent clinically significant absorption.*

NOTE: Only regular insulin may be injected IV. All other forms are suspensions and are contraindicated for IV use. All the above methods may be successful in treating ketoacidosis. Hourly observations of the patient's fluids, electrolytes (especially potassium), blood sugar, ketone levels, and arterial blood gases are essential to the proper treatment of ketoacidosis.

For maintenance therapy:

1. Newly diagnosed diabetic patients: after ketoacidosis and hyperglycemia have been controlled and the patient can tolerate oral feedings, determine the total amount of regular insulin needed in 24 hr. The usual initial dose in the nonketotic patient is 10 to 20 units of regular insulin SC. Subsequent doses administered ½ hr before meals and at bedtime are based on the blood glucose and urine glucose levels. After control is established, the patient is converted to intermediate-acting insulin administered in a dose 65% to 75% of the total dose of regular insulin required in 24 hr. Regular insulin is used as a supplement based on urine glucose levels. Adjustments in the intermediate-acting insulin will be necessary. Divided doses (two thirds in the morning, one third in the evening) or combination therapy using a mixture of insulin (see Table 13-2) may be required to maintain control, especially after the patient leaves the hsopital and has changes in exercise and diet.
2. Known diabetic patients: once ketoacidosis and hyperglycemia have been controlled and the patient can tolerate oral feedings, initiate maintenance therapy at one half to two thirds their previous dose of intermediate-acting or combination insulin. Supplemental regular insulin is given when indicated by blood sugar and urine glucose determinations. Adjust maintenance insulin until optimal control for the patient is achieved.

NOTE: "Control" of the hyperglycemia of diabetes in the hospital is usually easier than on an outpatient basis. Adjustments are almost always necessary after dismissal as a result of changes in exercise and diet. Some physicians will allow their patients to spill a 2+ to 3+ urine glucose while in the hospital so that after discharge a patient will spill a trace to 1+ as a result of change in routine. Other physicians will stabilize a patient to a trace to 1+ urine glucose while in the hospital and drop the insulin dosage 5 units on discharge. There is less change of a hypoglycemic reaction when using the second method, but regardless of which treatment program is used the discharged patient will have to be monitored frequently for medical and emotional adjustment to the new disease.

Special remarks and cautions

Insulin overdosage or decreased carbohydrate intake may result in hypoglycemia. Early symptoms may include nausea, hunger, headache, irritability, lethargy, ataxia, and mental confusion. The patient may also experience tremor, sweating and tachycardia. Severe hypoglycemia may result in convulsions and coma. If untreated, irreversible brain damage may occur. Hypoglycemia occurs most frequently when the administered insulin reaches its peak action. Hypoglycemia must be treated immediately. Mild symptomatology may be controlled by the oral administration of lump sugar, orange juice, carbonated cola beverages, or candy. Severe symptoms may be relieved by the administration of 5 to 25 g of dextrose (10 to 50 ml of dextrose 50%). The following conditions may predispose a diabetic patient to a hypoglycemic (insulin) reaction: improper measurement of insulin dosage, excessive exercise, insufficient food intake, concurrent ingestion of hypoglycemic drugs and discontinu-

_____
*Br. Med. J. **2:**687, 691, 694, 1974.

ance of drugs (see Drug interactions, p. 239), or conditions (infection, stress) causing hyperglycemia.

Allergic reactions manifested by itching, redness, and swelling at the site of injection are common occurrences in patients beginning insulin therapy. These reactions may be caused by modifying proteins in globin, NPH, or PZI insulin; the insulin itself (exogenous insulin amino acid content varies slightly from human insulin); the alcohol used to cleanse the injection site or sterilize the syringe; the patient's injection technique; or the intermittent use of insulin. Spontaneous desensitization frequently occurs within a few weeks, but changing to insulin without protein modifiers (the Lente series) or to insulins derived from another animal source, use of unscented alcohol swabs or disposable syringes and needles, and checking the patient's injection technique (inject at an angle, not perpendicularly) may reduce local irritation. Acute, whole body rashes and anaphylactic symptoms must be treated with antihistamines, epinephrine, and steroids. The animal source of the insulin should then be changed.

Rotation of injection sites is important. Atrophy or hypertrophy of subcutaneous fat tissue may occur at the site of frequent insulin injections. The hypertrophic areas tend to be used more frequently by diabetic patients because the fat pad becomes anesthetic. In addition to the adverse cosmetic effects, the absorption of insulin from these sites becomes significantly prolonged and erratic. Loss of diabetic control may result, particularly in brittle juvenile diabetes.

Insulin resistance is an infrequent complication in the control of diabetic symptoms. Acute resistance may develop if the patient acquires an infection or experiences serious trauma, surgery, or emotional disturbances. This type of resistance subsides with regression of the acute episode. Chronic insulin resistance may occur with the reinstitution of insulin therapy after a period of discontinuance. Resistance may be reduced by changing the animal source of the insulin, changing the use of glucocorticoids, or using specially prepared deal-anated or sulfated insulins.

Teaching the newly diagnosed diabetic patient to test for sugar content in the urine is essential for symptom-free control of the desease. A detailed discussion of the various products available for testing for glucosuria is beyond the scope of this chapter; however, there are a few points that should be mentioned.

1. Each method uses a different colorimetric system. Consequently, the " + " values for urine sugar concentration vary between products (Table 13-3). Note that a ½% urine glucose measures a 1 + using Clinitest, a 2 + using Diastix and Keto-Diastix, and a 3 + using Tes-Tape.

2. The patient should use a double-voided urine specimen, especially for the early morning determination. The second void provides a more accurate estimation of the urine glucose content at that time. It prevents the testing of glucose that may have accumulated over the last several hours.

3. When using Clinitest the patient should watch the reaction to see if the bright orange "pass through" phenomenon occurs. This is caused by a urine glucose

Table 13-3. A comparison of the values of urine glucose tests

| | | Percent | | | | | |
	Negative	1/10	1/4	1/2	3/4	1	2
Clinitest (5-drop method)	0		Trace	1 +	2 +	3 +	4 +
Diastix or Keto-Diastix	0	Trace	1 +	2 +		3 +	4 +
Tes-Tape	0	1 +	2 +	3 +			4 +

concentration of greater than 2%. If the patient is not observant, the final color will be misrecorded as a 2 + or 3 +. It is also important to read the results 15 sec after the boiling ceases. The color may begin to fade leading to a misinterpretation of the results.

4. Urine testing products should be stored properly. They are sensitive to temperature light, and humidity. If subpotency is suspected, the products can be tested by using Coca-Cola. A 4 + reading should result.

5. Clinitest tablets are poisonous and must not be taken internally. Treat ingestion with vinegar or lemon, grapefruit, or orange juice in large quantities. Follow with olive or mineral oil. The tablets should be handled by using the lid of the container.

6. Several drugs interfere with glucose urine testing products. See Table 13-4 for the false values that may occur. A "false positive" does not mean the results will automatically be a 4 +. The drug may induce small changes such as a 1 + registering as a 2 +. The opposite may occur with those drugs inducing false-negative values; a 3 + may be read as a 2 + or a 1 +. It may not record as a negative. These slight changes become significant to those patients who adjust their insulin dosages according to the glucose content in the urine (those using the "sliding" or "rainbow" scale).

A diabetic person whose urine glucose concentration is 4 + (2% or more) should also test the urine for ketones. If a patient has symptoms indicating ketoacidosis, but the results of Acetest tablets of Ketostix indicates no urine ketones, the patient should be observed carefully anyway, because these in vitro tests measure only acetone and acetoacetic acid. Beta-hydroxybutyric acid is not measured, although it is the major ketone responsible for ketoacidosis. Levodopa (Dopar) and phenazopyridine (Pyridium) may cause false-positive Labstix and Ketostix results. Paraldehyde may cause false-positive Acetest results. Ether anesthesia and overdoses of isopropyl alcohol, isoniazid, and insulin (or decreased carbohydrate intake) lead to true elevations of urine ketone levels.

Table 13-4. Drugs that may alter urine glucose determinations as a result of interference with the test procedure*

Drug	Clinitest	Tes-Tape, Diastix
Ascorbic acid (large doses)	False +	False −
Aminosalicyclic acid (PAS)	False +	
Azo Gantrisin (see Phenazopyridine)		
Cephalothin (Keflin)	False +	
Chloral hydrate (large doses)	False +	
Chloramphenicol (Chloromycetin)	False +	
Isoniazid (INH)	False +	
Ketones		False −
Levodopa, L-dopa (Dopar)	False +	False −
Metaxalone (Skelaxin)	False +	False −
Methyldopa (Aldomet) (2 g/day)	False +	False −
Nalidixic acid (NegGram)	False +	
Penicillin (large doses)	False +	
Phenazopyridine (Pyridium)		False + or −
Probenecid (Benemid)	False +	
Salicylates (40 to 90 grains/day)†	False +	False −
Sulfonamides	False +	
Tetracyclines	False +	

*From Hansten, P. D.: Drug interactions, ed. 3, Philadelphia, 1975, Lea & Febiger.
†8 to 18 325 mg tablets/day.

Pregnant diabetic women must be observed closely for changing insulin requirements. Insulin dosages increase especially in the last trimester of pregnancy. Following delivery, insulin requirements rapidly fall to prepregnancy levels.

Drug interactions

The following drugs may cause hyperglycemia, especially in prediabetic and diabetic patients. Insulin dosages may require adjustment.

Ethanol	Phenothiazines
Corticosteroids	Dextrothyroxine (Choloxin)
Epinephrine	Diazoxide (Hyperstat)
Oral contraceptives	Phenytoin (Dilantin)
Glucagon	Diuretics (thiazides, chlorthalidone)
Acetazolamide (Diamox)	Lithium carbonate
Salicylates	

The following drugs may cause hypoglycemia, decreasing insulin requirements in diabetic patients.

Ethanol	Salicylates
Anabolic steroids (Dianabol, Durabolin)	Acetaminophen (Tylenol)
Guanethidine sulfate (Ismelin)	Propranolol (Inderal)
Mono-amine oxidase inhibitors	

Although the mechanism is unknown, propanolol may produce hypoglycemia, especially in diabetic patients. The reaction may be particularly serious because propranolol may prevent signs of hypoglycemia (sweating, tachycardia).

GENERAL INFORMATION ON SULFONYLUREAS

The sulfonylureas are a class of compounds capable of producing hypoglycemia by stimulating the release of insulin from the beta cells in the pancreas. The exact mechanism is unknown. They are of no benefit in pancreatectomized patients and in juvenile onset diabetic patients; however, they are effective in maturity onset diabetic patients in whom the pancreas retains the capacity to secrete insulin.

Commercially available forms of sulfonylureas (Table 13-5) may be effective in the treatment of maturity onset diabetes mellitus that cannot be controlled by diet alone and if the patient is not prone to develop ketosis, acidosis, and/or infections. Patients most likely to benefit from treatment are those who have developed diabetes after 40 years of age and who require less than 40 units of insulin/day.

Special remarks and cautions

The University Group Diabetes Program (UGDP) study concluded that there may be a higher incidence of cardiovascular death in diabetic patients treated with oral hypoglycemic agents than in those treated by diet or insulin alone. The results of this study have been quite controversial, and further studies have as yet not refuted or confirmed the UGDP data. Until further studies are completed, it would be wise to initiate oral hypoglycemic therapy only in those patients whose diabetes truly can not be controlled by diet and weight reduction alone and where risks of insulin therapy outweigh its benefits.

Patients on oral hypoglycemic therapy are susceptible to hypoglycemia as those diabetic patients on insulin therapy. Consequently blood sugar levels and urine sugar levels must be monitored closely, especially in the early stages of therapy.

Patient education and dosage compliance as well as dietary restriction, exercise, and infection control are mandatory to ensure maintenance of therapy.

Individual dosage adjustment is essential for the successful use of oral hypoglycemic agents. A patient should be given a 1-month trial on maximum doses of the sulfonylurea being used before the patient can be considered a primary failure. If a patient represents a secondary failure (a patient initially controlled on oral agents), changing to an alternative sulfonylurea is occasionally successful.

Table 13-5. Comparison of the sulfonylureas

Characteristics	Acetohexamide (Dymelor)	Chlorpropamide (Diabinese)	Tolazamide (Tolinase)	Tolbutamide (Orinase)
Dosage range (g)	0.25-1.5 (single or divided dose)	0.1-0.5 (single dose)	0.1-0.25 (single or divided dose)	0.5-3 (divided dose)
Onset (hr)	1	1	4-6	0.5-1
Peak (hr)	3	—	—	3-5
Duration (hr)	12-24	72-96	10-15	—
Half-life (hr)	6	36	7	5
Metabolism	Liver (active)	80% liver	Liver (active)	Liver (inactive)
Excretion	>80% urine	20% unchanged in urine	Urine	>75% metabolites in urine
Dialysis	?	P-NO*	?	H-NO†

*Peritoneal dialysis.
†Hemodialysis.

If a patient develops severe hyperglycemia, acidosis, ketosis, severe infection, or undergoes a surgical procedure, the oral hypoglycemic should be discontinued temporarily while diabetic control is maintained with insulin.

Side effects of the sulfonylureas are infrequent and generally mild. The more common adverse reactions include allergic skin reactions (maculopapular, erythematous, and, occasionally, pruritus) and gastrointestinal symptoms (heartburn, fullness, nausea). Alcohol intolerance, manifested by facial flushing, pounding headache, feeling of breathlessness, and nausea, is occasionally noted, especially in patients being treated with chlorpropamide. This disulfiram-like reaction can be initiated by small amounts of alcohol in mouthwashes and other over-the-counter products with a hydroalcoholic base.

Sulfonylureas are not recommended for use in pregnant women or nursing mothers.

Drug interactions

The following drugs may produce hypoglycemia and may potentiate sulfonylureas. Propranolol may also mask some of the symptoms of hypoglycemia such as tachycardia and sweating. Dosage adjustment of the oral hypoglycemic may be necessary.

Ethanol
Methandrostenolone (Dianabol)
Chloramphenicol (Chloromycetin)
Warfarin (Coumadin)
Propranolol (Inderal)
Salicylates (aspirin)

Sulfisoxazole (Gantrisin)
Guanethidine sulfate (Ismelin)
Oxytetracycline (Terramycin)
MAO inhibitors (Marplan, Parnate, Eutonyl)
Phenylbutazone (Butazolidin)

The following drugs may antagonize the hypoglycemic effects of sulfonylureas, possibly requiring increased dosages of the oral hypoglycemic agent to maintain control of the diabetes.

Corticosteroids (prednisone)
Phenothiazines (chlorpromazine)
Diuretics (thiazides, chlorthalidone)
Oral contraceptives
Thyroid replacement therapy

Phenytoin (Dilantin)
Salicylates (aspirin)
Diazoxide (Hyperstat)
Lithium carbonate

CHAPTER FOURTEEN

Corticosteroids

General information on corticosteroids

GENERAL INFORMATION ON CORTICOSTEROIDS   AHFS 68:04

The corticosteroids are hormones secreted by the adrenal cortex. They are divided into two classes according to their structure and biologic activity. The activity of the mineralo-corticoids (desoxycorticosterone, aldosterone) is limited primarily to regulating water and electrolyte balance. The glucocorticoids (hydrocortisone, prednisone) regulate carbohydrate metabolism, but also affect most other physiologic processes.

The major glucocorticoid of the adrenal cortex is cortisol. The hypothalamic-pituitary axis regulates the secretion of cortisol by increasing or decreasing the output of corticotro-pin-releasing factor (CRF) from the hypothalamus. CRF stimulates the release of adreno-corticotropic hormone (ACTH) from the pituitary gland. ACTH then stimulates the adrenal cortex to secrete cortisol. As serum levels of cortisol increase, the amount of CRF secreted by the hypothalamus is decreased, resulting in diminished secretion of cortisol from the adrenal cortex.

Corticosteroids are used most frequently for their anti-inflammatory and antiallergic properties. While the underlying cause remains, the symptoms are suppressed. Corticosteroids nonspecifically inhibit inflammatory effects of many microorganisms, chemical or thermal irritants, allergens, and trauma. Although the precise mechanisms of action are unknown, steroids have been observed to inhibit the early inflammatory process (edema, capillary dilatation, migration of leukocytes into the inflamed area, and phagocytic activity), as well as the later processes (capillary proliferation, fibroblastic activity, deposition of colla-gen, and scar formation).

Corticosteroids are frequently used in rheumatic disorders (arthritis), collagen diseases (systemic lupus erythematosus), dermatologic disorders (pemphigus, exfoliative dermati-tis), allergic states (bronchial asthma, drug hypersensitivity reactions), gastrointestinal diseases (ulcerative colitis, regional enteritis), diagnostic testing, and cerebral edema.

Glucocorticoids are thought to be effective in the treatment of septic shock when (1) doses are massive, (2) therapy is initiated early, and (3) supportive therapy includes fluids, electrolytes, antibiotics, plasma expanders, and pressor agents. The proposed mechanisms by which glucocorticoids may be effective in the treatment of shock (in addition to those above) include a positive inotropic effect on the myocardium, a decrease in peripheral vascular resistance, and chemical inactivation of endotoxins.

Administrative considerations

Clinicians should have firm therapeutic goals prior to initiation of therapy. Once control has been established, dosage should be tapered to the lowest effective amount possible.

Continuous daily therapy is usually reserved for acute conditions (for example, trauma, burns, septic shock, systemic lupus erythematosus). For chronic disorders such as rheu-matoid disease or bronchial asthma enough steroid should be administered to allow func-tion, but usually not enough to provide complete symptomatic relief, since much higher dosages are often required.

The use of alternate-day therapy should be considered in chronic diseases treated with maintenance therapy. Patients receive a 2-day dosage in a single administration every other morning. This mode of administration may reduce side effects, particularly those of adrenal suppression. The theory of this method is that on the "off" days (when the patient receives no exogenous steroids), the patient has lower steroid blood levels, allowing a day of reacti-vation of the adrenal glands by the normal mechanism of CRF-ACTH and recovery of other

Table 14-1. Comparison chart of corticosteroid preparations*

USP name	Structure of synthetic analog	Trade names	Approximate equivalent dose (mg)	Anti-inflammatory potency	Mineralocorticoid potency	Usual starting dose (mg/day) Life-threat-ening illness	Usual starting dose (mg/day) Moderately severe illness
Hydrocortisone (cortisol)	—	—	20.0	1.0	1.0	—	80-120
Cortisone	—	Meticorten	25.0	0.8	0.8	—	100-150
Prednisone	delta-1-cortisone	Deltasone	5.0	3.0-5.0	0.8	50-100	20-30
Prednisolone	delta-1-cortisol	Meticortelone Hydeltra-T.B.A. Delta-Cortef	5.0	3.0-5.0	0.8	50-100	20-30
Triamcinolone	9-alpha fluoro-16-alpha-hydroxy-prednisolone	Aristocort Kenacort	4.0	3.0-5.0	0	40-80	16-24
Dexamethasone	9-alpha fluoro-16-alpha-methyl-prednisolone	Decadron Deronil Gammacorten Hexadrol	0.75	20.0-30.0	0	7.5-15.0	3.0-4.5
Methylprednisolone	6-alpha-methyl-prednisolone	Medrol	4.0	3.0-5.0	0	40-80	16-24
Fluprednisolone	6-alpha fluoro-prednisolone	Alphadrol	1.5	10.0-20.0	0	15-30	6-9
Betamethasone	9-alpha fluoro-16-beta-methyl-prednisolone	Celestone	0.6	20.0-30.0	0	6-12	2.4-3.6
Paramethasone	6-alpha fluoro-16-alpha-methyl-prednisolone 21-acetate	Haldrone Stemex	2.0	8.0-12.0	0	20-40	8-12
Meprednisone	16-beta-methyl-prednisone	Betapar	4	3.0-5.0	0	40-80	16-24

*From Boedeker, E. C., and Dauber, J. H., editors: Manual of medical therapeutics, ed. 21, Boston, 1974, Little, Brown and Co.

tissues from the metabolic effects of exogenous steroids. Steroids that are inactivated in less than 30 to 36 hr (that is, prednisone, prednisolone, methyl prednisolone) must be used to allow the body's own secretory mechanisms to prevail on the nontreatment days. The timing of dosage administration on the treatment days appears to be critical. The dose should be given in early morning to simulate the normal pattern of diurnal rhythm. In the normal individual ACTH accumulates in the circulation during sleep and produces peak serum levels of cortisol between 7 and 8 AM. By administering the shortacting steroid at about this time on the treatment day, the patient receives the benefit of high steroid serum levels that provide symptomatic relief. The high levels dissipate through normal metabolic mechanisms, allowing ACTH levels to accumulate through the night, which in turn stimulate the release of cortisol from the adrenal glands early in the morning of the nontreatment day.

When therapeutic dosages of steroids are administered for a week or longer, one must assume that endogenous cortisol production has been suppressed. Abrupt withdrawal of the glucocorticoids may result in adrenal insufficiency. Therapy should be withdrawn with gradual reductions in dosage. The length of time required to taper off glucocorticoids depends on the duration of treatment, the amount of the dosage, the mode of administration, and the corticosteroid being used. Symptoms of rapid taper include fever, malaise, muscle and joint pain, and possible exacerbation of the disease process being treated.

Special remarks and cautions

The glucocorticoids are very potent agents that produce many undesirable side effects as well as therapeutic benefits. Unless immediate life-threatening conditions exist, other methods of therapy should be given a good therapeutic trial before corticosteroid therapy is initiated. Many of the side effects of the steroids are related to dosage and duration of therapy.

Corticosteroids are quite valuable agents in the suppression of inflammation, but this action also eliminates the symptoms often necessary in monitoring the disease process and in evaluating the effectiveness of treatment. Corticoids may increase the susceptibility to infection, suppress skin sensitivity tests, and elevate serum amylase and blood glucose levels, while decreasing serum potassium and 24-hr ^{131}I thyroid uptake tests. Patients should be advised to avoid exposure to infections and to observe for evidence of recurring infections or delayed healing of wounds.

When glucocorticoids are administered over a prolonged period, the patient may display sodium and water retention, potassium depletion, and symptoms similar to Cushing's syndrome (hypersecretion of the adrenal cortex). These manifestations include hirsutism, cervicothoracic ("buffalo") hump, rounding of the face, hypertension, edema, amenorrhea, striae and thinning of the skin, hyperglycemia, hypokalemic, hypochloremic, metabolic alkalosis, and mental disturbances. Patients may also complain of increased appetite and weight gain, peptic ulcer, purpura, headache, and dizziness. Osteoporosis and vertebral compression are frequent serious complications in patients taking glucocorticoids for longer than a few months. Radiographic studies of the spine should be completed on a routine basis.

Glucocorticoids should be used with caution in the presence of diabetes mellitus (insulin therapy may require adjustment), hypertension, congestive heart failure, thrombophlebitis, infectious diseases, peptic ulcer disease, and tuberculosis.

Behavioral disturbances ranging from nervousness and insomnia to manic-depressive or schizophrenic psychoses and suicidal tendencies may develop, particularly with prolonged therapy. These psychotic manifestations are more likely to occur in patients with a previous history of mental instability.

Teratogenic effects have been reported in infants of women ingesting glucocorticoids during pregnancy. Glucocorticoids must be used only on a risk-versus-benefit basis during pregnancy as well as any other time.

Drug interactions

Although the mechanisms are only speculative, glucocorticoids may alter the coagulation status of patients ingesting oral anticoagulants such as warfarin (Coumadin). Anticoagulant therapy may have to be increased or decreased, depending on the response of the patient. The ulcerogenic potential of steroids requires even closer observation of anticoagulated patients.

Patients may require an increase in dosage of insulin or oral hypoglycemic agents as a result of the intrinsic hyperglycemic effects of glucocorticoids.

Although the mechanisms are unknown, estrogen administration retards the metabolism of hydrocortisone. This may allow reduction of the glucocorticoid dosage.

Corticosteroids may enhance potassium loss when administered with ethacrynic acid (Edecrin), furosemide (Lasix), and thiazide diuretics.

CHAPTER FIFTEEN

Antineoplastic agents

General information on cancer chemotherapy

GENERAL INFORMATION ON CANCER CHEMOTHERAPY

Cancer is a disorder of cellular growth. It is a collection of abnormal cells that generally proliferate more rapidly than do normal cells, lose the ability to perform specialized functions, invade surrounding tissues, and develop secondary growths in other tissues (metastases).

Cancer is a leading cause of death in the United States. Unfortunately the number of persons dying from malignant disease increases each year. Early diagnosis and treatment is still one of the most important factors in providing a more optimistic prognosis for those patients stricken with the many forms of neoplastic disease.

Treatment of cancer often requires a combination of surgery, radiation, and chemotherapy. Recent advancements in carcinogenesis, cellular and molecular biology, and tumor immunology have enhanced the role that antineoplastic agents may play in therapy. It is beyond the scope of this chapter to delve into the interrelationships of chemotherapy and neoplastic disease; however, a short discussion of the concepts of cancer chemotherapy will be presented. As a result of rapidly changing approaches to the treatment of specific malignancies and the changing nature of chemotherapeutic regimens, specific agents and dosages have not been discussed.

All cells, whether normal or malignant, pass through a similar series of phases during their lifetime, although the duration of time spent in each phase differs with the type of cell.

Mitosis (M) is that phase of cellular proliferation when the cell divides into two equal daughter cells. Phase G_1 follows mitosis and is considered a resting phase prior to the S phase, the stage of active DNA synthesis. G_2 is a postsynthetic phase wherein the cell contains a double complement of DNA. After a period of apparently minimal cellular activity in phase G_2, the M phase again divides the cell into two G_1 daughter cells. G_1 cells may advance again to the S phase or pass into a nonproliferative stage known as G_0. The time required to complete one cycle is called the "generation time."

Many antineoplastic agents are "cell-cycle specific"; that is, the drug is selectively toxic when the cell is in a specific phase of growth. Thus those malignancies most amenable to chemotherapy proliferate rapidly. "Cell-cycle nonspecific" drugs are active throughout the cell cycle and may be more effective against slowly proliferating neoplastic tissue. One implication of cell-cycle specificity is the importance of correlating the dosage schedule of anticancer therapy with the known cellular kinetics of that type of neoplasm. Drugs are usually administered when the cell is most susceptible to the cytotoxic effects of the agent. Table 15-1 lists the more common commercially available drugs, their dosage range, major toxicities, and major indications.

Pharmacology

Chemotherapeutic agents currently used are classified as (1) alkylating agents, (2) antimetabolites, (3) natural products, and (4) hormones. The mechanisms by which these agents cause cell death have not yet been fully determined.

Alkylating agents

The alkylating agents are highly reactive chemical compounds that unite with DNA molecules, causing cross-linking of DNA strands. The interstrand binding prevents the

Table 15-1. Cancer chemotherapeutic agents*

| Drug | Usual dosage | Toxicity | | Major indications |
		Acute	Delayed	
Alkylating agents				
Busulfan (Myleran)	2-8 mg/day for 2-3 weeks PO; stop for recovery; then maintenance	None	Bone marrow depression	Chronic granulocytic leukemia
Carmustine (BCNU)	As single agent: 100-200 mg/m^2 IV; over 1-2 hr infusion every 6-8 weeks In combination: 30-60 mg/m^2 IV Use gloves, since solution may cause skin discoloration	Nausea and vomiting; pain along vein of infusion	Granulocyte and platelet suppression Hepatic and renal toxicity	Brain, colon, breast, lung, Hodgkin's disease, lymphosarcoma, myeloma, malignant melanoma
Chlorambucil (Leukeran)	Start 0.1-0.2 mg/kg/day PO; adjust for maintenance	None	Bone marrow depression (anemia, leukopenia, and thrombocytopenia) can be severe with excessive dosage	Chronic lymphocytic leukemia, Hodgkin's disease, non-Hodgkin's lymphoma, trophoblastic neoplasms
Cyclophosphamide (Cytoxan)	40 mg/kg IV in single or in 2-8 daily doses or 2-4 mg/kg/day PO for 10 days; adjust for maintenance	Nausea and vomiting	Bone marrow depression, alopecia, cystitis	Hodgkin's disease and other lymphomas, multiple myeloma, lymphocytic leukemia, many solid cancers
Lomustine (CCNU)	130 mg/m^2 PO once every 6 weeks	Severe nausea and vomiting; anorexia	Thrombocytopenia, leukopenia, alopecia, confusion, lethargy, ataxia	Brain, colon, Hodgkin's disease, lymphosarcoma, malignant melanoma
Mechlorethamine (nitrogen mustard; HN$_2$, Mustargen)	0.4 mg/kg IV in single or divided doses	Nausea and vomiting	Moderate depression of peripheral blood count	Hodgkin's disease and other lymphomas, bronchogenic carcinoma
Melphalan (1-phenylalanine mustard; Alkeran)	0.25 mg/kg/day for 4 days PO; 2-4 mg/day as maintenance or 0.1-0.15 mg/kg/day for 2-3 weeks	None	Bone marrow depression	Multiple myeloma, malignant melanoma, ovarian carcinoma, testicular seminoma

Continued.

*Modified from Carter, S. K., and Kershner, L. M.: Pharmacy Times **41**(8):56, 1975.

Table 15-1. Cancer chemotherapeutic agents—cont'd

Drug	Usual dosage	Toxicity		Major indications
		Acute	Delayed	
Thiotepa (triethylene-thiophosphoramide)	0.2 mg/kg IV for 5 days	None	Bone marrow depression	Hodgkin's disease, bronchogenic and breast carcinomas
Antimetabolites				
Cytarabine hydrochloride (arabinosyl cytosine; Cytosar)	2-3 mg/kg/day IV until response or toxicity or 1-3 mg/kg IV over 24 hr for up to 10 days	Nausea and vomiting	Bone marrow depression, megaloblastosis	Acute leukemia
Fluorouracil (5-FU, FU)	12.5 mg/kg/day IV for 3-5 days or 15 mg/kg/week for 6 weeks	Nausea	Oral and gastrointestinal ulceration, stomatitis and diarrhea, bone marrow depression	Breast, large bowel, and ovarian carcinoma
Mercaptopurine (6-MP, Purinethol)	2.5 mg/kg/day PO	Occasional nausea and vomiting, usually well tolerated	Bone marrow depression, occasional hepatic damage	Acute lymphocytic and granulocytic leukemia, chronic granulocytic leukemia
Methotrexate (amethopterin; MTX)	2.5-5.0 mg/day PO; 0.4 mg/kg rapid IV daily 4-5 days (not over 25 mg) or 0.4 mg/kg rapid IV twice/week	Occasional diarrhea, hepatic necrosis	Oral and gastrointestinal ulceration, bone marrow depression (anemia, leukopenia, thrombocytopenia), cirrhosis	Acute lymphocytic leukemia, choriocarcinoma, carcinoma of cervix and head and neck area, mycosis fungoides, solid cancers
Thioguanine (6-TG)	2 mg/kg/day PO.	Occasional nausea and vomiting, usually well tolerated	Bone marrow depression	Acute leukemia
Plant alkaloids				
Vinblastine sulfate (Velban)	0.1-0.2 mg/kg/week IV or every 2 weeks	Nausea and vomiting, local irritant	Alopecia, stomatitis, bone marrow depression, loss of reflexes	Hodgkin's disease and other lymphomas, solid cancers
Vincristine sulfate (Oncovin)	0.01-0.03 mg/kg/week IV	Local irritant	Areflexia, peripheral neuritis, paralytic ileus, mild bone marrow depression	Acute lymphocytic leukemia, Hodgkin's disease and other lymphomas, solid cancers

Table 15-1. Cancer chemotherapeutic agents—cont'd

Drug	Usual dosage	Toxicity		Major indications
		Acute	*Delayed*	

Antibiotics

Drug	Usual dosage	Acute	Delayed	Major indications
Adriamycin (Doxorubicin)	60-90 mg/m^2 IV, single dose or over 3 days; repeat every 3 weeks up to total dose 500 mg/m^2	Nausea, red urine (not hematuria)	Bone marrow depression, cardiotoxicity, alopecia, stomatitis	Soft tissue, osteogenic and miscellaneous sarcomas, Hodgkin's disease, non-Hodgkin's lymphoma, bronchogenic and breast carcinoma, thyroid cancer
Bleomycin (Blenoxane)	10-15 mg/m^2 once or twice a week, IV or IM to total dose 300-400 mg	Nausea and vomiting, fever, very toxic	Edema of hands, pulmonary fibrosis, stomatitis, alopecia	Hodgkin's disease, non-Hodgkin's lymphoma, squamous cell carcinoma of head and neck, testicular carcinoma
Dactinomycin (actinomycin D; Cosmegen)	0.015-0.05 mg/kg/week (1-2.5 mg) for 3-5 weeks IV; wait for marrow recovery (3-4 weeks), then repeat course	Nausea and vomiting, local irritant	Stomatitis, oral ulcers, diarrhea, alopecia, mental depression, bone marrow depression	Testicular carcinoma, Wilms' tumor, rhabdomyosarcoma, Ewing's and osteogenic sarcoma, and other solid tumors
Mithramycin (Mithracin)	0.025-0.050 mg/kg every 2 days for up to 8 doses, IV	Nausea and vomiting, hepatotoxicity	Bone marrow depression (thrombocytopenia), hypocalcemia	Testicular carcinoma, trophoblastic neoplasms
Mitomycin C (Mutamycin)	0.05 mg/kg/day IV for 5 days	Nausea and vomiting, "flu-like syndrome"	Bone marrow depression, skin toxicity; pulmonary, renal, CNS effects	Squamous cell carcinoma of head and neck, lungs, and cervix; adenocarcinoma of the stomach, pancreas, colon, rectum; adenocarcinoma and duct cell carcinoma of the breast

Continued.

Table 15-1. Cancer chemotherapeutic agents—cont'd

Drug	Usual dosage	Toxicity — Acute	Toxicity — Delayed	Major indications
Streptozotocin	As single agent: 1.0-1.5 mg/m^2/week for 6 consecutive weeks with 4 weeks observation In combination: 400-500 mg/m^2 for 4-5 consecutive days with 6 weeks observation	Hypoglyce-mia	Moderate but transient renal and hepatic toxicity, hypoglycemia	Pancreatic islet cell tumors
Other synthetic agents				
Dacarbazine (DTIC-Dome; DIC)	4.5 mg/kg/day IV for 10 days; repeated every 28 days	Nausea and vomiting, "flu-like syndrome"	Bone marrow depression (rare)	Metastatic malignant melanoma
Hydroxyurea (Hydrea)	80 mg/kg PO single dose every 3 days or 20-30 mg/kg/day PO	Mild nausea and vomiting	Bone marrow depression	Chronic granulocytic leukemia
Mitotane (ortho para DDD o.p' DDD; Lysodren)	6-15 mg/kg/day PO	Nausea and vomiting	Dermatitis, diarrhea, mental depression	Adrenal cortical carcinoma
Procarbazine hydrochloride (Methyl hydrazine; ibenzmethyl-zin; Matulane)	Start 1-2 mg/kg/day PO; increase over 1 week to 3 mg/kg; maintain for 3 weeks, then reduce to 2 mg/kg/day until toxicity	Nausea and vomiting	Bone marrow depression, CNS depression	Hodgkin's disease, non-Hodgkin's lymphoma, bronchogenic carcinoma
Hormones				
Diethylstilbes-trol (DES)	15 mg/day PO (1 mg in prostate cancer)	None	Fluid retention, hypercalcemia, feminization, uterine bleeding; if during pregnancy, may cause vaginal carcinoma in offspring	Breast and prostate carcinomas
Dromostano-lone propionate (Drolban)	100 mg 3 times a week IM	None	Fluid retention, masculiniza-tion, hypercalcemia	Breast carcinoma
Ethinyl estradiol	3 mg/day PO	None	Fluid retention, hypercalcemia, feminization, uterine bleeding	Breast and prostate carcinomas
Fluoxymester-one	10-20 mg/day PO	None	Fluid retention, masculiniza-tion, cholestatic jaundice	Breast carcinoma

Table 15-1. Cancer chemotherapeutic agents—cont'd

Drug	Usual dosage	Toxicity		Major indications
		Acute	Delayed	
Hydroxyproges-terone capro-ate	1 g IM twice a week	None	None	Endometrial carcinoma
Medroxypro-gesterone acetate	100-200 mg/day PO; 200-600 mg twice a week	None	None	Endometrial carcinoma, renal cell, breast cancer
Prednisone	10-100 mg/day PO	None	Hyperadrenocorti-cism	Acute and chronic lymphocytic leukemia, Hodgkin's disease, non-Hodgkin's lymphomas
Testolactone (Teslac)	100 mg 3 times a week IM	None	Fluid retention, masculinization	Breast carcinoma
Testosterone enanthate	600-1200 mg/week IM	None	Fluid retention, masculinization	Breast carcinoma
Testosterone propionate	50-100 mg, IM 3 times a week	None	Fluid retention, masculinization	Breast carcinoma

separation of the double-coiled DNA molecule that is necessary for cellular division. Alkylating agents are cell-cycle nonspecific, being capable of combining with cellular components at any phase of the cell cycle. Generally speaking, the development of resistance to one alkylating agent imparts cross resistance to other alkylators.

Antimetabolites

The antimetabolites (subclassified as folic acid, purine, and pyrimidine antagonists) inhibit key enzymes in the biosynthetic pathways of DNA and RNA synthesis. Many of the antagonists are cell-cycle specific, killing cells during the S phase of cell maturation.

Natural products

1. Vinca alkaloids. Vincristine and Vinblastine are natural derivatives of the periwinkle plant. They are cell-cycle specific agents that block the formation of the mitotic spindle during mitosis, thus inhibiting cell division. Even though there is close structural similarity, cross resistance does not usually develop between the two agents.

2. Antibiotics. Through various mechanisms, the antibiotics bind with cellular DNA, preventing its replication as well as RNA synthesis, which is required for subsequent protein synthesis.

Hormones

Adrenocorticosteroids (usually prednisone) may be beneficial in treating lymphomas and acute leukemia because of their lympholytic effects and their ability to suppress mitosis in lymphocytes. Steroids are also used to help reduce edema secondary to radiation therapy and as palliative therapy in temporarily suppressing fever, sweats, and pain and in restoring, to some degree, appetite, lost weight, strength, and a sense of well-being in critically ill patients. With symptomatic relief, it is hoped that the patient's general physical condition may be improved sufficiently to permit further definitive therapy.

Estrogens and androgens are used in malignancies of sexual organs based on the assumption that these malignancies have hormonal requirements similar to those of nonmalignant sexual organs. Estrogens (usually diethylstilbestrol) are frequently used in prostatic carcinoma. There are regressions in the primary tumor and in soft tissue metastases, with significant symptomatic relief from the point of view of the patient. Androgens may be used in the treatment of metastatic breast cancer of any age group, and estrogens may be used in postmenopausal women with metastatic breast cancer.

Patients often may not complete a course of therapy because of the toxic effects of chemotherapeutic agents on normal as well as malignant cells. Malignant cells that were once susceptible may also develop a resistance to antineoplastic drugs. Several mechanisms may be involved, depending on the sites of action of the drug within the biochemical pathways of the cell. Theories about these mechanisms include a repair mechanism to damaged DNA molecules, altered permeability of the cell to the drug, and increased intracellular concentrations of protective chemicals.

Considerations in the treatment of neoplastic disease

Prior to the treatment of neoplastic disease, several factors must be considered:

1. A tissue diagnosis to determine the type, extent, and grade of the malignancy, its natural history, and the most current results of chemotherapeutic studies is essential in selecting the most effective therapeutic regimen.
2. The physiologic and psychologic status of the patient must be considered. Patients in a good nutritional state with adequate renal, hepatic, and bone marrow function generally respond to therapy with fewer complications.
3. Location of the treatment center should also be considered. Some hospitals may be capable of providing special supportive measures such as isolation rooms to help protect the patient while taking immunosuppressive agents.
4. An "endpoint" or goal for therapy should be established. Is the malignancy in a stage that is "curable," or is remission or palliation of symptomatology the goal? The goal will help determine the approach to therapy and which adverse effects of therapy may be considered "acceptable" while the patient is receiving therapy.

Unlike antimicrobial therapy, in vitro sensitivity studies prior to the initiation of chemotherapy are unavailable. The physician must rely on previously collected data used in similar tumors to select a course of therapy, using one or more agents that appear to be most effective.

The scheduling of dosages may be of crucial importance in achieving therapeutic benefit and diminishing toxic response. Based on cell-cycle kinetics, only cells in a specific stage of nucleic acid production will be affected by some chemotherapeutic agents. Depending on the type of malignant tissue and the agents being used, dosages may be best given by continuous infusion or daily single administration. Frequency of repetition of therapy for maintenance of remission will also affect the course of the disease and the clinical condition of the patient.

Once therapy is initiated, the drug must be given an adequate therapeutic trial. A mechanism must be used to measure the success of therapy (such as reduction in tumor size). Generally speaking, if there is an objective response to therapy, the same regimen should be used until there is little or no objective change while the patient is taking the drug.

While a drug is being observed for therapeutic benefit, it must also be monitored for toxic effects. There are no predetermined dosage schedules that are universally therapeutic, and dosage may change according to the patient's response.

Most chemotherapeutic agents are nonselective in their activity and have clinical effects on normal as well as on malignant cells. Normal cells of the bone marrow, gastrointestinal tract, gonads, and hair follicles also have rapid rates of growth and are most susceptible to the action of antineoplastic agents.

Bone marrow depression characterized by leukopenia, thrombocytopenia, and anemia is a common adverse effect of most chemotherapeutic agents. Increased susceptibility to infection and thrombocytopenic purpura may result. Observe for easy bruisability, coffee-ground emesis, tarry stools, hematuria, and bleeding gums. White blood cell and platelet counts and serum uric acid levels must be monitored routinely.

Stomatitis, manifested by erythema, ulcerations, or white patchy membranes can be very uncomfortable and may interfere with the patient's nutrition. An anesthetic mouthwash, soft-bristled toothbrush, good oral hygiene, and bland, nonirritating foods may be beneficial.

Cellular damage to the intestinal mucosa may be characterized by diarrhea, abdominal cramps, or bleeding. Stools should be checked periodically for occult blood.

Nausea, vomiting, and anorexia are particularly troublesome to the patient's nutritional status as well as physical well-being. Small frequent meals planned at prime tolerance time may help. Administering oral medications with meals as well as using antiemetics prior to therapy may be beneficial.

Skin lesions, incisions, and wounds should be closely examined on a routine basis. Cellular growth necessary for normal healing processes as well as normal defense mechanisms may be suppressed by chemotherapy.

Infection is a serious problem in these patients and susceptibility is generally higher in those with hematologic malignancies. Infections may result from lowered resistance caused by either depressed host immunity resulting from the cancer, steroid therapy, or depressed granulocyte levels resulting from chemotherapy or bone marrow metastases. These patients are also more susceptible to "opportunistic pathogens" such as candidiasis and aspergillosis. Patients with a previous positive skin test for tuberculosis are often started on prophylactic isoniazid therapy.

Patients must be observed closely for signs of infection (fever, sore throat, inflammation of cuts or abrasions) since many of the chemotherapeutic agents used alter clinical indications of infection. Analgesics (aspirin and acetaminophen) may also inadvertently suppress the fever response.

At the first sign of infection, urine, blood, and throat cultures should be obtained. Gram stains of the urine and throat cultures may give an indication of predominant microorganisms.

Antibiotic therapy based on the Gram stain and clinical judgment must often be initiated prior to the results of the cultures.

An area of patient care frequently neglected is the patient's emotional status. Information for the patient and family on matters of drug administration, expectations from therapy, and side effects should be discussed honestly. Hope of complete cure is usually unrealistic, while remission of symptoms and disease progression is more achievable. Patients and family should anticipate signs of fatigue and debilitation such as irritability, short attention span, and decreased pain threshold. Tell the patient what activity level to expect (shopping, occupational activities, driving) and how to plan and allow for frequent rest periods. Patients are usually interested in not what causes fatigue but rather what they can do in spite of it.

Long periods of therapy with frequent interruptions caused by adverse effects and short remissions may be expected to compound frustrations of both the patient and the family. Accept the patient's need to discuss feelings of anger, depression, and hopelessness. Verbal and nonverbal communications that convey feelings of interest and concern as well as positive progress in therapy help the patient retain a sense of dignity and self-respect.

CHAPTER SIXTEEN

Thyroactive agents

General information on thyroid therapy
Thyroid hormones
    Levothyroxine sodium
    Liothyranine sodium
    Liotrix
    Thyroglobulin
    Thyroid, USP
Antithyroid agents
    Methimazole
    Propylthiouracil

GENERAL INFORMATION ON THYROID THERAPY

The thyroid gland is an endocrine gland consisting of two oblong lobes connected by a narrow isthmus. In the mature adult it weighs between 25 and 35 g and is anatomically located in the anterior neck, overlying the larynx.

The gland is subdivided into pseudolobules made up of follicles or *acini*. The lumen of the acini contains a protein unique to the thyroid gland called "thyroglobulin." A primary function of thyroglobulin is the storage of triiodothyronine (T_3) and thyroxine (T_4, tetraiodothyronine), two hormones synthesized and secreted by the thyroid gland.

As with other endocrine glands, thyroid gland function is regulated by the hypothalamus and anterior pituitary gland. The hypothalamus secretes thyrotropin-releasing hormone (TRH), which stimulates the anterior pituitary gland to release thyroid-stimulating hormone (TSH thyrotropin). TSH mediates the synthesis and secretion of thyroid hormones from the thyroid gland. The release of TRH and TSH is controlled by complex feedback mechanisms that are based on demand for thyroid hormones and the circulating blood levels of T_3 and T_4.

Triiodothyronine and thyroxine regulate general body metabolism, more specifically, growth and maturation; CNS function; carbohydrate, protein, and lipid metabolism; fluid and electrolyte balance; thermal regulation, cardiovascular function; gastrointestinal activity; and lactation and reproduction. Imbalance in hormone production may interfere with the regulation of any of these metabolic processes.

An in-depth discussion of the diagnosis and treatment of thyroid dysfunction is beyond the scope of this chapter; however, guidelines for the use of pharmacologic agents used to treat thyroid disorders will be presented.

Drugs used to treat thyroid disorders fall into two categories: (1) those used to replace thyroid hormones in such deficiency states as nontoxic goiter, hypothyroidism, myxedema, chronic thyroiditis, and cretinism and (2) those antithyroid agents used to suppress synthesis of thyroid hormones in hyperthyroid states. Thyroid hormone replacements discussed in this chapter include levothyroxine (T_4), liothyronine (T_3), liotrix, thyroglobulin, and thyroid, USP. Thyrolytic agents discussed are propylthiouracil and methimazole.

Action and use of thyroid replacement hormone medication

See individual monographs: levothyroxine (pp. 258 and 259), liothyronine (p. 260), liotrix (pp. 261 and 262), thyroglobulin (p. 262) and thyroid, USP (p. 263).

Considerations in the treatment of hypothyroidism

Recognize that the patient's cooperation may initially be difficult to achieve. Patients with decreased thyroid function are often apathetic and lack ambition secondary to their disease. Inform the patient that treatment must be a gradual process and that it may require several weeks or months to achieve a normal (euthyroid) state.

One of the first indications of therapeutic effect in the adult hypothyroid patient will be a diuresis with loss of puffiness and weight. This generally occurs within the first 2 to 4 days after therapy is initiated. Over the next 2 weeks the patient will notice an increased appetite, heart rate, and activity level and a sense of well-being. Skin and hair abnormalities will resolve within several weeks.

Changes initiated by thyroid hormone replacement in pediatric patients include increased activity levels, rapid growth, initial weight loss, and loss of hair. Height, weight, sleeping pulse, and morning temperature reading are all parameters that may be used to monitor pediatric therapy.

Patients with cardiovascular disease, hypertension, diabetes mellitus, adrenal insufficiency, hyperadrenalism, and pituitary dysfunction must be observed closely when thyroid hormone dosage adjustments are made. Adjustment in other medications may also be required. Patients should be counseled to report any cardiac palpitations or chest pain immediately.

Adverse effects of thyroid replacement preparations are dose related and may occur 1 to 3 weeks after changes in therapy have been initiated. Symptoms that may occur include cardiac palpitations, arrhythmias, angina pectoris, tachycardia, weight loss, abdominal cramping and diarrhea, headaches, insomnia, menstrual irregularities, fever, and intolerance to heat. Symptoms may require a discontinuation of therapy. Patients may require up to a month without use of medication for toxic effects to fully dissipate. Therapy must be reinstituted at lower dosages after symptoms have abated.

Inadequate patient counseling frequently leads to noncompliance and the renewal of symptoms of hypothyroidism. The need for lifelong replacement therapy, a review of the symptoms of overdosage, and the importance of periodic reevaluation are facts that must be reinforced for successful therapy.

Action and use of antithyroid agents

Propylthiouracil (PTU) and methimazole are antithyroid agents that act by inhibiting the synthesis of T_3 and T_4. The drugs do not affect circulating hormone levels or hormones stored within the gland. Therefore there is usually a latent period of a few days to 2 weeks after antithyroid therapy has been initiated before symptoms improve. A euthyroid metabolic state is usually achieved within 6 to 8 weeks. Since PTU and methimazole do not alter the underlying thyroid disease therapy is either continued for 1 to 2 years at reduced dosages or at the same dosage but with levothyroxine (T_4) supplementation added to prevent hypothyroidism. The combination of PTU or methimazole and thyroxine helps control the symptoms of the ophthalmopathy that is characteristic of Graves' disease. After long-term therapy, antithyroid medication is gradually withdrawn to determine whether there has been a spontaneous remission of the underlying disease.

Propylthiouracil and methimazole also serve a role in preparing the hyperthyroid patient for thyroidectomy. Rendering the patient euthyroid prior to surgery reduces the risk of thyrotoxic crisis during and after surgery.

Considerations in the treatment of hyperthyroidism

Propylthiouracil and methimazole may rarely cause bone marrow suppression or a lupuslike syndrome, usually within the first few months of therapy. Patients should notify their physician if symptoms such as sore throat, enlargement of cervical lymph nodes, fever, rash, sore joints, or headache occur.

Propylthiouracil may rarely cause hypoprothrombinemia. Patients should be warned to report signs of bleeding such as easy bruisability, petechiae, purpura, ecchymoses, and bleeding gums immediately. These patients should be monitored particularly closely if receiving anticoagulant therapy.

The most common reaction (5%) that occurs with PTU and methimazole is a purpuric, maculopapular skin eruption. It often occurs during the first 2 weeks of therapy and usually resolves spontaneously without treatment. If pruritus becomes severe, a change to the other agent (PTU or methimazole) may be necessary. Cross-sensitivity is uncommon.

Evidence of therapeutic activity is usually seen within 2 to 3 weeks, although 6 to 8 weeks are required to return the patient to a euthyroid state. Early subjective indications are weight gain and reduced heart rate. Objectively the PBI and serum T_4 level will be reduced. A patient may participate in monitoring therapy by recording weight and pulse rate on a chart 2 or 3 times a week. Once the euthyroid state is attained, patients must be encouraged to remain on therapy as prescribed. Follow-up examinations and hematologic studies should be repeated every 2 to 3 months.

Hyperthyroidism during pregnancy may be treated with small dosages (100 to 300 mg) of propylthiouracil. PTU does cross the placenta and can induce hypothyroid goiter in the neonate, particularly when larger dosages are used. Thyroid hormone replacement therapy should not be given to prevent fetal goiter, since thyroid hormones do not cross the placenta and will increase antithyroid medication for the mother.

Both PTU and methimazole are secreted in breast milk. Postpartum patients receiving antithyroid therapy should not breast-feed their infants.

Drugs that may alter thyroid function tests

Lithium carbonate may cause a decrease in PBI, free thyroxine, and T_4 by column and an increase in ^{131}I uptake; however, the incidence of clinical hypothyroidism is very rare.

Phenytoin (Dilantin) displaces levothyroxine from protein-binding sites, causing decreases in PBI, T_4 by column, and T_4 by Murphy-Pattee. The T_3 resin uptake is occasionally elevated, while the ^{131}I uptake and free thyroxine index are normal.

Salicylates (6 to 8 g/day) may displace thyroxine from protein-binding sites, resulting in a decreased PBI, T_4 by Murphy-Pattee, and ^{131}I uptake and a slight increase in T_3 red cell uptake.

Although the mechanism of action is unknown, heparin administration results in an increase in free thyroxine levels and an increased T_3 uptake.

Para-aminosalicylic acid (PAS) reduces PBI and ^{131}I uptake by decreasing thyroxine production. The decrease in 24 hr ^{131}I uptake may last 2 weeks after PAS is discontinued.

Estrogens, including oral contraceptives, increase circulating proteins (thyroxine-binding globulin [TBG]), thus increasing circulating thyroxine levels. PBI, T_4 by column, and T_4 by Murphy-Pattee are increased and T_3 uptake is decreased, but ^{131}I thyroidal uptake is not affected. The alterations in laboratory tests may last for 2 to 4 weeks after discontinuation of therapy.

Phenylbutazone (Butazolidin, Azolid) competes with thyroxine for protein-binding sites. T_3 uptake is increased, and PBI and 24 hr ^{131}I thyroidal uptake are decreased.

Androgens and anabolic steroids may decrease TBG levels, resulting in a decrease in serum thyroxine and an increase in T_3 uptake. The 24 hr ^{131}I uptake is not affected.

Propylthiouracil (PTU) and methimazole (Tapazole) induce clinical hypothyroidism with reduced circulating thyroxine and T_3 uptake levels. The 24 hr ^{131}I thyroidal uptake may also be decreased.

Desiccated thyroid, levothyroxine, triiodothyronine, and liotrix, all products containing thyroid hormones, will alter thyroid function tests.

The protein-bound iodine (PBI) test measures the iodine content of precipitated protein as an indicator of the amount of bound thyroxine (T_4). The PBI may be falsely elevated by compounds containing iodides. (The T_4 by Murphy-Pattee method of measuring thyroxine is not altered by products containing iodides.) The following products have been reported to interfere with the PBI test:

Barium sulfate	Lugol's solution
Barium bromide	Suntan lotions
Diiodohydroxyquin (Diodoquin)	Antidandruff agents
Iodochlorhydroxyquin (Vioform)	Salt substitutes
Iodophor antiseptics (Betadine)	Cod liver oil
Cough syrups	Contrast media
Gargles	

Drug interactions associated with thyroid hormone replacement therapy

The toxicity of digitalis glycosides (digoxin, digitoxin, others) may be enhanced when thyroid therapy is initiated. Dosage adjustments with digitalis preparations are frequently necessary as a patient returns to a euthyroid state. Hypothyroid patients often require small dosages of digitalis, whereas hyperthyroid patients require high dosages because of rapid metabolic turnover in the hyperthyroid state.

Patients with hypothyroidism are "resistant" to warfarin (Coumadin) anticoagulant therapy and will require larger dosages of anticoagulant. If thyroid replacement therapy is initiated while the patient is receiving warfarin therapy, the patient should have frequent prothrombin time determinations and should be counseled to observe closely for signs of overanticoagulation. The dosage of warfarin may have to be reduced by one third to half over the next 1 to 4 weeks.

Estrogens (Premarin, oral contraceptives) increase the amount of circulating TBG. Those patients already receiving thyroid hormone replacement may require an increase in thyroid hormone, since the increase in TBG induced by estrogens may reduce the amount of free (active) thyroxine in circulation.

Cholestyramine (Questran) binds triiodothyronine and thyroxine in the gastrointestinal tract, preventing absorption and enterohepatic recirculation of thyroid hormones. Studies indicate that at least 4 hr should separate the administration of cholestyramine and thyroid hormones.

Patients with diabetes mellitus being treated with insulin or oral hypoglycemic agents should test urine for glucosuria and ketonuria more frequently when thyroid hormone replacement therapy is initiated. The hyperglycemic effects of thyroid therapy may require an increase in dosage of the antidiabetic agent.

Drug interactions associated with antithyroid therapy

Hyperthyroid patients with congestive heart failure require higher than normal dosages of digitalis glycosides (digitoxin, digoxin) to be effective. As an euthyroid state is approached, the dosages of digitalis must be reduced to prevent toxicity.

Thyrotoxic patients appear to metabolize warfarin (Coumadin) and clotting factors more rapidly than euthyroid patients. The anticoagulant response to warfarin should be monitored carefully in patients with thyrotoxicosis and the dosage adjusted as the thyroid status changes.

Thyroid hormones
LEVOTHYROXINE SODIUM
(Letter, Synthroid, others)

AHFS 68:36
CATEGORY Thyroid hormone

Action and use

Levothyroxine (L-thyroxine, T_4) is one of two primary hormones produced and secreted by the thyroid gland. It is partially metabolized to triiodothyronine (T_3, liothyronine), the other primary thyroid hormone, so that therapy with levothyroxine provides physiologic replacement of both thyroid hormones. Chemical purity, uniform potency, long half-life, and catabolic pathways make levothyroxine the drug of choice for hormone replacement in patients with an inadequately functioning thyroid gland (hypothyroidism).

Characteristics

Absorption: 50% to 60% (PO). Onset: 3 to 5 days (PO), 6 to 8 hr (IV). Duration: 6 to 10 days after discontinuation of therapy. Protein binding: 99.98% bound—80% to thyroxine-binding globulin (TGB), 15% to thyroxine binding prealbumin (TBPA), 4% to 5% to albumin. Half-life: euthyroid, 6 to 7 days; hypothyroid, 9 to 10 days; hyperthyroid, 3 to 4 days. Metabolism and excretion: 30% to 40% metabolized to triiodothyronine, 20% to 40% conjugated in liver and excreted in stool as sulfates and glucuronides.

Administration and dosage

NOTE: The age of the patient, severity of hypothyroidism, and other concurrent medical conditions will determine the initial dosage and the interval of time necessary before increasing the dosage. Hypothyroid patients are quite sensitive to replacement of thyroid hormones. Monitor patients closely for adverse effects.

NOTE: When transferring patients already stabilized on thyroid, USP to levothyroxine, 1 grain (60 mg) of thyroid, USP is approximately equivalent to 100 μg (0.1 mg) of levothyroxine. When converting a patient to levothyroxine, administer 50 μg (0.05 mg) of levothyroxine less than calculated. Thyroid, USP has variable potency. Adjust the dosage as necessary in 2 to 3 weeks.

Adult

PO 1. Normal, otherwise healthy adults with recent onset of hypothyroidism: initially, 100 μg (0.1 mg) daily. Reevaluate therapy in 30 days and adjust dosage in increments of 50 μg (0.05 mg) every 3 to 4 weeks. The average maintenance dosage range is 100 to 200 μg (0.1 to 0.2 mg)/day.

2. Patients with cardiovascular disease and long-standing hypothyroidism: initially, 25 μg (0.025 mg) daily. Increase the dosage by 25 μg (0.025 mg) every 3 to 4 weeks.

M—Generally not recommended due to erratic absorption.

V—Myxedema stupor or coma without severe heart disease: 200 to 500 μg (0.2 to 0.5 mg) on the first day, followed by 100 to 300 μg (0.1 to 0.3 mg) on the second day.

NOTE: Parenteral levothyroxine can be substituted for the PO dosage form when ingestion is unacceptable. When administering levothyroxine parenterally, one should be aware that PO absorption is incomplete. Therefore only 50% to 60% of the PO dosage should be administered IV. When reconstituting the levothyroxine powder, add 5 ml of 0.9% sodium chloride injection, USP to the vial. Do not use bacteriostatic water for injection because the bacteriostatic agent may interfere with complete dissolution. *Use immediately after dissolution and discard any unused portion.*

Pediatric

PO—Initially, 25 to 50 μg (0.025 to 0.05 mg) daily, with dosage increases of 25 to 50 μg (0.025 to 0.05 mg) every 2 weeks. The maintenance dosage may range from 0.3 to 0.4 mg daily.

IV—As for PO dosages; observe precautions for adult IV administration.

Special remarks and cautions

Laboratory tests commonly used to monitor levothyroxine therapy are the protein-bound iodine (PBI), the Murphy-Pattee T_4, and the T_3 resin uptake (T_3RU). A patient's clinical status must be assessed when thyroid function tests are interpreted. Variations in laboratory tests may indicate slight hyperthyroidism even though the patient is clinically euthyroid. Dosage should not be altered unless the patient displays symptoms of hyperthyroidism.

See General information on thyroid therapy (pp. 254 to 257).

Drug interactions

See General information on thyroid therapy (pp. 254 to 257).

LIOTHYRONINE SODIUM
(*Cytomel*)

AHFS 68:36
CATEGORY Thyroid hormone

Action and use

Liothyronine is a synthetic reproduction of triiodothyronine (T_3), one of two primary hormones synthesized by the thyroid gland. Triiodothyronine is about four times more potent in thyroid activity than thyroxine (T_4), the other biologically active thyroid hormone; however, circulating serum levels of T_3 are lower. Liothyronine has an onset of action more rapid than levothyroxine and is occasionally used as a thyroid hormone replacement when prompt activity is necessary. Liothyronine is also used as a diagnostic agent for thyroid function in the T_3 suppression test.

Characteristics

Absorption: 85% (PO). Onset: a few hours; maximal response in 2 or 3 days. Duration: 3 to 5 days after discontinuation of therapy. Protein binding: 99.8% to thyroxine-binding globulin (TBG), thyroxine-binding prealbumin (TBPA), and albumin. Half-life: euthyroid, 1 day; hypothyroid, up to 2 days; hyperthyroid, 0.6 day. Metabolism and excretion: deiodinated, inactive metabolites in urine and feces.

Administration and dosage

NOTE: Liothyronine therapy should not be used in patients with cardiovascular disease unless a rapid onset of activity is deemed essential. Initiate therapy at low dosages (see below) and observe patients particularly for tachycardia, palpitations, cardiac arrhythmias, and angina pectoris.

Adult

PO 1. Mild hypothyroidism: initially, 25 μg daily, with increases of 12.5 to 25 μg every 1 to 2 weeks. The usual maintenance dose is 25 to 75 μg daily. Occasionally 100 μg daily may be required.
2. Myxedema: initially, 5 μg daily, increased by 5 to 10 μg daily every 1 to 2 weeks. When 25 μg daily is attained, the dosage may be increased by 12.5 to 25 μg every 1 to 2 weeks. The usual maintenance dose is 50 to 100 μg daily.

Pediatric

PO 1. Initially, 5 μg daily, with increases of 5 μg every 4 to 5 days until the desired response is attained.
2. Maintenance:
   a. Infants: approximately 20 μg daily.
   b. Ages 1 to 3: approximately 50 μg daily.
   c. Over 3 years of age: as for adult dosage.

When transferring a patient from thyroid, levothyroxine. or thyroglobulin therapy to liothyronine therapy, discontinue the initial thyroid therapy and start liothyronine therapy at a low dosage. Liothyronine has a rapid onset of action, and the residual effects of the initial thyroid therapy may be evident for several weeks. Liothyronine, 25 μg, is equivalent to approximately 1 grain (60 mg) of desiccated thyroid or thyroglobulin and 0.1 mg (100 μg) of levothyroxine.

Special remarks and cautions

The PBI usually remains at levels below normal during full replacement therapy with liothyronine. Observe the clinical status of patients on liothyronine closely. Do not make dosage adjustments based solely on laboratory function tests.

See General information on thyroid therapy (pp. 254 to 257).

Drug interactions

See General information on thyroid therapy (pp. 254 to 257).

LIOTRIX

AHFS 68:36
CATEGORY Thyroid hormone

(Thyrolar, Euthroid)

Action and use

Liotrix is a combination of synthetically produced levothyroxine (T_4) and liothyronine (T_3) in a ratio of 4:1. Chemical purity, stability, and predictable potency are advantages of this combination product. These two thyroid hormones are marketed in this ratio because until a few years ago it was thought that the thyroid gland secreted these hormones in a ratio of 4:1. However, since it has been shown that a significant amount of active T_3 is produced from the peripheral catabolism of T_4, there is no longer a rationale for the use of this product.

Characteristics

See levothyroxine (pp. 258 and 259) and liothyronine (p. 260) for the specific characteristics of T_4 and T_3.

Administration and dosage

NOTE: Liotrix should not be used in patients with cardiovascular disease unless thyroid replacement is indicated. Initiate therapy at low dosages and observe patients particularly for tachycardia, palpitations, cardiac arrhythmias, and angina pectoris.

Adult

PO—Newly diagnosed or untreated hypothyroidism: initially, ¼ to ½ grain daily. Increase dosage by ¼ to ½ grain every 2 to 4 weeks. The maintenance dosage range is 1 to 3 grains daily.

Special remarks and cautions

Some individuals who are euthyroid while receiving liotrix complain of recurrent headaches. The dosage should be reduced in these patients. If the headaches persist or symptoms of hypoglycemia develop, another thyroid preparation should be substituted.

The PBI, T_3, and T_4 laboratory tests usually remain at levels in the normal range during

Table 16-1. Comparison of Thyrolar and Euthroid

Product (grains)	T_4/T_3 content	Approximate equivalence thyroid, USP (grains)
Thyrolar, ¼	12.5 μg/3.1 μg	¼
Thyrolar, ½	25 μg/6.25 μg	½
Euthroid, ½	30 μg/7.5 μg	½
Thyrolar, 1	50 μg/12.5 μg	1
Euthroid, 1	60 μg/15 μg	1
Thyrolar, 2	100 μg/25 μg	2
Euthroid, 2	120 μg/30 μg	2
Thyrolar, 3	150 μg/37.5 μg	3
Euthroid, 3	180 μg/45 μg	3
Thyrolar, 5	250 μg/62.5 μg	5

NOTE: Euthroid contains 20% more active T_3 and T_4 per approximate equivalent to Thyroid, USP than Thyrolar.

full replacement therapy with liotrix. Observe the clinical status of patients closely. Do not make any dosage adjustments based solely on laboratory function tests.

See General information on thyroid therapy (pp. 254 to 257).

Drug interactions

See General information on thyroid therapy (pp. 254 to 257).

THYROGLOBULIN
(*Proloid*)

AHFS 68:36
CATEGORY Thyroid hormone

Action and use

Thyroglobulin is a purified protein extract from hog thyroid glands. It contains the active thyroid hormones thyroxine (T_4) and triiodothyronine (T_3) in a ratio of 2.5:1. Its potency is adjusted to be equivalent to thyroid, USP, but it is considerably more expensive. Thyroglobulin is used clinically for thyroid hormone replacement therapy in patients with hypothyroidism.

Characteristics

See levothyroxine (pp. 258 and 259) and liothyronine (p. 260) for the specific characteristics of T_4 and T_3.

Administration and dosage

NOTE: Thyroglobulin should not be used in patients with cardiovascular disease unless thyroid replacement is indicated. Initiate therapy at low dosages (see below) and observe patients particularly for tachycardia, palpitations, cardiac arrhythmias, and angina pectoris.

Adult

PO
1. Mild hypothyroidism with no other apparent disorders: initially, 65 mg (1 grain) daily, with increases of 30 mg (0.5 grain) every 1 to 2 weeks. The maintenance dosage range is 30 to 200 mg (0.5 to 3 grains) daily.
2. Cardiovascular disease: 15 to 30 mg (0.25 to 0.5 grain) daily, with increases of 15 to 30 mg (0.25 to 0.5 grain) every 2 weeks.

Special remarks and cautions

The PBI usually remains at levels in the normal range during full replacement therapy with thyroglobulin. Observe the clinical status of patients closely. Do not make dosage adjustments based solely on laboratory function tests.

See General information on thyroid therapy (pp. 254 to 257).

Drug interactions

See General information on thyroid therapy (pp. 254 to 257).

THYROID, USP
(Various)

AHFS 68:36
CATEGORY Thyroid hormone

Action and use

Thyroid, USP (desiccated thyroid) is derived from pig, beef, and sheep thyroid glands. It contains the active thyroid hormones thyroxine (T_4) and triiodothyronine (T_3) in a ratio of about 2:1. There is some variation in potency, since the content of iodine and T_4 and T_3 vary slightly. Thyroid, USP is the oldest thyroid hormone replacement available and the least expensive. Due to its lack of purity, uniformity, and stability, it is generally not the drug of choice for the initiation of thyroid replacement therapy.

Administration and dosage

NOTE: Thyroid, USP should not be used in patients with cardiovascular disease unless thyroid replacement is indicated. Initiate therapy at low dosages (see below) and observe patients particularly for tachycardia, palpitations, cardiac arrhythmias, and angina pectoris.

Adult

PO 1. Mild hypothyroidism with no other apparent disorders: initially, 60 mg (1 grain) daily, with increases of 60 mg every month until the desired result is obtained. The maintenance dosage range is 30 to 200 mg (0.5 to 3 grains) daily.
    2. Myxedema or cardiovascular disease: initially, 15 mg (0.25 grain) daily, with increases of 15 mg every 2 weeks to a total dosage of 60 mg (1 grain) daily. The patient should continue to receive this dosage for 1 month and then be reassessed for further dosage adjustment. The usual maintenance dosage is 30 to 200 mg (0.5 to 3 grains) daily.

Pediatric

PO—As for adults with myxedema. Maintenance dosages may be greater than those for adults.

Special remarks and cautions

The PBI usually remains at levels in the normal range during full replacement therapy with thyroid, USP. Observe the clinical status of patients closely. Do not make any dosage adjustments based solely on laboratory function tests.

See General information on thyroid therapy (pp. 254 to 257).

Drug interactions

See General information on thyroid therapy (pp. 254 to 257).

Antithyroid agents
METHIMAZOLE
(*Tapazole*)

AHFS 68:36
CATEGORY Antithyroid agent

Action and use

Methimazole is an antithyroid agent used in the treatment of hyperthyroidism. For further information, see General information on thyroid therapy (pp. 254 to 257).

Characteristics

Onset of clinical activity: dependent on thyroid hormone storage levels. Half-life: 6 to 8 hr. Metabolism: extensive. Excretion: in urine. Dialysis: unknown.

Administration and dosage
Adult

PO   1. Initial daily dosage:
    a. Mild hyperthyroidism: 5 mg every 8 hr.
    b. Moderate to severe hyperthyroidism: 10 to 15 mg every 8 hr.
    c. Severe hyperthyroidism: 20 mg every 8 hr.
   2. Maintenance daily dosage: 5 to 15 mg.

Pediatric

PO   1. Initial daily dosage: 0.4 mg/kg divided into 3 doses and administered every 9 hr.
   2. Maintenance daily dosage: approximately half the initial dosage.

Special remarks and cautions

See General information on thyroid therapy (pp. 254 to 257).

Drug interactions

See General information on thyroid therapy (pp. 254 to 257).

PROPYLTHIOURACIL
(Propacil)

AHFS 68:36
CATEGORY Antithyroid agent

Action and use

Propylthiouracil (PTU) is a thyrolytic agent used in the treatment of hyperthyroidism. For further information, see General information on thyroid therapy (pp. 254 to 257).

Characteristics

Onset: rapid absorption (PO); onset of clinical activity dependent on thyroid hormone storage levels. Half-life: less than 2 hr. Metabolism: extensive. Excretion: in urine. Dialysis: unknown.

Administration and dosage
Adult

PO—Initially, 100 to 150 mg every 6 to 8 hr. Dosage range: to 900 mg daily (150 mg every 4 hr). The maintenance dosage is 50 mg 2 or 3 times daily.

Pediatric
Ages 6 to 10

PO—Initially, 50 to 150 mg daily. The maintenance dosage is 50 to 100 mg daily, dependent on response.

Over 10 years of age

PO—Initially, 150 to 300 mg daily. The maintenance dosage is as for ages 6 to 10.

Special remarks and cautions

See General information on thyroid therapy (pp. 254 to 257).

Drug interactions

See General information on thyroid therapy (pp. 254 to 257).

CHAPTER SEVENTEEN

Agents used in the treatment of gout

Allopurinol
Colchicine
Probenecid
Sulfinpyrazone

ALLOPURINOL
(Zyloprim)

AHFS 92:00
CATEGORY Xanthine oxidase inhibitor

Action and use

Allopurinol is used in the treatment of hyperuricemia. In contrast to the uricosuric agents (probenecid, sulfinpyrazone) that enhance the excretion of uric acid, allopurinol inhibits the enzyme xanthine oxidase, reducing the formation of uric acid from xanthine and hypoxanthine. Xanthine and hypoxanthine are then excreted unchanged in the urine. Allopurinol is indicated for use in the long-term management of the primary hyperuricemia of gout and the secondary hyperuricemia of antieoplastic therapy. It is not effective in treating acute attacks of gouty arthritis.

Characteristics

Onset: serum levels of uric acid start falling within 2 to 3 days after therapy is initiated. Duration: serum levels of uric acid return to pretreatment levels within 7 to 10 days after discontinuation of therapy. Protein binding: 0%. Half-life: allopurinol, 2 to 3 hr; oxipurinol, 18 to 30 hr. Metabolism: allopurinol is metabolized by xanthine oxidase to oxipurinol (active). Dialysis: unknown.

Administration and dosage

For primary hyperuricemia:

Adult

PO—Initially, 100 mg daily. Increase the daily dosage by 100 mg/week until the serum urate level falls to 60 mg/100 ml or a maximum dosage of 800 mg daily is achieved. The average maintenance dose is 300 mg daily. Allopurinol may be better tolerated if it is taken after meals.
Dosage must be reduced in patients with renal failure (see chart below).

Creatine clearance (ml/min)	Recommended dosage
10-20	200 mg daily
<10	100 mg daily
<3	100 mg every 36-48 hr

For secondary hyperuricemia during antineoplastic therapy:

Adult

PO—600 to 800 mg daily for 2 or 3 days.

Pediatric

Under 6 years of age

PO—150 mg daily.

Ages 6 to 10

PO—300 mg daily.

    Readjust therapy after 48 hr.

NOTE: Initiate allopurinol therapy 1 or 2 days before starting oncological chemotherapy. Urine output should be maintained at 2 to 3 L/day. Alkalinization of the urine may also be beneficial.

Special remarks and cautions

    The frequency of gouty attacks may increase during the first six to twelve months of therapy. During these attacks, continue allopurinol therapy without changing dosages. Treat the attack with full therapeutic courses of colchicine or other anti-inflammatory agents. Alkalinization of the urine increases the solubility of urates, reducing the possibility of renal stone formation.

    Therapy should be discontinued immediately if any form of skin rash should develop. Skin rashes may be an early indication of hypersensitivity reactions and may occur months or years after therapy has begun.

    Hepatotoxicity manifested by hepatomegaly, hepatitis, and jaundice with abnormal liver function tests (SGOT, SGPT, alkaline phosphatase) have occurred. Symptoms are reversible on discontinuation of therapy. Liver function tests should be performed before initiating therapy and periodically thereafter, especially during the first few months of therapy.

    Blood dyscrasias manifested by anemia, thrombocytopenia, and granulocytopenia have been reported. Periodic blood cell counts should be performed before initiating therapy and periodically thereafter, especially during the first few months of therapy.

    Allopurinol is contraindicated in patients with idiopathic hemochromatosis. The manufacturer also states that iron salts should not be administered to patients who are receiving allopurinol therapy.

    Allopurinol should not be administered to pregnant or nursing women. The effects of xanthine oxidase inhibition on the fetus and infant are not known.

Drug interactions

    Allopurinol inhibits the metabolism of azathioprine (Imuran) and mercaptopurine (Purinethol). When initiating therapy with azathioprine or mercaptopurine, start at one fourth to one third of the normal dosage and adjust subsequent dosages to the patient's response.

    Allopurinol may increase the frequency of bone marrow depression in patients receiving cyclophosphamide. The mechanism of action is unknown. When concomitant therapy is used, monitor patients closely for bone marrow depression.

    Allopurinol may prolong the half-life of the oral hypoglycemic agent chlorpropamide (Diabinese). The patient should be advised of signs of hypoglycemia (faintness, pallor, diaphoresis, increased irritability, seizures, or coma). Reduction of the dosage of chlorpropamide may be required.

    Allopurinol may prolong the half-life of dicumarol. This interaction has not been shown to take place with warfarin (Coumadin); however, patients receiving both allopurinol and warfarin must be observed closely for signs of hemorrhage (bruises, bleeding gums, hematuria, or petechial hemorrhages).

    There has been an increased incidence of rash reported in patients receiving concomitant therapy with ampicillin and allopurinol. If a rash occurs, evaluate patient carefully for penicillin and allopurinol hypersensitivity.

COLCHICINE

AHFS 92:00
CATEGORY Unclassified

Action and use

Colchicine is a unique agent known for two centuries to be effective in the treatment of acute attacks of gouty arthritis. It has mild anti-inflammatory but no analgesic activity.

Colchicine evokes several pharmacologic responses such as hypothermia, respiratory depression, vasoconstriction, and gastrointestinal stimulation. It is an antimitotic agent, arresting cell division in metaphase by blocking spindle formation. It inhibits migration of granulocytes (white blood cells) to inflamed tissue and reduces urate crystal deposition in inflamed joints, but its mechanism of action in the treatment of gouty arthritis has not been completely determined. It does not enhance renal excretion of uric acid or reduce its concentration in the blood.

Because of its broad pharmacologic activity, colchicine has been used investigationally in the treatment of neoplastic and inflammatory diseases but is currently a drug of choice only for preventing and aborting acute attacks of gouty arthritis.

Characteristics

Absorption: well absorbed after administration (PO). Protein binding: 31%. Half-life: plasma, 20 min; leukocytes, several days. Metabolism: deacetylated in the liver. Excretion: 10% to 30% renal excretion, remainder by fecal elimination. Dialysis: unknown.

Administration and dosage
Adult

PO   1. Acute gout: initially, 0.5 to 1.2 mg, followed by 0.6 mg every 1 to 2 hr until pain subsides or nausea, vomiting and diarrhea develop. A total dosage of 4 to 10 mg may be required. Joint pain and swelling begin to subside within 12 hr and are usually gone within 48 to 72 hr following initiation of therapy. After the acute attack, 0.5 to 0.6 mg should be administered every 6 hr for a few days to prevent relapse. Do not repeat high-dosage therapy for at least 3 days.

2. Prophylaxis for recurrent gout: 0.5 to 0.6 mg every 1 to 3 days depending on the frequency of gouty attacks.

IV—Acute gout: initially, 2 mg diluted in 20 ml saline solution, administered slowly over 5 min, and followed by 0.5 mg every 6 to 12 hr to a maximum of 4 mg in 24 hr. If pain recurs, daily doses of 1 to 2 mg may be administered for several days. Do not repeat high-dosage therapy for at least 3 days. *Avoid extravasation.*

SC OR IM—*Do not administer SC or IM.* Severe local reactions may occur.

NOTE: Use with extreme caution in elderly or debilitated patients and in those patients with impaired renal, cardiac, or gastrointestinal function.

Special remarks and cautions

Nausea, vomiting, and diarrhea are common adverse effects of colchicine therapy. Discontinue therapy when gastrointestinal symptoms develop. Symptoms tend to be less severe when IV therapy is used. Antidiarrheal agents such as diphenoxylate (Lomotil), loperamide (Imodium), or paregoric may be required to control severe diarrhea. Black tarry stools or bright red blood in the stools may indicate gastrointestinal bleeding and should be reported immediately.

Although it occurs infrequently, chronic administration of colchicine may result in bone marrow depression, leading to agranulocytosis, thrombocytopenia, and aplastic anemia.

Drug interactions

Although not specifically a drug-drug interaction, salicylates should be used with caution in patients suffering from gouty arthritis. Salicylates reduce the solubility and renal tubular secretion of urates.

PROBENECID
(Benemid, Probalan)

AHFS 40:40
CATEGORY Uricosuric agent

Action and use

Probenecid is a sulfonamide derivative that increases uric acid excretion by inhibiting renal tubular reabsorption of uric acid. Probenecid is used in the long-term management of hyperuricemia associated with gout and gouty arthritis.

Probenecid also blocks the secretion of weak organic acids into the proximal and distal renal tubules. This activity can be used to advantage clinically by blocking the secretion of penicillins and cephalosporins into the urine. Antibiotic plasma concentrations are maintained at higher levels for a longer duration, allowing more effective antibiotic therapy with less frequent dosage administration. Combination therapy with probenecid and a penicillin antibiotic is routinely used in the treatment of *N. gonorrhoeae.*

Characteristics

Peak plasma levels: 2 to 4 hr. Protein-binding: greater than 75%. Half-life: 4 to 17 hr. Metabolism: liver to several active metabolites. Excretion: 5% to 10% unchanged, 90% to 95% as metabolites, in urine. Dialysis: unknown.

Administration and dosage

For hyperuricemia:

PO—Initially, 250 mg twice daily for 1 week, then 500 mg twice daily. Dosage may be increased by 500 mg every few weeks to a maximum of 2 to 3 g daily. Probenecid may be administered with food or milk to diminish gastric irritation.

NOTE: Do not start probenecid therapy during an attack of acute gout; wait 2 to 3 weeks before initiating treatment.

Patient fluid intake should be maintained at 2 to 3 L/day.

Do not administer to patients with a creatine clearance of less than 40 ml/min or a BUN greater than 40 mg/100 ml.

Do not administer to patients with a history of blood dyscrasias or uric acid kidney stones.

In combination with penicillins or cephalosporins:

Adult

PO—500 mg 4 times daily.

Pediatric (2 to 14 years of age)

PO—25 mg/kg initially, followed by 10 mg/kg 4 times daily. Children weighing more than 50 kg may receive the adult dosage.

For acute, uncomplicated gonorrhea:

1. Probenecid, 1 g PO, plus 4.8 million units of IM aqueous procaine penicillin G injected at 2 different sites.
2. Probenecid, 1 g PO, plus 3.5 g of ampicillin PO.

Special remarks and cautions

The frequency of gouty attacks may increase during the first 6 to 12 months of therapy. During these attacks, continue probenecid therapy without changing dosages. Treat the acute attack with full therapeutic regimens of colchicine or other anti-inflammatory agents. Alkalinization of the urine increases the solubility of urates, reducing the possibility of renal stone formation.

Gastrointestinal complaints are the most common adverse effects of probenecid therapy. About 8% of patients will suffer from anorexia, nausea, and vomiting. Use with caution in patients with a history of peptic ulcer disease.

Hypersensitivity reactions manifesting as fever, pruritus, and rashes occur in about 5% of patients. Discontinue probenecid therapy.

A false-positive reaction for glucose in the urine may occur with Clinitest tablets, but not with Tes-tape.

There are no reports of adverse effects to either mother or fetus when probenecid is used during pregnancy.

Drug interactions

Probenecid may reduce the renal excretion of nitrofurantoin, diminishing its effectiveness as a urinary anti-infective agent as well as increasing the potential for toxicity.

Probenecid may prolong the half-life of oral hypoglycemic agents (chloropromide, tolbutamide). Reduction of the dosage of the oral hypoglycemic may be required, and the patient should be advised of signs of hypoglycemia (faintness, pallor, diaphoresis, increased irritability, seizures, or coma).

Probenecid may block the renal excretion of indomethacin (Indocin) dapsone (Avlosulfon), sulfinpyrazone (Anturane), and para-aminosalicylic acid (PAS), increasing the possibility of adverse effects from these agents. Dosage reduction may be all that is necessary to reduce toxicity while maintaining therapeutic activity.

Salicylates inhibit the uricosuric activity of probenecid. Any more than an occasional small dose of salicylate should be avoided in patients receiving probenecid.

Antineoplastic therapy frequently elevates serum uric acid levels. Probenecid is *not* recommended in these patients because of the possibility of their developing uric acid stones in the kidneys.

SULFINPYRAZONE
(Anturane)

AHFS 40:40
CATEGORY Uricosuric agent

Action and use

Sulfinpyrazone is a renal tubular blocking agent. It inhibits the reabsorption of urate from the proximal renal tubules, increasing the urinary excretion of uric acid and decreasing serum urate levels. Sulfinpyrazone is used in the long-term management of hyperuricemia associated with gout and gouty arthritis.

Sulfinpyrazone also inhibits platelet adhesiveness and prolongs platelet life. Studies are now under way to determine whether sulfinpyrazone is effective in the prevention of thromboembolic diseases such as angina pectoris, transient ischemic attacks, and myocardial infarction.

Characteristics

Peak plasma levels: 1 to 2 hr. Duration: 4 to 10 hr. Protein-binding: 98%. Half-life: 1 to 9 hr. Metabolism: liver, active and inactive metabolites. Excretion: 95% excreted in urine as unchanged drug, active and inactive metabolites. Dialysis: unknown.

Administration and dosage

PO—Initially, 100 to 200 mg 2 times daily during the first week of therapy. The maintenance dosage is usually 200 to 400 mg twice daily. Sulfinpyrazone may be administered with food or milk to diminish gastric irritation.

NOTE: Do not start sulfinpyrazone therapy during an attack of acute gout. Wait 2 to 3 weeks before initiating therapy.

Patient fluid intake should be maintained at 2 to 3 L/day.

Do not administer to patients with a creatinine clearance of less than 40 ml/min or a BUN greater than 40 mg/100 ml.

Do not administer to patients with a history of blood dyscrasias or uric acid kidney stones.

Special remarks and cautions

The frequency of gouty attacks may increase during the first 6 to 12 months of therapy. During these attacks, continue sulfinpyrazone therapy without changing dosages. Treat the acute attack with full therapeutic regimens of colchicine or other anti-inflammatory agents. Alkalinization of the urine increases the solubility of urates, reducing the possibility of renal stone formation.

Gastrointestinal complaints are the most common adverse effects of sulfinpyrazone therapy. Use with caution in patients with a history of peptic ulcer disease.

Hypersensitivity reactions manifesting as fever, pruritus, and rashes occur in less than 3% of patients. Sulfinpyrazone therapy should be discontinued. Patients who have developed hypersensitivities to oxyphenbutazone (Oxalid, Tandearil) or phenylbutazone (Azolid, Butazolidin) should not be placed on sulfinpyrazone therapy. All are pyrazolone derivatives and carry cross-sensitivities.

Serious and fatal blood dyscrasias including anemia, agranulocytosis, and thrombocytopenia have been associated with sulfinpyrazone therapy. Although the development of blood dyscrasias is quite rare, periodic differential blood counts are recommended.

Drug interactions

Sulfinpyrazone may reduce the renal excretion of nitrofurantoin, diminishing its effectiveness as a urinary anti-infective agent as well as increasing the potential for toxicity.

Salicylates inhibit the uricosuric activity of sulfinpyrazone. Patients receiving sulfinpyrazone therapy should refrain from using salicylates.

Antineoplastic therapy frequently elevates serum uric acid levels. Sulfinpyrazone is *not* recommended in these patients because of the possibility of their developing uric acid stones in the kidneys.

CHAPTER EIGHTEEN

Oral contraceptives

General information on oral contraceptives

GENERAL INFORMATION ON ORAL CONTRACEPTIVES

Oral (hormonal) contraception is one of the most common forms of artificial birth control now in use in the United States; it is used by approximately one third of all women between 18 and 44 years of age.

There are two types of oral hormonal contraceptives in general use: (1) the combination pill, which is taken for 21 days of the menstrual cycle and contains both an estrogen and a progestin and (2) the "mini-pill," which is taken every day and contains only a progestin. The approximately 24 "combination"-type oral contraceptives currently available contain one of five progestins (norethynodrel, norethindrone, norethindrone acetate, ethynodiol diacetate, or norgestrel) and either of two estrogens (ethinyl estradiol or mestranol). The progestin-only pills contain either norethindrone or norgestrel.

Estrogens and progestins, to some extent, induce contraception by inhibiting ovulation. The estrogens block pituitary release of follicle-stimulating hormone (FSH), preventing the ovary from developing a follicle from which the ovum is released. Progestins inhibit pituitary release of lutenizing hormone (LH), the hormone responsible for release of the ovum from the follicle.

Other mechanisms play an ancillary role in preventing conception. Estrogens and progestins (1) alter cervical mucus by making it thick and viscous, inhibiting sperm migration; (2) alter mobility of uterine and oviduct muscle, reducing transport of both sperm and ovum; and (3) alter the endometrium, impairing implantation of the fertilized ovum.

The mini-pills or progestin-only pills represent a relatively new direction in oral contraceptive therapy. Many of the adverse effects of combination-type contraceptives are due to the estrogen component of the tablet. For those patients particularly susceptible to adverse effects of estrogen therapy, the mini-pill provides an alternative. Women who might prefer the mini-pill are those with a history of migraine headaches, hypertension, mental depression, weight gain, and breast tenderness and those who want to breastfeed postpartum. The mini-pill is not without its disadvantages, however. Between 30% and 40% of patients of the mini-pill continue to intermittently ovulate. Birth control is maintained by progestin activity on cervical mucus, uterine and fallopian transport, and implantation. There is a slightly higher incidence of both uterine and ectopic (tubal) pregnancy. Dysmenorrhea, manifested by irregular periods, infrequent periods, and spotting between periods, is common among women taking the mini-pill.

Adverse effects associated with oral contraceptive therapy

Two decades of clinical experience have shown that birth control pills (BCP) are not as "safe" as indicated by earlier studies. Use of oral contraceptives must be considered in light of the potential risks and complications stemming from pregnancy. There are (1) minor side effects, (2) major adverse effects, and (3) contraindications to use associated with oral contraceptives.

About 40% of patients using BCP will suffer some side effects. Hormones such as estrogens and progestins have many other actions that affect nearly every organ system within the body. It is beyond the scope of this general introduction to list every adverse effect associated with oral contraceptives. Only the more frequent minor side effects and the major adverse effects are listed (Table 18-1).

Table 18-1. Pill side effects: a time framework*

Worse in first 3 months	Over time: steady-constant	Worse over time	Worse after discontinuation
Nausea plus dizziness	Headaches during 3 weeks that pills are being taken	Headaches during week pills are not taken	Infertility, amenorrhea; hypothalmic and endometrial‡ suppression, and miscalculation of the expected date of confinement
Thrombophlebitis (venous)	Arterial thromboembolic events, blurred vision, stroke†	Weight gain	One form of acne
Leg veins	Anxiety, fatigue, depression	Monilial vaginitis	Hair loss—alopecia
Pulmonary emboli†	Thyroid function studies	Periodic missed menses while on oral contraceptives	
Pelvic vein thrombosis†	Elevated PBI	Chloasma†	
Retinal vein thrombosis†	Depressed T₃ resin uptake	Myocardial infarction†	
Cyclic weight gain edema	Susceptibility to amenorrhea after discontinuation of pill	Spider angiomata	
Breast fullness, tenderness	Change in cervical secretions—mucorrhea	Growth of myoma	
Breakthrough bleeding	Decrease in libido	Predisposition to gallbladder disease	
Elevated serum lipid levels even to the extent of pancreatitis	Autophonia, chronic dilatation of eustachian tubes rather than cyclic opening and closing	Hirsutism	
Abnormal glucose tolerance test†	Acne	Decreased menstrual flow	
Contact lenses fail to fit because of fluid retention		Small uterus, pelvic relaxation, cystocele, rectocele, atropic vaginitis	
Abdominal cramping		Cystic breast changes	
Suppression of lactation		Photodermatitis—sunlight sensitivity with hypopigmentation	
Failure to understand correct use of oral contraceptives; pregnancy		One form of hair loss—alopecia	
		Hypertension	
		Focal hyperplasia of liver and hepatic adenomas	

*From Hatcher, R. A., et al.: Contraceptive technology, 1978-1979, ed. 9, New York, 1978, Halstead Press.
†May be irreversible or produce permanent damage.
‡To avoid this complication in many patients, advise women desiring to become pregnant to discontinue pills 3-6 months prior to desired pregnancy.

Table 18-2. Pill side effects: hormone etiology*

Estrogen excess	Progestin excess	Androgen excess	Estrogen deficiency	Progestin deficiency
Nausea, dizziness	Increased appetite and weight gain (noncyclic)	Increased appetite and weight gain	Irritability, nervousness	Late breakthrough bleeding
Edema and abdominal or leg pain with cyclic weight gain	Tiredness and fatigue and feeling weak	Hirsutism	Hot flushes	Heavy menstrual flow and clots
Leukorrhea	Depression and decrease in libido	Acne	Uterine prolapse	Delayed onset of menses following last pill
Increase in leiomyoma size	Oily scalp, acne	Oily skin, rash	Early and midcycle spotting	
Chloasma	Loss of hair	Increased libido	Decreased amount of menstrual flow	
Uterine cramps	Cholestatic jaundice	Cholestatic jaundice	No withdrawal bleeding	
Irritability	Decreased length of menstrual flow	Pruritus	Decreased libido	
Increase female fat disposition	Hypertension(?)		Diminished breast size	
Cervical exotrophia	Headaches between pill packages		Dry vaginal mucosa and dyspareunia	
Contact lenses fail to fit	Monilial vaginitis cervicitis		Headaches	
Telangiectasia	Increase in breast size (areolar tissue)		Depression	
Vascular type headache	Breast tenderness without fluid retention			
Hypertension(?)	Decreased carbohydrate tolerance			
Lactation suppression				
Headaches while taking pills				
Cystic breast changes				
Breast tenderness with fluid retention				
Thrombophlebitis				
Cerebrovascular accidents				
Hepatic adenoma				

*From Hatcher, R. A., et al.: Contraceptive technology, 1978-1979, ed. 9, New York, 1978, Halstead Press.

The most common side effects are related to the dose of estrogen and progestin in each product. The patient should return for reevaluation and a possible change in product if many early effects have not resolved by the third month. Nausea, headaches, weight gain, spotting, decreased menstrual flow, missed periods, mood changes, depression, fatigue, chloasma, yeast infection, vaginal itching or discharge, and changes in libido are all relatively common side effects. See Table 18-2 for those adverse effects that tend to be dose related.

Disease states that may be aggravated by continued use of oral contraceptives are hypertension (it may require 3 to 6 months to reverse hypertension after BCP are discontinued), gallbladder disease, diabetes mellitus, severe varicose veins, seizure disorders, oligomenorrhea or amenorrhea, and rheumatic heart disease.

The list of absolute contraindications to the use of oral contraceptives is somewhat variable depending on the clinician and the particular case history of each patient. However, patients with any of the following conditions should strongly consider other forms of contraception: a history of thromboembolic disease, stroke, malignancy of breast or reproductive system, renal or liver disease, severe mental depression, suspected pregnancy, and repeated contraceptive failure.

Administration and dosage

See Table 18-3 for products and range of hormone concentrations available. The estrogenic component of the combination-type pills is responsible for most of the major and minor side effects associated with oral contraceptive therapy. The FDA has recommended that therapy be initiated with a product containing a lower dose of estrogen. Side effects must be reviewed in relation to individual case histories, but many physicians initiate therapy to individual case histories, but many physicians initiate therapy with Norinyl 1 + 50 or Ortho Novum 1/50. Therapy and therefore products may be adjusted based on incidence of side effects.

Combination oral contraceptives: patient instructions

When to start the pill: start the first pill on the first Sunday after your period begins. Take one pill daily, at the same time daily, until the pack is gone. If using a 21-day pack, wait one week and restart on the next Sunday. If using a 28-day pack, start a new pack the day after finishing the last pack. Use another form of birth control (condoms, foam) during this first month. You may not be fully protected by the pill during this first month.

Missed pills: if you miss *one* pill, take it as soon as you remember it; take the next pill at the regularly scheduled time. If you miss *two* pills, take two pills as soon as you remember, and two the next day. Spotting may occur when two pills are missed. Use another form of birth control (condoms, foam) until you finish this pack of pills. If you miss *three or more* pills, start using another form of birth control immediately. Start a new pack of pills on the next Sunday even if you are menstruating. Discard your old pack of pills. Use other forms of birth control through the next month after missing three or more pills.

Missed pills and skipped periods: return to your physician for a pregnancy test.

Skipping one period but no missed pills: it is not uncommon for a woman to occasionally miss a period when on the pill. Start the next pack on the appropriate Sunday.

Spotting for two or more cycles: see your physician.

Periodic examinations: a yearly examination should include tests for blood pressure, pelvic examination, urinalysis, breast examination, and Papanicolaou smear.

Discontinuing the pill for conception: because of a possibility of birth defects, discontinue the pill 3 months before attempting pregnancy. Use other methods of contraception for these 3 months.

Duration of oral contraceptive therapy: many physicians prefer to have their patients discontinue the pill for 3 out of every 18 months. This allows the body to return to a normal cycle. Be sure to use other forms of contraception during this time. Long-term use (3 or more years) must be determined on an individual basis.

Table 18-3. Oral contraceptives

Brand name	Progestin					Estrogen		Other
	Norethindrone (mg)	Norethindrone acetate (mg)	Norgestrel (mg)	Ethynodiol diacetate (mg)	Norethynodrel (mg)	Ethinyl estradiol (µg)	Mestranol (µg)	
Combination-type*								
Brevicon (21, 28)†	0.5					35		
Demulen (21, 28)				1		50		
Enovid, 5 mg (20)					5		75	
Enovid-E (20, 21)					2.5		100	
Loestrin 1/20 (21, 28)		1				20		
Loestrin 1.5/3.0 (28)		1.5				30		
Lo/Ovral (21)			0.3			30		
Modicon (21, 28)	0.5					35		
Norinyl 1 + 50 (21, 28)	1						50	
Norinyl 1 + 80 (21, 28)	1						80	
Norinyl, 2 mg (21)	2						100	
Norlestrin 1/50 (21, 28)		1				50		
Norlestrin Fe 1/50 (28)		1				50		75 mg ferrous fumarate
Norlestrin 2.5/50 (21, 28)		2.5				50		
Ortho-Novum 1/50 (21, 28)	1						50	
Ortho-Novum 1/80 (21, 28)	1						80	
Ortho-Novum-2	2						100	
Ortho-Novum-10	10						60	
Ovcon-35 (28)	0.4					35	35	
Ovcon-50 (28)	1						50	
Ovral (21, 28)			0.5			50		
Ovulen (20, 21, 28)				1			100	
Progestin only‡								
Micronor (35)	0.35							
Nor-QD (42)	0.35							
Ovrette (28)			0.075					

*Products contain 20 or 21 hormone tablets/package.
†21 hormone tablets/package plus 7 inert tablets.
‡Products contain all active hormone tablets.

Side effects to be reported as soon as possible: severe headaches, dizziness, blurred vision, leg pain, shortness of breath, chest pain, and acute abdominal pain. Although these side effects are usually of minor consequence, absence of serious adverse effects must be confirmed.

NOTE: When being seen by a physician or dentist for other reasons, be sure to mention that you are currently taking oral contraceptives.

Mini-pill: patient instructions

Starting the mini-pill: start on the first day of menstruation. Take 1 tablet daily, every day, regardless of when your next period is. Tablets should be taken at about the same time every day.

Missing 1 pill: take it as soon as you remember, and take your next pill at the regularly scheduled time. Use another form of birth control until your next period.

Missing 2 pills: take one of the missed pills immediately and take your regularly scheduled pill that day on time. The next day, take the regularly scheduled pill as well as the other missed pill. Use another method of birth control until your next period.

Missed periods: some women note changes in the time as well as duration of their periods while using mini-pills. These changes are to be expected. If menses occurs every 28 to 30 days, ovulation may still be occurring. For maximal safety, use alternate forms of contraception on days 10 through 18. If irregular bleeding occurs every 25 to 45 days, ovulation is probably not occurring on a regular basis. You may feel more comfortable if you use other forms of contraception with the mini-pill or discuss switching to an estrogen-containing (combination) contraceptive.

If you have taken all tablets correctly, but do not have a period for over 60 days, speak to your physician concerning a pregnancy test.

NOTE: Sudden, severe abdominal pain, with or without nausea and vomiting, should be reported to your physician immediately. There is a higher incidence of ectopic pregnancy with the mini-pill, since ovulation is not inhibited in all women.

Side effects to be reported as soon as possible: severe headaches, dizziness, blurred vision, leg pain, shortness of breath, chest pain, and acute abdominal pain. Although these side effects are usually of minor consequence, absence of serious adverse effects must be confirmed.

Duration of oral contraceptive therapy: many physicians prefer to have their patients discontinue the pill for 3 out of every 18 months. This allows the body to return to a normal cycle. Be sure to use other forms of contraception during this time. Long-term use (3 or more years) must be determined on an individual basis.

Discontinuing the pill for conception: because of a possibility of birth defects, discontinue the pill 3 months before attempting pregnancy. Use other methods of contraception for these 3 months.

NOTE: When being seen by a physician or dentist for other reasons, be sure to mention that you are currently taking oral contraceptives.

Special remarks and cautions

Prior to initiating therapy the patient should have a complete physical examination that includes blood pressure, pelvic and breast examination, Papanicolaou smear, urinalysis, and hemoglobin or hematocrit.

Patients planning elective surgery should discontinue oral contraceptive therapy 2 weeks prior to surgery. Studies indicate that there is an increased incidence of postsurgical thrombosis in patients taking oral contraceptives.

There is some evidence suggesting that the hormones used as oral contraceptives may carry tetratogenic risks. Therefore if pregnancy is suspected, a pregnancy test should be completed and contraceptive therapy should be discontinued as soon as possible. It is also recommended that patients stop taking the pill 3 months before pregnancy is planned.

Combination-type BCP tend to reduce the volume of breast milk produced and shorten the duration of lactation. For those mothers wishing to breast-feed, low-dose estrogen combination pills or progestin-only mini-pills should be used.

No adverse effects secondary to hormone therapy have been noted in infants of nursing mothers using oral contraceptives. However, many clinicians recommend that mothers use other forms of contraception so that infants are not exposed to potentially harmful side effects from ingestion of hormones.

Laboratory tests altered by oral contraceptive therapy

The acute onset of pancreatitis with elevated serum amylase levels has been reported in several patients following the initiation of oral contraceptive therapy.

Oral contraceptive therapy tends to lower serum cholesterol levels in those patients with baseline cholesterol levels greater than 200 mg/100 ml. Elevations in serum cholesterol levels have been reported in those patients with baseline levels of about 160 mg/100 ml.

Abnormal glucose tolerance tests have been reported many times. However, the significance must be determined on an individual patient basis. The mechanism is not known, and variables appear to depend on estrogen content, duration of therapy, and patients.

Estrogens, including oral contraceptives, increase circulating proteins (TBG), thus increasing circulating thyroxine levels. PBI, T_4 by column, and T_4 by Murphy-Pattee are increased and T_3 uptake is decreased, but ^{131}I thyroidal uptake is not affected. The alterations in laboratory tests may last for 2 to 4 weeks after discontinuation of therapy.

Oral contraceptives decrease the urinary excretion of 17-hydroxycorticosteroids, 17-ketosteroids, and 17-ketogenic steroids.

Drug interactions

Oral contraceptives may increase the activity of clotting factors in the blood. Those patients requiring oral anticoagulation may need increased dosages of warfarin (Coumadin) to maintain anticoagulation.

Although it rarely occurs, patients with seizure disorders may have increased seizure activity while receiving oral contraceptives.

Although the mechanism of action is unknown, estrogens may inhibit phenytoin (Dilantin) metabolism, resulting in phenytoin toxicity.

Phenobarbital appears to increase the rate of metabolism of estrogens. Patients receiving low estrogen-content birth control pills may not have adequate contraceptive coverage if they are also taking barbiturates on a regular basis.

Estrogens, by unknown mechanisms, appear to diminish the metabolism of hydrocortisone. Patients receiving both estrogens and hydrocortisone should be observed for evidence of excessive hydrocortisone effects.

Patients who have no thyroid function and who start on BCP may require an increase in their thyroid hormone replacement dosage. Estrogens tend to increase serum thyroxine-binding globulin (TBG), leaving less unbound, active thyroxine in circulation. Do not alter thyroid therapy unless the patient shows clinical signs of hypothyroidism.

The contraceptive efficacy of oral contraceptives when taken with rifampin may be impaired. Alternative contraceptive methods should be considered.

Local anesthetics

General information on local anesthetics

GENERAL INFORMATION ON LOCAL ANESTHETICS

Local anesthetics are synthetic compounds that when applied in appropriate concentrations, block nerve conduction in the area of application. Two major advantages of local anesthetics are that (1) all types of nervous tissue are affected, and (2) their action is reversible; their use is followed by complete recovery in nerve function with no residual damage to nerve fibers or cells.

Local anesthetics apparently prevent depolarization (and therefore prevent propagation of nerve impulses) by displacing calcium ions from binding sites on the nerve cell membrane. Loss of bound calcium inhibits permeability of the cell membrane to sodium ions. The influx of sodium ions is necessary for depolarization of the nerve membrane and propagation of the action potential or nerve impulse.

The primary uses of parenteral local anesthetics include:

Spinal anesthesia: injection into the spinal theca or subarachnoid space, blocking nerve impulses in the sensory roots (pain, temperature, touch), sympathetic and parasympathetic fibers, and motor nerves.

Epidural anesthesia: injection of anesthetic into the epidural space (between the dura mater and the vertebral canal). Although somewhat similar to spinal anesthesia, an epidural block differs from a subarachnoid block in time of onset, duration, dose, and extent of anesthesia.

Regional nerve blocks: injection into the vicinity of a specific nerve such as the pudendal nerve for obstetric procedures or a nerve plexus such as the brachial plexus for anesthesia of the arm, hand, and fingers.

Infiltration anesthesia: intradermal or subcutaneous injection of anesthetic to anesthetize nerve endings in a localized area.

Characteristics of local anesthetics

Local anesthetics for parenteral administration are the water-soluble salts (usually hydrochloride) of lipid-soluble substances. Each drug has its own specific pharmacologic properties that determine the duration of action, potency, and toxicity of the agent. The duration of anesthesia is dependent on the time that the drug is in contact with nerve tissue, the pH of the solution, and the electrolyte status of the tissue. After injection it is that fraction of the drug that is present as the lipid-soluble free base at the pH of the extracellular fluid that is active. A lowering of the pH by inflammation greatly decreases the amount of active free base present. Conversely, alkalinization enhances drug penetration and onset of activity. Many local anesthetics inherently cause vasodilatation, which will shorten the contact time and duration of action of local anesthetics. Local anesthetics are frequently administered in combination with vasoconstrictors, such as epinephrine, to prolong the duration of action.

Other factors that influence anesthetic activity include the diameter of the nerve fiber and the extent of myelination of the nerve. Larger nerves require greater amounts of anesthetic because of a larger surface area with more pores to be blocked. Local anesthetics also work only on unmyelinated neurons; nodes are more distant and require a larger volume and concentration of anesthetic to block an adequate number of nodes to render the neurons inexcitable.

From a structural standpoint there are two classes of local anesthetics: the ester type and amide type (Table 19-1). The ester-type anesthetics are metabolized primarily in the

Table 19-1. A comparison of local anesthetics

Drug	Anesthesia	Percent concentration	Onset (min)	Duration (hr)	Maximum dose (mg)	Comments
Ester type						
Chloroprocaine hydrochloride (Nesacaine)	Infiltration; peripheral or sympathetic nerve block; epidural	1-2 / 1-2 / 2-3	6-12	1/2-1	800	Do not autoclave; do not use as spinal anesthetic
Procaine hydrochloride (Novocain)	Infiltration; peripheral or sympathetic nerve block; epidural; spinal	0.5 / 1.2 / 2 / 10	2-5	1	1000	Produces vasodilatation. Do not exceed 14 mg/kg/dose
Tetracaine hydrochloride (Pontocaine)	Topical; epidural; spinal	0.5-2 / 0.15 / 0.2-0.3	15	1 1/2-3	75	Slowest rate of metabolism of ester-type anesthetics
Amide type						
Bupivacaine hydrochloride (Marcaine)	Infiltration; peripheral or sympathetic nerve block; epidural	0.25 / 0.25 / 0.5 / 0.5-0.75	4-17	3-17 / 6-9	400	Do not repeat doses more often than every 3 hr; accumulation occurs with multiple doses. Has lowest degree of placental transfer of local anesthetic

Drug	Clinical use	(1)	(2)	(3)	(4)	Remarks
Dibucaine hydrochloride (Nupercaine)	Spinal	0.5	10-15	6	10	Produces vasodilatation
Etidocaine hydrochloride (Duranest)	Infiltration; peripheral or sympathetic nerve block; epidural	0.5 0.5-1 0.5-1	2-8	4-13	400	Very rapid onset of action Maximum single dose: 400 mg May repeat in 2-3 hr
Lidocaine hydrochloride (Xylocaine)	Topical; infiltration; peripheral or sympathetic nerve block; epidural; spinal	2-4 1 1-2 5	1	$1\frac{1}{2}$ $1\frac{1}{2}$-2	300	Also used as an antiarrhythmic agent
Mepivacaine hydrochloride (Carbocaine)	Infiltration; peripheral or sympathetic nerve block; epidural; caudal	0.5-1 1-2 1-2 1-2	7-15	2-$2\frac{3}{10}$ $1\frac{3}{5}$-$2\frac{9}{10}$	400	Accumulation occurs with multiple doses No vasodilatory effect on injection
Prilocaine hydrochloride (Citanest)	Infiltration; peripheral or sympathetic nerve block; epidural	1-2 2-3 2-3	?	2-$2\frac{3}{5}$	600	May produce methemoglobinemia, resulting in hypoxia Do not use in patients with anemia or methemoglobinemia Maximum single dose: 600 mg May repeat in 2 hr

plasma by pseudocholinesterases and esterases in the liver. Patients susceptible to prolonged duration of action are those with atypical pseudocholinesterases or hepatic dysfunction. Microsomal enzymes within the liver metabolizes local anesthetics of the amide type. Both the ester and the amide types are excreted primarily as metabolites in the urine.

Administration and dosage

The dosage of local anesthetics varies with the anesthetic procedure, the degree of anesthesia required, and the individual patient response. The smallest dosage and lowest concentration required to produce the desired effect should be used. See Table 19-1 for the concentrations generally used and the maximum dosages that should be administered. Resuscitative equipment should be immediately available to treat adverse reactions should they occur.

Local anesthetic solutions containing preservatives should not be used for spinal or epidural anesthesia. Partially used bottles of anesthetic that do not contain preservatives should be discarded immediately after use.

Special remarks and cautions

It is essential that when local anesthetics are to be injected, the plunger of the syringe is pulled back first to determine blood return. Do not inject local anesthetics if there is blood return.

Local anesthetics eventually pass into the vascular system and are distributed to all tissues within the body. Adverse effects to other organ systems include:

1. Central nervous system: early signs of toxicity are stimulant in nature. Anxiety, apprehension, nervousness, confusion, disorientation, and seizure activity may be followed by CNS depression manifested by drowsiness, sedation, unconsciousness, and respiratory arrest.
2. Cardiovascular system: cardiovascular effects are usually seen only after high systemic concentrations have been achieved. After absorption, local anesthetics may cause direct myocardial depression, arterial vasodilatation, and autonomic nerve blockade that may result in bradycardia, cardiac arrhythmias, hypotension, and cardiac arrest. When anesthetics are administered by epidural or subarachnoid routes, cardiovascular and respiratory effects may be secondary to the effects of these agents on the vasomotor center in the medulla.
3. Rare allergic or hypersensitivity reactions manifested by skin rashes, edema, and status asthmaticus may occur. Most allergic reactions are associated with the ester type anesthetics (Table 19-1). Reactions to the amide type are very infrequent, and cross-sensitivity between the two types of anesthetics is quite rare.

Patients with hepatic disease, myasthenia gravis, cardiac or respiratory disease, hyperthyroidism, and other neuromuscular disorders are more susceptible to the toxic effects of local anesthetics. Particular attention to the selection of the agent and the route and dosage used is required.

Possible localized and systemic adverse effects of vasoconstrictors (such as epinephrine) must always be considered when they are used in conjunction with local anesthetics. Vasoconstrictors must not be used when local anesthesia of the penis, nose, fingers, ears, or toes is required. Mepivacaine and prilocaine produce little or no vasodilatation and usually do not require the use of vasoconstrictors.

Drug interactions

Local anesthetics that are derivatives of para-aminobenzoic acid (PABA) such as benzocaine, procaine, and tetracaine may antagonize the antibacterial activity of sulfonamides (Gantrisin, Gantanol, Bactrim, Septra). Anesthetics that may be substituted instead include lidocaine and dibucaine.

Patients with glaucoma who are treated with echothiopate iodide (Phospholine iodide) may develop lower levels of circulating pseudocholinesterase. These patients are susceptible to prolonged anesthesia from the ester-type anesthetics.

CHAPTER TWENTY

Skeletal muscle relaxants

General information on neuromuscular
blocking agents
Pancuronium bromide
Succinylcholine chloride

Tubocurarine chloride
Dantrolene sodium
Methocarbamol

GENERAL INFORMATION ON NEUROMUSCULAR BLOCKING AGENTS

Neuromuscular blocking agents, also known as skeletal muscle relaxants, have a long history. South American Indians have used crude extracts (known generically as curare) from plants for centuries as arrow poisons. Use of neuromuscular blocking agents as adjuvants to anesthesia during surgery, however, has evolved only over the last 30 years. Neuromuscular blocking agents are now used extensively as muscle relaxants during surgical procedures to allow milder levels of anesthesia to be employed.

Neuromuscular blocking agents act by interrupting the transmission of impulses from motor nerves to muscles at the skeletal neuromuscular junction. These agents have no CNS activity and do not alter the patient's level of consciousness, memory, or pain threshold.

All neuromuscular blocking agents are quaternary ammonium compounds; however, the apparent mechanisms by which sensitivity to acetylcholine (the neurotransmitter released from the nerve terminal membrane) is reduced subdivide this category of drugs into two classes: (1) the competitive or nondepolarizing agents such as tubocurarine chloride and pancuronium bromide and (2) the depolarizing agents, represented by succinylcholine chloride.

The competitive neuromuscular blocking agents bind to the acetylcholine receptor site on the postjunctional membrane, competitively inhibiting the released acetylcholine from contacting the receptors on the postjunctional membrane, thus preventing depolarization and muscle contraction. The acetylcholine released into the synaptic cleft is rapidly metabolized to acetate and choline by the enzyme acetylcholinesterase. Recent investigations indicate that the competitive blockers also reduce the amount of acetylcholine released from the nerve terminal membrane.

Depolarizing agents also induce paralysis by blocking the acetylcholine receptors of the postjunctional membrane. However, the initial effect is to depolarize the membrane, resulting in a brief period of fine muscular contractions or fasciculations, followed by paralysis.

Selection of a neuromuscular blocking agent is dependent on (1) the pharmacokinetic properties of a particular drug, (2) the mechanism of action of the drug at the neuromuscular junction and at other sites, (3) the length of the surgical procedure, (4) the anesthetic to be used, and (5) conditions of the patient that might alter response to the blocking agent. Anesthesiologists frequently use a combination of premedicants, neuromuscular blocking agents, and anesthesia to produce a "balanced" anesthesia appropriate for the patient and the required surgery.

Special remarks and cautions

The human body contains at least three different types of neuromuscular junctions. They differ in the size and shape of nerve terminals and postjunctional membranes, the density of neuromuscular junctions per muscle, and the amount of metabolic enzymes present. Therefore a differential response to neuromuscular blocking agents by different muscle groups is to be expected. The muscles of the eyelids are the most easily paralyzed, while the last muscles to become affected are usually the intercostal muscles and the diaphragm. There is considerable overlapping of these effects, however, and even small doses may depress respiration. Patients receiving neuromuscular blocking agents often require assisted ventilation and must be observed closely for evidence of inadequate respiratory effort.

Neuromuscular blocking agents may have significant effects on the autonomic nervous system. See the individual monographs for specific cardiovascular effects of each agent.

All neuromuscular blocking agents cause some release of histamine. The relative potential for histamine release is (1) tubocurarine, (2) succinylcholine, and (3) decamethonium, with gallamine and pancuronium being the least potent. Histamine release may cause bronchospasm, bronchial and salivary secretions, flushing, edema, and urticaria.

Electrolyte imbalance may have a profound effect on the depth and duration of neuromuscular blockade. Competitive blockers may be potentiated by hypokalemia. Hypocalcemia, hyponatremia, and hypermagnesemia may potentiate both competitive and depolarizing agents.

A fall in body temperature enhances the duration and intensity of depolarizing agents, but diminishes the effect of the competitive agents. Higher dosages of tubocurarine or pancuronium may be necessary with hypothermia, but may be excessive when the patient's temperature rises.

Patients with hepatic, pulmonary, or renal impairment or neurologic disorders such as myasthenia gravis, spinal cord injury, or multiple sclerosis must be fully evaluated to assess their ability to tolerate neuromuscular blocking agents. Much smaller dosages are often necessary when these diseases are present. Neonates and elderly patients also require adjustments in dosage because of the insensitivity of their neuromuscular junctions. Their volumes of distribution also differ from those of children and young adults.

Reversal of neuromuscular blockade

The blockade induced by the competitive neuromuscular blocking agents may be antagonized by acetylcholinesterase inhibitors. When enzyme inhibitors are used, acetylcholine accumulates in the synaptic cleft, competing with the blocking agent for receptor sites on the postjunctional membrane. Agents that may be used are neostigmine methylsulfate (Prostigmin), pyridostigmine bromide (Mestinon, Regonol) and edrophonium chloride (Tensilon). Atropine must usually be administered with neostigmine or pyridostigmine to block bradycardia, hypotension, and salivation induced by these agents.

The early blockade induced by succinylcholine is not reversible. Cholinesterase inhibitors may actually prolong it. Fortunately the early succinylcholine blockade is of short duration and thus does not require reversal.

Drug interactions

General anesthetics (ether, fluroxene [Fluoromar], methoxyflurane [Penthrane], enflurane [Ethrane], halothane [Fluothane], and cyclopropane) produce muscle relaxation by both CNS depression and neuromuscular junctional blockade. General anesthetics (except nitrous oxide) may thus add to or potentiate neuromuscular blocking agents.

Competitive and depolarizing neuromuscular blocking agents may be used to either antagonize or potentiate blockade:

1. Sub-blocking dosages of tubocurarine or pancuronium are occasionally administered to prevent muscle fasciculations induced by succinylcholine.
2. Small dosages of succinylcholine may be administered to facilitate neuromuscular transmission during the recovery phase from a competitive blocking agent.
3. A synergistic blocking effect results when a competitive blocker is administered after a depolarizing agent.

Aminoglycoside antibiotics (kanamycin, gentamicin, neomycin, and streptomycin [possibly amikacin and tobramycin, although as yet unreported]) act synergistically with neuromuscular blocking agents to enhance blockade. Cases have been reported to occur up to 48 hr after recovery. IV calcium administration reverses the blockade.

The central respiratory depressant effects of narcotic analgesics may add to the respiratory depressant effects of the neuromuscular blocking agents.

Propranolol (Inderal) has been reported to prolong the activity of neuromuscular blocking agents.

Quinidine and quinine potentiate both competitive and depolarizing muscle relaxants. Patients requiring quinidine after surgery must be observed closely for unresponsiveness and apnea.

PANCURONIUM BROMIDE
(*Pavulon*)

AHFS 12:20
CATEGORY Skeletal muscle relaxant

Action and use

Pancuronium bromide is a synthetic, competitive (nondepolarizing) neuromuscular blocking agent. It differs from other competitive blocking agents in that it has little or no histamine-releasing effect, does not block sympathetic ganglia (and therefore does not cause hypotension or bronchospasm), and has vagolytic effects on the heart, resulting in a rise in pulse rate of about 20%, a 10% to 20% rise in systolic blood pressure, and an increase in cardiac output. Pancuronium bromide may be used to produce skeletal muscle relaxation in surgical procedures, to aid in mechanical ventilation in patients with status asthmaticus, and to control spasms in electroconvulsive therapy.

See also General information on neuromuscular blocking agents (pp. 283 to 285).

Characteristics

Onset: 3 to 5 min (IV). Duration: dose related; supplemental dosages increase the magnitude and duration of blockade. Protein binding: insignificant. Metabolism: minimal. Excretion: single doses lost by redistribution to nonreactive tissues, multiple doses excreted unchanged primarily by glomerular filtration; when renal impairment is present, larger portions are excreted via the bile.

Administration and dosage

NOTE: There is wide patient variation in response to neuromuscular blocking agents. Dosages must be individualized based on the length of surgery, anesthetics used, and the clinical condition of the patient. The following dosages are to be used as guidelines only.

Adult

IV—Initially, 40 to 100 µg/kg. Additional doses of 10 µg/kg may be administered every 20 to 60 min to maintain skeletal muscle relaxation.

Pediatric
Neonates

IV—Initially, 40 to 100 µg/kg. Additional doses of 20 to 40 µg/kg may be administered as needed.

Children

IV—Initially, 40 to 100 µg/kg. Additional doses of 16 to 20 µg/kg may be administered as needed.

Special remarks and cautions

The cardiac effects and excess salivation may be blocked by atropine.
See General Information on neuromuscular blocking agents (pp. 283 to 285).

Drug interactions

See General Information on neuromuscular blocking agents (pp. 283 to 285).

SUCCINYLCHOLINE CHLORIDE
(Anectine, Quelicin, SUX-CERT)

AHFS 12:20
CATEGORY Skeletal muscle relaxant

Action and use

Succinylcholine is a short-acting depolarizing neuromuscular blocking agent. Other pharmacologic actions attributed to the use of succinylcholine include histamine release and bronchospasm; vagal stimulation with resultant bradycardia, hypotension, and cardiac arrhythmias; and increased gastric and salivary secretions. Because of its short duration of action, succinylcholine is particularly useful in providing muscular relaxation for procedures such as endoscopies, endotracheal intubation, manipulations, and electroconvulsive therapy. See also General information on neuromuscular blocking agents (pp. 283 to 285).

Characteristics

Onset: within 30 sec (IV). Duration: dissipation within 10 min. Protein binding: insignificant. Metabolism: rapidly by plasma pseudocholinesterase. Excretion: up to 10% unchanged in urine, metabolites eventually excreted in urine.

Administration and dosage

NOTE: There is wide patient variation in response to neuromuscular blocking agents. Dosages must be individualized based on the length of surgery, the anesthetics used, and the clinical condition of the patient. The following dosages are to be used as guidelines only.

Adult

IV—Short procedures (2 to 4 min): 40 to 60 mg (0.75 to 1 mg/kg). Supplemental doses of 20 to 30 mg may be given as required.

IV INFUSION—Prolonged procedures: 0.5 to 5 mg/min, depending on the response and requirements of the patient. Dilute 500 to 1000 mg in 500 ml of dextrose 5%, saline solution, or Lactated Ringer's solution.

Pediatric
Neonates

IV—Initially, 1 to 2 mg/kg, followed by supplementary doses of 0.25 to 0.5 mg as required. The total dosage should not exceed 50 mg.

Children

IV—Initially, 1 mg/kg, followed by supplemental doses of 0.3 mg/kg.

Special remarks and cautions

The vagal activity and secretory effects of succinylcholine may be blocked by premedication with atropine.

An idiosyncratic response of prolonged neuromuscular blockade is occasionally seen after normal dosages of succinylcholine. About 1 person in 2800 has a genetic abnormality that causes the production of an atypical pseudocholinesterase that only slowly metabolizes succinylcholine. Prolonged muscle relaxation results when succinylcholine is administered to these patients. Plasma pseudocholinesterase levels may also be decreased in patients with hepatocellular disease, malnutrition, severe anemia, or severe dehydration.

Administration of succinylcholine causes an abrupt rise in intraocular pressure that may be hazardous to patients with glaucoma or penetrating wounds of the eye. A small dose of a competitive neuromuscular blocking agent prior to the use of succinylcholine can prevent the rise in intraocular pressure.

Succinylcholine should be used with caution in patients with bone fractures. Initial muscle fasciculations may cause additional trauma. Small doses of a competitive neuromuscular blocking agent may be used to abolish the initial fasciculations.

Succinylcholine may cause release of intracellular potassium into the plasma. Patients most susceptible to developing hyperkalemia are those with burns, trauma, spinal cord injuries, and degenerative muscle diseases and those with cardiac arrhythmias that may result from potassium ion shift in digitalized patients.

See also General information on neuromuscular blocking agents (pp. 283 to 285).

Drug interactions

Patients with glaucoma who are treated with echothiophate iodide (Phospholine iodide) may develop lower levels of pseudocholinesterase. These patients are susceptible to prolonged muscle relaxation if succinylcholine is administered.

Caution should be used in administering succinylcholine to patients also receiving cyclophosphamide (Cytoxan) or promazine (Sparine). Case reports suggest that these agents may reduce cholinesterase levels, prolonging the action of succinylcholine.

See also General information on neuromuscular blocking agents (pp. 283 to 285).

TUBOCURARINE CHLORIDE

AHFS 12:20
CATEGORY Skeletal muscle relaxant

Action and use

Tubocurarine chloride is the oldest skeletal muscle relaxant in clinical use. It was first used as a muscle relaxant with anesthesia in 1942. Tubocurarine is classified as a competitive (nondepolarizing) neuromuscular blocking agent. Other pharmacologic actions include varying degrees of sympathetic blockade, resulting in hypotension and mild tachycardia, and occasional bronchospasm secondary to histamine release. It is also occasionally used to aid in the diagnosis of myasthenia gravis.

See also General information on neuromuscular blocking agents (pp. 283 to 285).

Characteristics

Onset: maximum within 5 min (IV). Duration: dependent on the total dosage and the number of doses administered, the anesthetic used, and the depth of anesthesia; single doses usually begin to subside in 20 to 30 min. Protein binding: 40% to 45%. Metabolism: hepatic. Excretion: 33% to 75% unchanged in urine, up to 11% in bile, in 24 hr.

Administration and dosage

NOTE: There is wide patient variation in response to neuromuscular blocking agents. Dosage must be individualized based on the length of surgery, anesthetics used, and the clinical condition of the patient. The following dosages are to be used as guidelines only.

Adult

IV—Initially, 15 to 30 mg (or 100 to 300 μg/kg) with supplementary doses of 5 to 10 mg at 45- to 60-min intervals. Administer each injection over 60 to 90 min.

Pediatric

IV—Initially, 0.1 mg/lb (0.045 mg/kg).

Special remarks and cautions

If severe hypotension occurs, treat with IV fluids and sympathomimetic agents such as dopamine.

Patients with liver disease often require higher dosages of tubocurarine.

See General information on neuromuscular blocking agents (pp. 283 to 285).

Drug interactions

See General information on neuromuscular blocking agents (pp. 283 to 285).

DANTROLENE SODIUM
(Dantrium)

AHFS 12:20
CATEGORY Skeletal muscle relaxant

Action and use

Dantrolene is a muscle relaxant that acts directly on the skeletal muscle. It is thought that dantrolene decreases the release of calcium from the sarcoplasmic reticulum, causing a decreased response of the muscle to electrical stimulation, thus diminishing the force of muscle contraction. The drug has no effect on electrical activity and does not affect the rate of acetylcholine production or release. Dantrolene is used to control the spasticity of chronic disorders such as cerebral palsy, multiple sclerosis, spinal cord injury, and stroke syndrome. It has also been used investigationally in the treatment of malignant hyperthermia associated with the use of general anesthesia.

Characteristics

Absorption: 35% (PO). Plasma half-life: 7 to 9 hr. Metabolism: liver by microsomal enzymes. Excretion: primarily in urine as metabolites.

Administration and dosage
Adult

PO—Initially, 25 mg daily. Dosage may be increased in increments of 25 mg every 4 to 7 days until therapeutic response is attained or side effects demand dosage reduction or discontinuation. The manufacturer suggests incremental changes of 25 to 100 mg 2 to 4 times daily. Some patients may require up to 200 mg 4 times daily; however, doses over 400 mg daily are rarely necessary.

Pediatric

NOTE: Not recommended in children under 5 years of age.
PO—0.5 mg/kg 3 to 4 times daily, then by increments of 0.5 mg/kg up to 3.0 mg/kg 2, 3, or 4 times daily. Do not exceed 400 mg daily.
NOTE: Dantrolene may cause hepatotoxicity as evidenced by abnormal liver function tests and symptomatic hepatitis. The incidence of hepatic disease appears to be greater in those patients taking over 400 mg daily, those taking other medications, those with previous liver disease, and those over 35 years of age and in women. Hepatitis occurs most frequently between the third and twelfth months of therapy. Therapy should be discontinued if no significant benefit is derived after 45 days of therapy.

Special remarks and cautions

Common side effects of dantrolene include muscle weakness, drowsiness, dizziness, lightheadedness, nausea, diarrhea, malaise, and fatigue. These adverse effects are generally transient and often dose related. Dantrolene is a drug with a wide variety of possible side effects. Its use must be weighed against the clinical improvement of and the toleration of adverse effects by the patient.

As a muscle relaxant, dantrolene must be used with caution in patients with obstructive lung disease or severely impaired cardiac function due to myocardial disease.

Counseling must include warning the patient of possible photosensitivity. Patients should avoid unnecessary exposure to sunlight.

The safety of dantrolene in pregnancy is not known. It should not be used in nursing mothers.

Drug interactions

Other drugs that may cause sedation may enhance the drowsiness and sedation occasionally seen in patients receiving dantrolene.

Although no direct cause-and-effect relationship has been established, hepatotoxicity has occurred more frequently in women over 35 years of age receiving concomitant estrogen therapy.

METHOCARBAMOL
(Robaxin)

AHFS 12:20
CATEGORY Skeletal muscle relaxant

Action and use

Methocarbamol is a CNS depressant traditionally suggested for use in acute, painful musculoskeletal conditions such as muscle tension and pains associated with anxiety states. The mechanism of action is not known, although research studies indicate that methocarbamol does not directly relax skeletal muscle. Many clinicians conclude that muscle relaxation is due to the sedative properties of the drug.

Characteristics

Onset: 30 min (PO), immediate (IV). Half-life: 1 to $2\frac{1}{5}$ hr. Metabolism: liver. Excretion: unknown.

Administration and dosage
Adult

PO—Initially, 1.5 g 4 times daily for the first 48 to 72 hrs. The maintenance dosage is 4 g daily in 3 to 6 divided doses.

SC—Not recommended.

IM—Initially, up to 1 g every 8 hr. Do not exceed 3 g daily for more than 3 consecutive days. Do not infuse more than 500 mg/gluteal region.

IV—As for IM administration. Administer undiluted at a rate no faster than 300 mg/min to minimize side effects. The patient should be recumbent during and for 10 to 15 min following the injection. Methocarbamol may be diluted to not more than 1 g in 250 ml of dextrose 5% for infusion.

NOTE: Avoid extravasation; observe patient closely for phlebitis and pain at the injection site. Do not administer IV for more than 3 consecutive days. Do not administer parenterally to patients with impaired renal function, since the diluent, polyethylene glycol-300, may be nephrotoxic.

Pediatric

Not recommended in children under 12 years of age.

Special remarks and cautions

As with most CNS depressants, common side effects include drowsiness, dizziness, and lightheadedness. Patients should be warned against engaging in activities requiring mental alertness.

Allergic manifestations such as urticaria, pruritus, rash, and conjunctivitis with nasal congestion may occur in patients receiving methocarbamol. Such reactions may be successfully treated with antihistamines, epinephrine, and corticosteroids.

Use with caution in patients with seizure disorders such as epilepsy. Seizure activity has been reported during IV administration.

Patients taking methocarbamol should be told that their urine may turn brown, black, or green on standing.

Safe use of methocarbamol in pregnancy and lactation has not been proven, and its use is not recommended in these conditions.

Drug interactions

The CNS depressant effects of antihistamines, analgesics, anesthetics, tranquilizers, and sedative-hypnotic agents may potentiate the sedative effects of methocarbamol.

Biologic agents

General information
Immune serum globulin (human), USP
Pneumococcal vaccine, polyvalent
Rubella virus vaccine, live
Tetanus immune globulin (human), USP

Tetanus antitoxin, USP
Tetanus toxoid, USP
DTP (diphtheria and tetanus toxoids and pertussis vaccine)

GENERAL INFORMATION

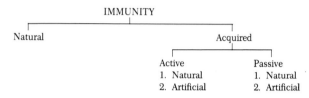

Definitions

A. Natural immunity: immunity present at birth. It does not include any mechanisms to develop immunity during the life of the individual.

B. Acquired: immunity derived from an exogenous source.
  1. Active: immunity developed by an individual in response to the introduction of antigenic substances into the body. Immunity develops slowly, but is long lasting.
    a. Natural: immunity developed secondary to an infection (for example, measles).
    b. Artificial: immunity produced by stimulating body defense mechanisms to produce antibodies to specific antigens injected into the body (for example, influenza virus or mumps vaccines).
  2. Passive: immunity developed by introducing specific antibodies produced from another source into the body. Immunity is produced quickly, but is not long lasting.
    a. Natural: an example is antibodies passed to a neonate from the blood of the mother.
    b. Artificial: injection of biologics (for example, tetanus antitoxin, tetanus immune globulin) that contain antibodies to a specific organism.

C. Antibody: protein substance developed by the body as a protective mechanism in response to the presence of an antigen.

D. Antigen: a foreign substance that includes the formation of antibodies.

E. Antitoxins: a specific antibody harvested from animals that have been injected repeatedly with a toxin (that is, diphtheria antitoxin, tetanus antitoxin, botulism antitoxin).

F. Human immune globulin: solution of globulins derived from human blood that contains many antibodies normally present in adult human blood (measles, pertussis, tetanus, poliomyelitis).

G. Toxoids: modification of a toxin to reduce or eliminate the poisonous properties while retaining the antigenic properties that are capable of producing antibodies (that is, diphtheria toxoid, tetanus toxoid).

H. Toxins: bacterial waste products considered poisonous. When injected, they act as antigens, resulting in the production of antibodies called antitoxins (that is, diagnostic diphtheria toxin).

I. Vaccines: living, attenuated, or killed viruses, killed rickettsiae, or killed bacteria that are

Table 21-1. Recommended schedule for active immunization of normal infants and children*

2 months	DTP†	TOPV‡
4 months	DTP	TOPV§
6 months	DTP	
1 year		Tuberculin test‖
15 months	Measles,¶ rubella¶	Mumps¶
1½ years	DTP	TOPV
4-6 years	DTP	TOPV
14-16 years	Td#—repeat every 10 years	

*From American Academy of Pediatrics: Report of the committee on infectious diseases, ed. 18, Evanston, Ill., Copyright American Academy of Pediatrics 1977.

†DTP—diphtheria and tetanus toxoids combined with pertussis vaccine.

‡TOPV—trivalent oral poliovirus vaccine. This recommendation is suitable for breast-fed as well as bottle-fed infants.

§A third dose of TOPV is optional but may be given in areas of high endemicity of poliomyelitis.

‖Frequency of repeated tuberculin tests depends on risk of exposure of the child and on the prevalence of tuberculosis in the population group. For the pediatrician's office or outpatient clinic, an annual or biennial tuberculin test, unless local circumstances clearly indicate otherwise, is appropriate. The initial test should be done at the time of or preceding the measles immunization.

¶May be given at 15 months as measles-rubella or measles-mumps-rubella combined vaccines.

#Td—combined tetanus and diphtheria toxoids (adult type) for those more than 6 years of age, in contrast to diphtheria and tetanus (DT) toxoids, which contain a larger amount of diphtheria antigen. For tetanus toxoid at time of injury: For clean, minor wounds, no booster dose is needed by a fully immunized child unless more than 10 years have elapsed since the last dose. For contaminated wounds, a booster dose should be given if more than 5 years have elapsed since the last dose.

NOTE: Because the concentration of antigen varies in different products, the manufacturer's package insert should be consulted regarding the volume of individual doses of immunizing agents.

Because biologics are of varying stability, the manufacturer's recommendations for optimal storage conditions (e.g., temperature, light) should be carefully followed. Failure to observe these precautions may significantly reduce the potency and effectiveness of the vaccines.

used to stimulate the production of antibodies (that is, smallpox, rabies, influenza virus, poliomyelitis, measles, mumps vaccines).

Administration and dosage

See individual monographs on biologic agents.

See Tables 21-1 and 21-2 for pediatric immunization schedules.

Special remarks and cautions

Prior to administration of any biologic agent, histories of allergies and tests for sensitivity should be completed. Since biologic agents are protein and foreign to the body, sensitivity ranging from erythema and fever to urticaria, angioedema, respiratory distress (including dyspnea and bronchospasm), and anaphylaxis have occurred.

Biologic agents should not be administered IV because of the potential for serious hypersensitivity reactions. Epinephrine 1:1000 and other emergency drugs and equipment should be readily available in the event that severe systemic reactions should develop.

Vaccines should not be administered to patients taking corticosteroids. Steroids may interfere with the antibody response to the vaccine, inhibiting the production of active immunity by the vaccine.

Immunizations should usually be deferred during acute febrile illness.

Table 21-2. Primary immunization for children not immunized in early infancy*†

Under 6 years of age		6 years of age and over	
First visit	DTP, TOPV, tuberculin test	First visit	Td, TOPV, tuberculin test
Interval after first visit		Interval after first visit	
1 month	Measles,‡ mumps, rubella	1 month	Measles, mumps, rubella
2 months	DTP, TOPV	2 months	Td, TOPV
4 months	DTP§	8 to 14 months	Td, TOPV
10 to 16 months or preschool	DTP, TOPV	Age 14-16 years	Td—repeat every 10 years
Age 14-16 years	Td—repeat every 10 years		

*From American Academy of Pediatrics: Report of the committee on infectious diseases, ed. 18, Evanston, Ill., Copyright American Academy of Pediatrics 1977.

†Physicians may choose to alter the sequence of these schedules if specific infections are prevalent at the time. For example, measles vaccine might be given on the first visit if an epidemic is under way in the community.

‡Measles vaccine is not routinely given before 15 months of age (see Table 21-1).

§Optional.

Patients should be informed about what type of biologic agent is being administered. They should be informed of the reasons for use and the associated reactions that might occur. Patients should be encouraged to report any adverse response to immunizations. A record of immunization should also be completed and given to the patient, indicating the date, the biologic agent used, the site of injection, and the dosage.

Interruptions in the schedule of immunizations of infants and children, with a delay between doses, does not interfere with the final immunity achieved. The series need not be started over, regardless of the length of time elapsed.

Observe expiration dates of the agents and store at proper temperature.

IMMUNE SERUM GLOBULIN (HUMAN), USP   AHFS 80:04

Immune serum globulin (human) contains the antibodies present in normal blood. It is indicated for the modification or prevention of measles (rubeola), german measles, chickenpox (varicella), infectious hepatitis (hepatitis A), and for patients deficient in gamma globulin or of specific immunoglobulins.

Administration and dosage

IM 1. Measles (rubeola):
    Modification: 0.02 ml/lb (0.009 ml/kg).
    Prevention: 0.1 ml/lb (0.045 ml/kg).
    With vaccine: 0.01 ml/lb (0.0045 ml/kg).
  2. German measles (rubella):
    Prevention in pregnant women in first trimester: 20 to 30 ml.
  3. Chickenpox (varicella):
    Modification: 0.1 to 0.6 ml/lb (0.045 to 0.27 ml/kg) up to 20 to 30 ml.
  4. Infectious hepatitis:
    Prevention: 0.01 to 0.05 ml/lb (0.0045 to 0.0225 ml/kg) to be repeated at 4- to 6-month intervals when there is repeated or continued exposure.
    Store at 2° C to 8° C (36° F to 46° F). Do not freeze.
NOTE: See General information on biologic agents (pp. 292 to 294).

PNEUMOCOCCAL VACCINE, POLYVALENT

(*Pneumovax*)

Polyvalent pneumococcal vaccine is a solution containing antigenic capsular polysaccharides from 14 types of pneumococcal microorganisms. The vaccine provides active immunity against the 14 most common pneumococcal organisms that currently cause over 80% of pneumococcal infections. No protection is provided against other types of pneumococcal disease or other bacterial infections.

Pneumococcal vaccine is recommended for patients over the age of 2 who are at high risk from pneumococcal infection. Patients who should be considered for immunization are those with chronic debilitating diseases, institutionalized patients, those convalescing from severe illness, and those over 50 years of age. Revaccination should be no more frequent than every 3 years.

Administration and dosage
Adult and pediatric (over 2 years of age)

sc or IM—0.5 ml.

Special remarks and cautions

Use in pregnancy is not recommended because the effects on the fetus are unknown.

See General information on biologic agents (pp. 292 to 294).

RUBELLA VIRUS VACCINE, LIVE

(*Various*)

Rubella virus vaccine is administered to provide active immunity against rubella (German measles). The vaccine is not effective in the prevention of rubeola (measles), nor is it of any benefit when administered to patients after they have been exposed to rubella virus.

Administration and dosage

sc—0.5 ml.

Before reconstitution, store at 2° to 8° C (35° to 46° F). Protect from light.

Use only the diluent supplied by the manufacturer to reconstitute the vaccine.

Use the reconstituted vaccine as soon as possible. Protect from light and store at 2° to 8° C (35° to 46° F). Discard if not used within 8 hr of reconstitution.

The color of the reconstituted solution may vary from red to pink to yellow. It may be administered if crystal clear.

Special remarks and cautions

Rubella virus vaccine *must not* be administered to pregnant women or those who may become pregnant within the following 3 months. Multiple teratogenic effects are associated with naturally acquired rubella virus infections, although the possible effects of the vaccine on fetal development are unknown at this time.

Rubella virus vaccine should be administered with caution in patients who have shown previous allergic reactions to neomycin, chicken or duck feathers or eggs, dogs, or rabbits. Epinephrine should be available for immediate use should an anaphylactoid reaction occur.

It is not uncommon for patients, especially older women, to experience symptoms of joint and muscle stiffness and pain and peripheral numbness and tingling within 4 weeks after administration of the vaccine. Patients may be assured that the symptoms are transient and that there are no long-term complications.

See General information on biologic agents (pp. 292 to 294).

TETANUS IMMUNE GLOBULIN (HUMAN), USP   AHFS 80:04

Tetanus immune globulin is a solution of gamma globulin pooled from venous plasma of individuals hyperimmunized to tetanus. Each vial (and prefilled syringe) contains 250 units of tetanus antibody.

Human antitetanus globulin is used to provide immediate passive immunization for patients exposed to the risk of tetanus. The administration of 250 units provides protective levels of antibody for several weeks. Tetanus toxoid may be administered concurrently to allow the patient to develop active immunity to tetanus while deriving short-term protection from tetanus immune globulin.

Administration and dosage
Adult

IM—250 units.

Pediatric

IM—4 units/kg.

Store at 2° to 8° C (36° to 46° F). Do not freeze.

NOTE: See General information on biologic agents (pp. 292 to 294).

TETANUS ANTITOXIN, USP   AHFS 80:04

Tetanus antitoxin is a sterile solution of the refined and concentrated proteins, primarily globulins, containing antibodies obtained from the blood plasma of a healthy animal, usually the horse, that has been immunized with tetanus toxin or toxoid, thus producing antitoxin antibodies.

Tetanus antitoxin may be used in the treatment and prophylaxis of tetanus, creating passive immunity. It is recommended for use, however, only if tetanus immune globulin (human) is not available. Antitoxins are derived from animal sources and contain foreign proteins that may initiate an allergic reaction.

TETANUS TOXOID, USP
AHFS 80:08

Tetanus toxoid is a sterile solution of the formaldehyde-treated products of growth of the tetanus bacillus (*Clostridium tetani*). Treatment with formaldehyde and heat causes modification of the toxins, resulting in loss of toxic effects but with retention of the property for inducing active immunity. Adequate dosages provide active immunity against tetanus.

Administration and dosage

IM—0.5 ml of tetanus toxoid, USP 4 weeks apart, with a booster at 9 months and subsequent boosters every 10 years.

NOTE: *Shake well before administration.* See General information on biologic agents (pp. 292 to 294).

DTP (DIPHTHERIA AND TETANUS TOXOIDS AND PERTUSSIS VACCINE)
AHFS 80:08

DTP is used for simultaneous active immunization against diphtheria, tetanus, and pertussis. (It is not recommended for use in children over 6 years of age.) The combination product reduces the number of necessary injections and does not impair the resultant immunity.

Primary immunization may be started as early as 2 months of age.

Administration and dosage

IM 1. Primary immunization: 3 doses of 0.5 ml each, 4 to 6 weeks apart.
2. Reinforcing dose: 0.5 ml, 1 year after third primary immunization dose.
3. A second reinforcing dose is recommended upon entering school.
Store at 2° to 8° C (36° to 46° F). Do not freeze.

NOTE: *Shake thoroughly.* See General information on biologic agents (pp. 292 to 294).

Miscellaneous agents

Atropine sulfate	*Loperamide hydrochloride*
Benztropine	*Naloxone hydrochloride*
Calcium chloride	*Oxytocin*
Cimetidine	*Physostigmine salicylate*
Clofibrate	*Probucol*
Diphenoxylate hydrochloride	*Sodium bicarbonate*
Ipecac	*General information on laxatives*

ATROPINE SULFATE

AHFS 12:08
CATEGORY Anticholinergic

Action and use

Atropine sulfate blocks the cholinergic response by competitively binding to the acetylcholine receptor site. This reduces vagal tone, enhances atrioventricular conduction, and accelerates the cardiac rate. It also suppresses perspiration, saliva, bronchial mucus and gastric secretion and produces mydriasis. Atropine sulfate is indicated for the treatment of sinus bradycardia with a pulse of less than 60 beats/min when accompanied by PVCs or a systolic blood pressure of less than 90 mm Hg. It is also used in AV block with bradycardia. Other uses of atropine include control of secretions and spasm of smooth muscle during surgery and the symptomatic treatment of organophosphate insecticide poisoning.

Administration and dosage
Adult

IM—0.3 to 1.2 mg.
IV—0.3 to 1.2 mg (usual dose: 0.5 mg) bolus; may be repeated in 4 to 5 min if pulse rate is less than 60 beats/min.

Pediatric

PO—0.01 mg/kg; may repeat every 2 hours as needed. The maximum single dose is 0.4 mg.
SC or IM—As for PO administration.

Special remarks and cautions

The total dosage of atropine sulfate should not exceed 2 mg except in cases of third degree AV block and the treatment of organophosphate insecticide poisoning, when larger dosages may be required.

Side effects often include dry mouth with thirst and dysphagia, flushing, dizziness, blurred vision and photophobia, tachycardia, and urinary retention.

Indications of atropine toxicity include anxiety, delirium, disorientation, hallucinations, hyperactivity, convulsions, and respiratory depression.

Drug interactions

Enhanced anticholinergic effects may occur with tricyclic antidepressants (amitriptyline [Elavil], imipramine [Tofranil], doxepin [Sinequan]), haloperidol (Haldol), procainamide (Pronestyl), quinidine, antihistamines, and meperidine (Demerol).

BENZTROPINE
(Cogentin)

AHFS 12:08
CATEGORY Anticholinergic

Action and use

Benztropine is an anticholinergic, antihistaminic agent used to help control the symptoms of parkinsonism (tremor; drooling; rigidity in gait, posture, and balance; and masklike facies). It may also be effective in controlling extrapyramidal effects caused by other drugs such as phenothiazines.

Administration and dosage

PO 1. Parkinsonism: usual dosage is 1 to 2 mg daily, with a range of 0.5 to 6 mg/day. Therapy should be initiated at low doses, 0.5 to 1 mg daily, and increased in increments of 0.5 mg every 5 to 6 days because of its accumulative activity.
2. Drug-induced extrapyramidal disorders: 1 to 4 mg 1 to 2 times daily usually provides relief in 1 to 2 days.

IM—Acute drug-induced extrapyramidal disorders: 1 to 2 mg. If the symptoms return, repeat the dosage. After parenteral doses, PO administration 1 to 2 mg 2 times daily usually prevents recurrence.

IV—As for IM administration.

Special remarks and cautions

Dry mouth, blurred vision, nausea, and nervousness may develop and become severe enough to require dosage adjustment. Patients may also complain of constipation, numbness of the fingers, listlessness, and depression.

With higher dosages mental confusion and visual hallucinations may occur. In patients being treated for mental disorders with phenothiazines or reserpine, psychiatric symptoms may be exacerbated, and antiparkinsonian drugs can precipitate a toxic psychosis.

After long-term therapy with phenothiazines, patients may develop tardive dyskinesia. Benztropine is usually not effective against these symptoms (involuntary movement of the mouth and face with frequent smacking of the lips with thrusting tongue movement) and in some instances may aggravate this adverse effect.

Benztropine may produce anhidrosis, a decrease or absence of secretion of sweat. This adverse effect may be seen in hot weather, in older, chronically ill patients, in alcoholics, and in those patients who have CNS disorders. Dosage may have to be diminished to allow body heat equilibration.

Benztropine may aggravate narrow-angle glaucoma and is not recommended for use in patients with this disease.

Benztropine probably should not be used in pregnancy and may diminish lactation in the nursing mother.

Drug interactions

Benztropine may display additive anticholinergic effects (dry mouth, constipation, urinary retention, blurred vision) when administered with antihistamines, phenothiazines, trihexiphenidyl (Artane), meperidine (Demerol), and other agents with anticholinergic activity.

CALCIUM CHLORIDE

AHFS 68:24

Action and use

Calcium chloride increases myocardial contractility, prolongs systole, and enhances ventricular excitability. It is useful in profound cardiovascular collapse (for example, electromechanical dissociation where QRS complexes are observed without an adequate pulse). It may be useful in restoring an electrical rhythm in instances of asystole and may enhance electrical defibrillation.

Administration and dosage

IV—2.5 to 5 ml of 10% calcium chloride (3.4 to 6.8 mEq Ca^{2+}). Rate is 1 to 2 ml/min. When required, calcium chloride boluses may be repeated every 10 min.

Special remarks and cautions

Digitalis and calcium ions are synergistic in their inotropic and toxic effects. Use with extreme caution in digitalized patients.

Calcium gluconate provides less ionizable calcium per unit volume. If it is used the dose should be 10 ml of a 10% solution (4.8 mEq Ca^{2+}). Calcium gluceptate, 5 ml (4.5 mEq Ca^{2+}) may also be used.

Drug interactions

Beware of injecting calcium chloride and sodium bicarbonate concurrently or immediately following each other. Rinse the line briefly to avoid precipitation.

CIMETIDINE
(Tagamet)

AHFS 56:40
CATEGORY H₂ receptor antagonist

AHFS 56:40
CATEGORY H_2 receptor antagonist

Action and use

Cimetidine is the first histamine H_2 receptor antagonist approved by the Food and Drug Administration for use in the United States. Cimetidine inhibits the action of histamine on specific H_2 receptors of parietal cells of the stomach, reducing gastric acid output. It has no apparent effect on gastric motility, emptying time, or biliary or pancreatic secretion. Cimetidine is now being used extensively in the management of duodenal ulcers and pathologic hypersecretory conditions such as Zollinger-Ellison syndrome and for the prevention and treatment of stress ulcers.

Characteristics

Onset: 20 to 30 min (PO). Peak activity: 45 to 75 min (PO). Duration: 4 to 5 hr. Protein binding: 15% to 20%. Metabolism: hepatic to two inactive metabolites. Half-life: 2 hr (normal renal function), $2^9/_{10}$ hr (CCR = 20 to 50 ml/min), $3^7/_{10}$ hr (CCR = less than 20 ml/min), 5 hr (anephric patients). Excretion: 50% to 70% unchanged in urine, 20% to 40% as metabolites in urine, 10% in feces. Dialysis: yes, H.

Administration and dosage
Adult

PO—300 mg 4 times daily with meals and at bedtime. Dosage increases should be made by increasing the frequency of administration. Do not exceed 2.4 g daily.

IV—300 mg every 6 hours. Dilute in 20 ml of saline solution or dextrose 5% and administer over 1 to 2 min *or* dilute in 100 ml of IV fluid and infuse over 15 to 20 min.

NOTE: Initial recommended dosage for patients with impaired renal function is 300 mg every 12 hr.

Pediatric

Cimetidine is not recommended in patients under 16 years of age.

Special remarks and cautions

Adverse reactions reported with use of cimetidine are usually quite mild. Mental confusion, slurred speech, and disorientation are associated with the use of high dosages in patients with renal dysfunction and patients over 50 years of age. Mild bilateral gynecomastia and breast soreness may occur on long-term use (greater than 1 month), but resolves after discontinuation of therapy. Other adverse effects include transient hyperthermia, maculopapular rashes, urticaria, muscular pain, and transient neutropenia.

Safe use in pregnancy has not been established.

Drug interactions

No significant drug interactions have been reported.

CLOFIBRATE
(*Atromid S*)

AHFS 24:06
CATEGORY Antilipemic agent

Action and use

Clofibrate is an antilipemic agent structurally unrelated to other antilipemic agents. It is particularly effective in reducing elevated serum triglyceride levels and is therefore used to treat types III, IV, and V hyperlipoproteinemias. Clofibrate appears to have several sites of action; its mechanisms of action are largely unknown.

Characteristics

Primary activity is due to a metabolite, chlorophenoxyisobutyric acid (CPIB). Onset: 2 to 5 days. Protein binding (CPIB): 95%. Half-life (CPIB): 54 hr. Excretion: in urine, 60% as glucuronide.

Administration and dosage

PO—2 g daily divided into 2 to 4 doses. Administer with meals to reduce stomach upset. NOTE: Prior to initiating therapy, attempts should be made to control serum triglycerides by weight reduction and dietary control. Serum cholesterol and triglyceride levels should be measured prior to and every 2 weeks during initial therapy. After 3 months of therapy, the patient should be fully reevaluated to determine whether further therapy is justified.

Special remarks and cautions

Gastrointestinal complaints of nausea, vomiting, flatulence, and abdominal cramping and diarrhea occur most frequently. Most symptoms are mild and diminish with continued therapy.

Other rare adverse effects include drowsiness, weakness, skin reactions, cardiac arrhythmias, decreased libido in men, and "flu-like symptoms" (muscle aches, soreness, and cramping).

Use clofibrate with caution in patients with hepatic and renal disease. Dosage adjustment may be required if the decision is made to continue therapy.

Do not use in pregnant or lactating women. Animal studies indicate that fetal enzyme immaturity inhibits metabolism of clofibrate. In patients who plan to become pregnant, clofibrate should be withdrawn several months before conception.

Drug interactions

Clofibrate displaces warfarin (Coumadin) from protein-binding sites. If concomitant therapy is indicated, start warfarin at half the normal dosage and adjust the dosage according to the prothrombin time.

Clofibrate may induce hypoglycemic episodes by blocking the renal excretion of the oral hypoglycemic agent chlorpropamide (Diabinese).

Furosemide (Lasix) and clofibrate may compete for similar protein-binding sites. Observe patients receiving both agents for increased clinical response and/or toxicity from either agent.

DIPHENOXYLATE HYDROCHLORIDE

AHFS 56:08; C-V
CATEGORY Antidiarrheal agent

(Lomotil)

Action and use

Diphenoxylate is a synthetic narcotic derivative that diminishes intestinal smooth muscle spasm, thus inhibiting gastrointestinal motility. Lomotil is a combination product containing diphenoxylate, 2.5 mg, and atropine, 0.025 mg. The atropine is added in subtherapeutic dosages to prevent deliberate abuse. Lomotil is used for the symptomatic relief of acute nonspecific diarrhea.

Characteristics

Onset of action: 45 to 60 min. Peak activity: 2 hr. Duration: 3 to 4 hr. Half-life: $2\frac{1}{2}$ hr. Metabolism: to diphenoxylic acid (active) and hydroxydiphenoxylic acid. Excretion: primarily fecal.

Administration and dosage
Adult

PO—Initially, 2 tablets or 10 ml of Lomotil liquid 4 times daily. After control is achieved, reduce the dosage as needed to maintain control (usually 1 tablet 4 times daily).

Pediatric (2 to 12 years of age)

NOTE: Do not use in patients under 2 years of age. Pediatric patients are more susceptible to atropine overdosage.
1. Initial dosage: (Lomotil liquid):

Ages 2 to 5 years

PO—4 ml 3 times daily.

Ages 5 to 8 years

PO—4 ml 4 times daily.

Ages 8 to 12 years

PO—4 ml 5 times daily.
2. After control is achieved, reduce the dosage to half the initial dosage.

Special remarks and cautions

Overdosage of Lomotil results in symptoms related to narcotic analgesic overdosage (diphenoxylate) and atropine toxicity. The full effects of overdosage may not be apparent until 24 to 30 hr after the agent was taken. Early manifestations may include symptoms of atropism such as tachycardia, dry mouth, nose, and throat, flushing, and hyperthermia. Symptoms progress to include drowsiness, hypotonia, hyporeflexia, nystagmus, miosis, and convulsions followed by respiratory depression and total apnea.

All cases of diarrhea should be investigated fully, and specific treatment instituted as soon as possible. Lomotil, an antimotility drug, is indicated only for *symptomatic* control of diarrhea. Do not use in (1) acute diarrhea when bacterial pathogens are suspected, since medications that slow intestinal motility may delay clearance of infecting organisms from the bowel; (2) antibiotic-induced colitis, since it may prolong the disorder; and (3) severe, acute attacks of ulcerative colitis, since antimotility drugs may cause a paralytic ileus with overdilatation of the bowel (toxic megacolon).

Treatment consists of gastric lavage, close observation for at least 48 hr, use of naloxone (Narcan) to reverse respiratory depression, and mechanical ventilatory assistance. Patients may require multiple doses of naloxone because of its short duration of activity. Urinary bladder catheterization may also be necessary because of urinary retention.

Side effects reported during diphenoxylate therapy are usually gastrointestinal in nature and may be related to the condition being treated. Nausea, vomiting, and abdominal distention are common side effects. Other side effects reported include sedation, dizziness, tachycardia, numbness of extremities, blurred vision, weakness, and mental depression.

Allergic manifestations including pruritus, urticaria, and angioneurotic edema have been reported.

Use with caution in patients with cirrhosis or other liver disease. Hepatic coma has been reported following administration of Lomotil to these patients.

Repeated use may lead to tolerance, dependence, and addiction. Evaluate the *patient's* response to this antidiarrheal product and suggest a change to another form of antidiarrheal product when indicated.

Lomotil should be used with caution in pregnant and lactating women. Effects on the fetus are unknown. Diphenoxylate and atropine are excreted in breast milk.

Drug interactions

The depressant effects of diphenoxylate are additive with those of general anesthetics, phenothiazines, tranquilizers, sedative-hypnotics, tricyclic depressants, antihistamines, and other CNS depressants, including alcohol.

IPECAC

AHFS 56:20
CATEGORY Emetic

Action and use

Syrup of ipecac is used to induce vomiting in cases of poisoning by orally ingested drugs and other chemicals.

Characteristics

Onset: 15 to 45 min.

Administration and dosage

PO—15 to 30 ml syrup of ipecac. Administer with copious amounts of fluid.
NOTE: Do *not* use fluid extract of ipecac. It is as much as 14 times more potent than the syrup.

Special remarks and cautions

Do not use emetics in deeply sedated or unconscious patients. Emetics are not active when medullary centers are depressed. Patients may also aspirate gastric contents.

Emetics should not be used in patients who are convulsing or who have ingested a convulsant or corrosives such as alkali (lye), strong acids, strychnine, and strong petroleum distillates (kerosene, gasoline, paint thinner, cleaning fluid).

Toxic effects include sweating, tachycardia, hypotension, dyspnea, and weakness.

Drug interactions

No specific interactions have been reported.

LOPERAMIDE HYDROCHLORIDE
(*Imodium*)

AHFS 56:08; C-V
CATEGORY Antidiarrheal agent

Action and use

Loperamide hydrochloride is a new synthetic orally active antidiarrheal agent. Loperamide slows peristalsis of the gastrointestinal tract by acting directly on cholinergic and noncholinergic nerve receptors in the intestinal wall. The intestinal transit time is prolonged, resulting in greater fecal viscosity and bulk density with reduced loss of fluids and electrolytes. It has been effective in providing symptomatic relief of acute, nonspecific diarrhea and chronic diarrhea associated with inflammatory bowel disease, and in reducing the volume of discharge from ileostomies.

Characteristics

Peak serum levels: 4 hr (PO). There are no published studies on the relationship between plasma levels and clinical response or on whether the delayed transit time caused by loperamide affects its own absorption. Half-life: 7 to 15 hr. Excretion: unchanged in feces, 10% unchanged in urine (PO). The metabolic pathways in humans for the remainder of the drug have not been delineated.

Administration and dosage
Adult

PO 1. Acute diarrhea: initially, 2 capsules (4 mg), followed by 1 capsule (2 mg) after each unformed stool. Daily dosage should not exceed 8 capsules (16 mg). If clinical improvement does not occur within 48 hr, loperamide should be discontinued.
   2. Chronic diarrhea: initially, 2 capsules (4 mg), followed by 1 capsule (2 mg) after each unformed stool until diarrhea is controlled. The average daily maintenance dosage is 2 to 4 capsules (4 to 8 mg)/day.

Pediatric

Safe use in children under 12 years of age has not been established.

Special remarks and cautions

Side effects reported during loperamide therapy have usually been gastrointestinal in nature and may be related to the condition being treated. Constipation is the most frequent adverse effect. Nausea, abdominal pain, dizziness, and dry mouth have occasionally occurred.

All cases of diarrhea should be investigated fully, and specific treatment instituted as soon as possible. Loperamide, an antimotility drug, is indicated only for *symptomatic* control of diarrhea. Do not use in (1) acute diarrhea when bacterial pathogens are suspected, since medications that slow intestinal motility may delay clearance of infecting organisms from the bowel; (2) antibiotic-induced colitis, since loperamide may prolong the disorder; and (3) severe, acute attacks of ulcerative colitis, since antimotility drugs may cause a paralytic ileus with overdilatation of the bowel (toxic megacolon).

Physical dependence has not been observed in humans; however, it has developed in laboratory animals.

Safe use during pregnancy and lactation has not been established.

Drug interactions

No specific drug interactions with loperamide have been reported.

NALOXONE HYDROCHLORIDE

(Narcan)

AHFS 28:10

CATEGORY Narcotic antagonist

Action and use

Naloxone is a semisynthetic narcotic antagonist. It antagonizes respiratory depression induced by natural and synthetic narcotics, pentazocine (Talwin), and propoxyphene (Darvon). When administered to patients who have not recently received narcotics, there is no further respiratory depression, psychomimetic effects, circulatory changes, or other pharmacologic activity. Naloxone is a drug of choice for treatment of respiratory depression when the causative agent is unknown.

Characteristics

Onset: 1 to 2 min (IV), 3 to 5 min (IM or SC). Duration: 3 to 5 hr (dose dependent). Metabolic fate: unknown.

Administration and dosage
Adult

IM—0.4 mg (1 ml). If immediate response is not obtained, the dose may be repeated every 2 to 3 min for 2 to 3 doses.

IV or SC—As for IM administration.

Pediatric

IM—10 μg/kg. The dosage may be repeated every 2 to 3 min for 2 or 3 times.

IV or SC—As for IM administration.

Special remarks and cautions

Because of a relatively short duration of action, naloxone may have to be readministered as the effects of the antagonist subside and those of the narcotic return.

Naloxone is not effective in the treatment of respiratory depression caused by sedatives, hypnotics, anesthetics, or other nonnarcotic CNS depressants.

In patients dependent on opiates, naloxone may precipitate a withdrawal syndrome, the severity of which depends on the dose of the naloxone and the degree of dependence.

Safe use of naloxone during pregnancy has not been determined.

Drug interactions

There are no drug interactions other than that of the antagonist activity toward opiates, pentazocine, and propoxyphene.

OXYTOCIN
(Pitocin, Syntocinon)

AHFS 76:00
CATEGORY Oxytocic

Action and use

Oxytocin is a hormone produced in the hypothalamus and stored in the posterior pituitary gland (neurohypophysis). It has selective stimulatory effects on the smooth muscle of the uterus, blood vessels, and mammary myoepithelium. Oxytocin apparently induces and augments muscular contractility by increasing the permeability of muscle cell membranes to sodium ions, increasing the number of contracting myofibrils. The dosage required to initiate muscular contractions is dependent on the excitability of the muscle tissue. A very low level of muscular activity is present in the human uterus during the first and second trimesters of pregnancy, and the uterus is fairly resistant to the effects of oxytocin. As the third trimester progresses, however, uterine excitability increases significantly, and active labor may be initiated with relatively small doses of exogenous oxytocin.

Oxytocin is the current drug of choice for inducing labor at term and for augmenting uterine contractions during the first and second stages of labor. Oxytocin is routinely administered immediately postpartum to control uterine atony and postpartum hermorrhage. Oxytocin may also be applied intranasally to promote milk ejection and treat breast engorgement during lactation.

Characteristics

Onset of uterine activity: 3 to 7 min (IM), immediate (IV). Duration of uterine activity: 2 to 3 hr (IM), 45 to 60 min (IV). Plasma half-life: 3 to 5 min. Metabolism: lactating mammary gland, liver, kidneys, placenta, uterus. Excretion: small amounts excreted unchanged in urine.

Administration and dosage

For induction of labor:

IV INFUSION—Initial rate: 1 to 2 mU/min. It is strongly recommended that an infusion pump be used to help control the rate of oxytocin infusion. Most pregnancies close to term will respond well to 2 to 10 mU/min. Rarely will a patient require more than 20 mU/min. Those patients at 32 to 36 weeks of gestation often require 20 to 30 mU/min or more to develop a laborlike contractility pattern. Rates of infusion should not be altered more frequently than every 20 to 30 min. It is frequently necessary to reduce or discontinue the infusion as spontaneous uterine activity develops and labor progresses.

For augmentation of labor:

IV INFUSION—Occasionally a labor that started spontaneously may not progress satisfactorily. Labor may be augmented by oxytocin infusions at rates of 0.5 to 2 mU/min.

For milk ejection:

INTRANASAL OXYTOCIN (40 units/ml)—1 spray or 3 drops may be instilled into 1 or both nostrils 2 to 3 min before nursing or pumping of the breasts. The patient should sit upright if using nasal spray and recline if using nasal drops.

Special remarks and cautions

Most clinicians now recommend that fetal monitors be used during infusions of oxytocin. Overdosage of oxytocin may cause hyperstimulation of the uterus, resulting in tetanic contractions with possible abruptio placentae, cervical lacerations, impaired uterine blood flow, and fetal trauma and hypoxia manifested by fetal bradycardia, tachycardia, and arrhythmias.

Oxytocin has some minor antidiuretic activity. When administered in large dosages or over prolonged periods with electrolyte-free solutions, water intoxication manifested by drowsiness, listlessness, headache, confusion, anuria, edema, and seizure activity may develop.

Side effects that may occur include nausea, vomiting, hypotension, tachycardia, and cardiac arrhythmias.

Drug interactions

Anesthetics used during labor and delivery may modify the cardiovascular effects (blood pressure, heart rate) of oxytocin.

PHYSOSTIGMINE SALICYLATE

AHFS 12:08
(Antilirium)   CATEGORY Anticholinesterase agent

Action and use

Physostigmine enhances cholinergic activity by inhibiting cholinesterase, the enzyme that destroys acetylcholine. Consequently parasympathetic activity is sustained by physostigmine administration. Physostigmine is used as an antidote for reversing most of the cardiovascular (tachycardia, arrhythmias) and CNS effects (delirium, coma) of overdosage with tricyclic antidepressants (amitriptyline [Elavil], imipramine [Tofranil], doxepin [Sinequan) and belladonna alkaloids (atropine, scopolamine).

Characteristics

Onset: 3 to 8 min. Duration: 30 to 60 min.

Administration and dosage
Adult

IV 1. Therapeutic trial: 2 mg slowly at a rate of 1 mg/min. A second dose of 1 to 2 mg may be repeated in 20 min if there is no response.
    2. Therapeutic dose: 1 to 4 mg slowly as life-threatening symptoms recur.
IM—As for IV administration.

Pediatric

IV 1. Therapeutic trial: 0.5 mg slowly over 1 min. Repeat at 5-min intervals if no cholinergic effects are produced and there are no therapeutic effects. Maximum dosage is 2 mg.
    2. Therapeutic dose: the lowest effective trial dose.

NOTE: Physostigmine overdosage may result in cholinergic crisis. Overdosage may be manifested by excessive salivation and sweating, pupil constriction, nausea, vomiting, bradycardia, tachycardia, hypertension, hypotension, confusion, convulsions, coma, and paralysis. Treat with mechanical respiration, frequent bronchial aspiration, and atropine, 2 to 4 mg IV every 3 to 10 min until symptoms reverse. Atropine, however, will not reverse muscular weakness and respiratory depression. Pralidoxime chloride (Protopam) may be useful in treating this adverse effect.

Special remarks and cautions

Side effects of physostigmine usually result from enhanced parasympathetic activity caused by the blockade of acetylcholine's metabolic enzyme. They include salivation, sweating, lacrimation, nausea, vomiting, diarrhea, irregular pulse, and palpitations. The dosage should be reduced if they become prominent.

Physostigmine should be used with caution in patients with epilepsy, parkinsonism, or bradycardia.

Physostigmine should be used with extreme caution in patients with asthma, diabetes, cardiovascular disease, or mechanical obstruction of the intestinal or urogenital tract.

Physostigmine crosses the placental barrier. It should only be used in pregnant women when the benefit of therapy outweighs the risk to the mother and the fetus.

Drug interactions

Physostigmine exaggerates the activity of other cholinergic agents such as bethanechol (Urecholine), methacholine (Mecholyl), and edrophonium (Tensilon).

Physostigmine may potentiate muscular paralysis induced by depolarizing neuromuscular blocking agents (decamethonium [Syncurine] and succinylcholine [Anectine]).

Physostigmine may antagonize muscular paralysis induced by nondepolarizing neuromuscular blocking agents (gallamine [Flaxedil], pancuronium [Pavulon], and tubocurarine).

PROBUCOL
(Lorelco)

AHFS 24:06
CATEGORY Antilipemic agent

Action and use

Probucol is used to reduce elevated serum cholesterol levels in patients with primary type II hyperlipoproteinemia. Effects on serum triglyceride levels are variable. The mechanism of action is unknown, and therapy should be instituted only after dietary therapy has failed to reduce elevated cholesterol levels adequately.

Characteristics

Probucol is poorly absorbed from the gastrointestinal tract, and 3 months of therapy may be required before significant reduction in serum cholesterol levels is noted. Elimination is biphasic; initial phase half-life is 24 hr, second phase half-life is about 20 days. Metabolic fate is unknown.

Administration and dosage

PO—500 mg twice daily administered *with* meals.

Special remarks and cautions

Diarrhea may occur in about 10% of patients. Flatulence, nausea, and vomiting may also occur, but they are usually mild and subside with continued administration. Hyperhydrosis (excessive perspiration) and foul-smelling sweat have also been reported. Of patients in clinical trials, 2% discontinued therapy because of side effects.

Prior to initiation of therapy, hypercholesterolemia must first be treated by weight reduction and dietary control. Serum cholesterol and triglyceride levels should be measured prior to and during therapy. After 6 months of therapy, the patient must be reevaluated to determine whether further therapy is justified.

Safe use of probucol in pregnant or lactating patients has not been established.

Drug interactions

No specific drug interactions have been reported.

SODIUM BICARBONATE

AHFS 40:08
CATEGORY Alkalinizing agent

Action and use

As an alkalinizing agent, sodium bicarbonate increases plasma bicarbonate, buffers excess hydrogen ion, and increases blood pH. It is used to treat metabolic acidosis as a result of a variety of conditions including renal disease, diabetes, circulatory insufficiency caused by shock or dehydration, and cardiac arrest. It is also indicated in barbiturate intoxication and salicylate or methyl alcohol poisoning.

Administration and dosage

IV—Initial dose: 1 mEq/kg bolus, followed by 1 ampule (50 ml = 1 mEq/ml) every 5 to 10 min as dictated by the patient's condition.

Special remarks and cautions

It is recommended that, in hospitalized patients, further administration of sodium bicarbonate be governed by arterial blood gas and pH measurement.

Be aware of other drugs running in the same IV line. Many drugs used in critical medicine are unstable in alkaline media (for example, calcium chloride, calcium gluconate, dopamine hydrochloride, and penicillin G).

GENERAL INFORMATION ON LAXATIVES
Classification

Saline: hypertonicity of the saline cathartic increases liquid in the colon.

Irritants or stimulants: increase intestinal tract motor activity.

Bulk-producing products: absorb imbibed water, adding bulk and moisture to the feces, thus causing distention and elimination.

Emollients: lubricate the intestinal tract and soften feces.

Fecal softeners: penetrate and soften fecal masses through the action of the contained wetting agents.

Contraindications

Do not administer when nausea, vomiting, abdominal pain, or other symptoms of appendicitis are present.

Do not administer when fecal impaction exists or when there is intestinal obstruction, hemorrhage, severe spasm, diarrhea, or intestinal perforation.

Warnings and precautions

Use laxatives with caution in presence of inflamed or irritable colon.

Rectal bleeding or failure to respond to enema therapy may indicate a serious condition that may have to be treated surgically.

Persons with a hernia, severe hypertension, or cardiovascular disease and those who are about to undergo or who have undergone surgery for hemorrhoids or other anorectal disorders should not strain at the stool. In such cases an emollient fecal-softening laxative is indicated.

Table 22-1. Laxative active ingredients

Product	Stimulant	Saline	Bulk-forming	Emollient	Fecal softener
Agoral	Phenolphthalein	—	—	Mineral oil	—
Colace	—	—	—	—	Dioctyl sodium sulfosuccinate
Dialose	—	—	Sodium carboxy-methylcellulose	—	Diocytl sodium sulfosuccinate
Dialose Plus	Casanthranol	—	Sodium carboxy-methylcellulose	—	Diocytl sodium sulfosuccinate
Doxidan	Danthron	—	—	—	Diocytl sodium sulfosuccinate
Dulcolax	Bisacodyl	—	—	—	—
Haley's M-O	—	Milk of magnesia	—	Mineral oil	—
Peri-Colace	Casanthranol	—	—	—	Dioctyl sodium sulfosuccinate
Phillip's Milk of Magnesia	—	Milk of magnesia	—	—	—
Sufak	—	—	—	—	Dioctyl calcium sulfosuccinate
X-Prep	Standardized senna concentrate	—	—	—	—

Common medical abbreviations

A

A	Assessment (POMR)
A_2	Aortic second sound
$A_2 > P_2$	Aortic sound larger than second pulmonary sound
AAL	Anterior axillary line
Ab	Abortion
Abd	Abdomen, abdominal
ABE	Acute bacterial endocarditis
ABG	Arterial blood gases
ACD	Anterior chest diameter
ADH	Antidiuretic hormone
ADT	Alternate day therapy
AF	Atrial fibrillation; acid fast
AFB	Acid fast bacteria; acid fast bacilli
A/G	Albumin to globulin ratio
AGN	Acute glomerular nephritis
AHF	Antihemophilic factor
AHFS	American Hospital Formulary Service
AHG	Antihemophilic globulin
AI	Aortic insufficiency
AJ	Ankle jerk
AK	Above knee (amputation)
ALD	Alcoholic liver disease
ALL	Acute lymphocytic leukemia
ALS	Amyotrophic lateral sclerosis
AMA	Against medical advice
AMI	Acute myocardial infarction
ANA	Antinuclear antibodies
AODM	Adult onset diabetes mellitus
A & P	Anterior and posterior; auscultation and percussion
ASAP	As soon as possible
AP	Apical pulse, anteroposterior
APB	Atrial premature beats
AS	Anal sphincter; arteriosclerosis
ASCVD	Arteriosclerotic cardiovascular disease
ASHD	Arteriosclerotic heart disease
ASO	Anti-streptolysin titer; arteriosclerosis obliterans
ATN	Acute tubular necrosis
AV	Arteriovenous; atrioventricular
A & W	Alive and well

B

BAL	British anti-lewisite (dimercaprol)
bands	Banded neutrophils
BBB	Bundle branch block; blood brain barrier
BBT	Basal body temperature
BE	Barium enema; base excess
BEI	Butanol-extractable iodine
bili	Bilirubin
BJ	Biceps jerk; bone and joint
BK	Below knee (amputation)
BLB	A type of oxygen mask
BLOBS	Bladder observation
BM	Bowel movement; basal metabolism
BMR	Basal metabolic rate
B & O	Belladonna and opium
BP	Blood pressure; British Pharmacopoeia
BPH	Benign prostatic hypertrophy
BRP	Bathroom privileges
BS	Bowel sounds; breath sounds
BSO	Bilateral salpingoophorectomy
BSP	Bromsulphalein
BT	Breast tumor; brain tumor
BTL	Bilateral tubal ligation
BTFS	Breast tumor frozen section
BU	Bodansky unit
BUN	Blood urea nitrogen
BVL	Bilateral vas ligation
BW	Body weight
Bx	Biopsy

C

C	Centigrade, Celsius
C_2	Second cervical vertebra
CA	Carbonic anhydrase
Ca	Cancer, calcium
C & A	Clinitest and Acetest
CAD	Coronary artery disease
CBC	Complete blood count
CC	Chief complaint
CCR	Creatinine clearance
CCU	Coronary Care Unit
Ceph floc	Cephalin flocculation
CF	Complement fixation
CHF	Congestive heart failure
CHO	Carbohydrate
Chol	Cholesterol
CI	Color index; contraindication
CK	Check
CLL	Chronic lymphocytic leukemia
CNS	Central nervous system
COAP	Cyclophosphamide, Oncovin, Ara-C, Prednisone
C/O	Complains of
Cong	Congenital
COP	Cyclophosphamide, Oncovin, Prednisone
COPD	Chronic obstructive pulmonary disease
CPK	Creatine phosphokinase
C & P	Cystoscopy and pyelography
CP	Cerebral palsy; cleft plate
CPR	Cardiopulmonary resuscitation
CR	Cardiorespiratory
CRF	Chronic renal failure
CRP	C-reactive protein
CS	Coronary sclerosis
C & S	Culture and sensitivity
CSF	Cerebrospinal fluid
C sect	Cesarean section
CT	Circulation time
CV	Cardiovascular; costovertebral angle
CVA	Cerebrovascular accident
CVP	Central venous pressure
CX	Cervix, cervical
CXR	Chest x-ray

D

DC (D/C)	Discontinue
D & C	Dilatation and curretage
DD	Differential diagnosis
DDD	Degenerative disc disease
DIC	Disseminated intravascular coagulation
Diff	Differential blood count
DJD	Degenerative joint disease
DM	Diabetes mellitus
DOA	Dead on arrival
DOE	Dyspnea on exertion
DPT	Diphtheria, pertussis, and tetanus
DSD	Dry sterile dressing
DT	Delirium tremens
DTR	Deep tendon reflex
Dx	Diagnosis
D_5W	Dextrose 5% in water

E

E	Enema
EBL	Estimated blood loss
ECF	Extracellular fluid
ECG	Electrocardiogram
ECT	Electroconvulsive therapy
ECW	Extracellular water
EDC	Expected date of confinement (obstetrics)
EEG	Electroencephalogram
EENT	Eyes, ears, nose, throat
EFA	Essential fatty acids
EH	Enlarged heart
EKG	Electrocardiogram
EM	Electron microscope
EMG	Electromyography
ENT	Ears, nose, and throat
ER	Emergency Room
ESR	Erythrocyte sedimentation rate (sed rate)
EST	Electroshock therapy
EUA	Examine under anesthesia

F

F	Fahrenheit
FB	Finger breadths; foreign bodies
FBS	Fasting blood sugar
FEV_1	Forced expiratory volume in one second
FF	Filtration fraction
FFA	Free fatty acids
FH	Family history

FLK	Funny looking kid
FP	Family practice; family planning
FSH	Follicle-stimulating hormone
FTA	Fluorescent treponemal antibody
FUO	Fever of undetermined origin
Fx	Fracture; fraction

G

G	Gravida
GA	General appearance
GB	Gallbladder
GC	Gonococcus; gonorrhea
GFR	Glomerular filtration rate
GI	Gastrointestinal
G6PD	Glucose-6-phosphate dehydrogenase
G-P-	Gravida-; para-
GU	Genitourinary
GYN	Gynecology

H

H	Hypodermic; heroin
HA	Headache
HAA	Hepatitis-associated antigen
HBP	High blood pressure
Hct	Hematocrit
HCVD	Hypertensive cardiovascular disease
HEENT	Head, eyes, ears, nose, throat
Hgb	Hemoglobin
HHD	Hypertensive heart disease
HO	House officer
HOB	Head of bed
HPF	High power field
HPI	History of present illness
HSA	Human serum albumin
HTN	Hypertension
HTVD	Hypertensive vascular disease
Hx	History

I

IASD	Intra-atrial septal defect
IBC	Iron binding capacity
IBI	Intermittent bladder irrigation
ICF	Intracellular fluid volume
ICM	Intracostal margin

ICS	Intercostal space
ICU	Intensive Care Unit
ICW	Intracellular water
ID	Initial dose; intradermal
I & D	Incision and drainage
IDU	Idoxuridine
I & O	Intake and output
IHSS	Idiopathic hypertrophic subaortic stenosis
IM	Intramuscular
Imp	Impression
Int	Internal
IP	Intraperitoneal
IPPB	Intermittent positive pressure breathing
ISW	Interstitial water
ITh	Intrathecal
IU	International unit
IUD	Intrauterine device (contraceptive)
IVP	Intravenous pyelogram
IVPB	Intravenous piggyback
IVSD	Intraventricular septal defect

J

JRA	Juvenile rheumatoid arthritis
JVD	Jugular venous distention

K

K^+	Potassium
KO	Keep open
17-KS	17-Ketosteroids
KUB	Kidney, ureter, and bladder
K.W.	Keith Wagner (ophthalmoscopic findings)

L

L_2	Second lumbar vertebra
LA	Left atrium
Lap	Laparotomy
LATS	Long-acting thyroid stimulator
LBBB	Left bundle branch block
LCM	Left costal margin
LD	Longitudinal diameter (of heart)
LDH	Lactic dehydrogenase
LDL	Low density lipoproteins
LE	Lupus erythematosus
LFT's	Liver function tests

LHF	Left heart failure
LKS	Liver, kidneys, and spleen
LLE	Left lower extremity
LLL	Left lower lobe
LLQ	Left lower quadrant (abdomen)
LMD	Local medical doctor
LML	Left middle lobe (lung)
LMP	Last menstrual period
LOA	Left occipital anterior
LOM	Limitation of motion
LOP	Left occipital posterior
LP	Lumbar puncture
lpf	Low power field
LUQ	Left upper quadrant
LVH	Left ventricular hypertrophy
L & W	Living and well
LWCT	Lee-White clotting time
lytes	Electrolytes

M

M	Murmur
M^2	Square meters of body surface
M_1	First mitral sound
MCH	Mean corpuscular hemoglobin
MCHC	Mean corpuscular hemoglobin concentration
MCL	Midclavicular line
MCV	Mean corpuscular volume
MF	Myocardial fibrosis
MH	Marital history; menstrual history
MI	Myocardial infarction; mitral insufficiency
MIC	Minimum inhibitory concentration
MJT	Mead Johnson tube
ML	Midline
MOM	Milk of Magnesia
MS	Morphine sulfate; multiple sclerosis; mitral stenosis
MSL	Midsternal line

N

N	Normal; Negro
NAD	No acute distress; no apparent distress
NG	Nasogastric
NM	Neuromuscular

NPN	Nonprotein nitrogen
NPO	Nothing by mouth
NR	No refill
NS	Normal saline
NSFTD	Normal spontaneous full-term delivery
NSR	Normal sinus rhythm
NTG	Nitroglycerin
NVD	Nausea, vomiting, diarrhea; neck vein distention
NYD	Not yet diagnosed

O

Oz	Oxygen
O	Objective data (POMR)
OB	Obstetrics; occult blood
OOB	Out of bed
OOBBRP	Out of bed with bathroom privileges
OD	Overdose
OR	Operating room
OT	Occupational therapy

P

P	Plan (POMR), pulse
P & A	Palpation and auscultation
PA	Posteroanterior
PAT	Paroxysmal atrial tachycardia
PBI	Protein-bound iodine
PC	After meals
PCN	Penicillin
PCV	Packed cell volume (hematocrit)
PE	Physical examination
PEEP	Positive and expiratory pressure
PEG	Pneumoencephalogram
PERRLA	Pupils equal, round, react to light and accommodation
PH	Past history
PI	Present illness
PID	Pelvic inflammatory disease
PIE	Pulmonary infiltration with eosinophilia
PKU	Phenylketonuria
PMH	Past medical history
PMI	Point of maximal impulse or maximum intensity
PMN	Polymorphonuclear neutrophil
PMT	Premenstrual tension

PND	Paroxysmal nocturnal dyspnea
PNX	Pneumothorax
POMR	Problem-oriented medical record
Postop	After surgery
PO	By mouth
PP	Postpartum; postprandial
PPD	Purified protein derivative
PPL	Penicilloyl-polylysine conjugate
P & R	Pulse and respiration
Preop	Before surgery
PT	Physical therapy; prothrombin time
PTA	Prior to admission
PUD	Peptic ulcer disease
PVC	Premature ventricular contraction
PZI	Protamine zinc insulin

R

R	Respiration
RA	Rheumatoid arthritis; right atrium
RBC	Red blood cell
RBF	Renal blood flow
RCM	Right costal margin
RF	Rheumatoid factor
RHD	Rheumatic heart disease; renal hypertensive disease
RISA	Radioactive iodine serum albumin
RLL	Right lower lobe
RLQ	Right lower quadrant
RO	Rule out
ROM	Range of motion
ROS	Review of systems; review of symptoms
RPF	Renal plasma flow; relaxed pelvic floor
RQ	Respiratory quotient
RR	Recovery room; respiratory rate
RSR	Regular sinus rhythm
RTA	Renal tubular acidosis
RTN	Renal tubular necrosis
RUL	Right upper lobe
RUQ	Right upper quadrant
RV	Right ventricle
RVH	Right ventricular hypertrophy

S

S	Subjective data (POMR)
S_1	First heart sound
S_2	Second heart sound
SA	Sinoatrial
SBE	Subacute bacterial endocarditis
SC	Subclavian, subcutaneous
Sed rate	Erythrocyte sedimentation rate
Segs	Segmented neutrophils
SGOT	Serum glutamic oxaloacetic transaminase
SGPT	Serum glutamic pyruvic transaminase
SH	Social history; serum hepatitis
SID	Sudden infant death
SL	Sublingual
SLE	Systemic lupus erythematosus
SLDH	Serum lactic dehydrogenase
SMA	Serial multiple analysis
SOAP	Subjective, objective, assessment plan (POMR)
SOB	Shortness of breath
S/P	Status post
SR	Sedimentation rate (ESR)
SSE	Saline solution enema; soapsuds enema
SSPE	Subacute sclerosing panencephalitis
STD	Skin test dose
STS	Serologic test for syphilis
SVC	Superior vena cava

T

T	Temperature
T_3	Triiodothyronine
T_4	Thyroxin
T & A	Tonsillectomy and adenoidectomy
TAH	Total abdominal hysterectomy
TAO	Thromboangiitis obliterans
TB	Tuberculosis
TBW	Total body water
TD	Transverse diameter (of heart)
TEDS	Elastic stockings
TIA	Transient ischemic attack
TIBC	Total iron-binding capacity

TKO	To keep open
TLC	Tender loving care
TM	Tympanic membrane
TP	Total protein; thrombophlebitis
TPI	*Treponema pallidum* immobilization
TPN	Total parenteral nutrition
TPR	Temperature, pulse, and respiration
TRA	To run at
T-set	Tracheotomy set
TSH	Thyroid stimulating hormone
TUR	Transurethral resection
TV	*Trichomonas vaginalis*

U

UA (U/A)	Urinalysis
U & C	Urethral and cervical
UCHD	Unusual childhood diseases
UGI	Upper gastrointestinal
URI	Upper respiratory infection
UTI	Urinary tract infection

V

V	Vein
Vag hyst	Vaginal hysterectomy
VAH	Veteran's Administration Hospital
VC	Vena cava
VCU	Voiding cystourethrogram
VDRL	Venereal Disease Research Laboratories (for syphilis)
VF	Ventricular fibrillation
VMA	Vanillylmandelic acid
VP	Venous pressure
VPC	Ventricular premature contraction
VS	Vital signs
VSD	Ventricular septal defect
VT	Ventricular tachycardia

W

W	White; widow
WBC	White blood cell; white blood count
WDWN-WF	Well developed, well nourished, white female
WDWN-WM	Well developed, well nourished, white male
WNL	Within normal limits
Wt	Weight

Derivatives of medical terminology

adeno-	gland	*lipo-*	fat
adreno-	adrenal gland	*litho-*	stone
-algia	pain	*lympho-*	lymph
angio-	vessel	*macro-*	large
arterio-	artery	*masto-*	breast
arthro-	joint	*medius*	middle
auto-	self	*megalo-*	huge
broncho-	bronchus	*meningo-*	meninges
brachy-	short	*metra-, metro-*	uterus
brady-	slow	*micro-*	small
carcino-	cancer	*myco-*	fungus
cardio-	heart	*myelo-*	bone marrow; spinal cord
cele-	herniation		
-centesis	puncture	*myo-*	muscle
chole-	bile	*necro-*	death
chondro-	cartilage	*neo-*	new
costo-	ribs	*nephro-*	kidney
cranio-	head	*neuro-*	nerve
cysto-	bladder	*oculo-*	eye
cyto-	cell	*oligo-*	few
derma-	skin	*-oma*	tumor
diplo-	double	*oophoro-*	ovary
-ectomy	out	*orchio-, orchido-*	testes
edem-	swell	*os*	mouth; bone
entero-	intestines	*-osis*	condition
erythro-	red	*osteo-*	bone
gastro-	stomach	*-ostomy*	opening
glomerulo-	glomerulus	*-otomy*	into
glyco-	sweet	*patho-*	disease
hem-, hemato-	blood	*phago-*	eat
hepato-	liver	*phlebo-*	vein
-hesion	join together	*-phobia*	fear
hetero-	different	*pilo-*	hair
homo-	same	*-plegia*	paralysis
hydro-	wet, water	*pneumo-*	lungs; air
hystero-	uterus	*procto-*	rectum
ileo-	ileum	*ptosis*	fall
-itis	inflammation	*pyelo-*	pelvis of kidney
jejuno-	jejunum	*pyo-*	pus
laparo-	loin or flank	*rhino-*	nose
laryngo-	larynx	*-rrhagia*	burst forth
leuko-	white	*-rrhaphy*	suture

rrhea	flow; discharge	*thyro-*	thyroid
sero-	serum	*tom-*	cut
splanchno-	viscera	*tricho-*	hair
spleno-	spleen	*uretero-*	ureter
-stasis	stop	*urethro-*	urethra
stoma-	mouth	*uro-*	urine
tachy-	fast; swift	*vaso-*	vessel
thrombo-	clot	*veno-*	vein

Prescription abbreviations

aa, a̅a̅	of each (equal parts)		o.u.	both eyes
a.c.	before meals		p.c.	after meals
ad	to; up to		p.r.n.	as needed
ad lib	as much as desired		q	every
b.i.d.	twice daily		qd	once daily
c̄, c	with		q.i.d.	four times daily
caps	capsules		qod	every other day
d	day		s̄	without
et	and		sig.	label
ext	an extract		ss	one-half
fl	fluid		stat	at once
gtt	a drop		t.i.d.	three times daily
h.s.	at bedtime		ung	ointment
o.d.	right eye		ut dict.	as directed
o.s.	left eye			

Mathematic conversions

Abbreviations

kg = kilograms	ng = nanograms	mEq = milliequivalent
g = grams	m = meter	μm = micron
mg = milligrams	cm = centimeter	L = liter
μg = micrograms	mm = millimeter	ml = milliliter

Metric system	Common system
WEIGHT	**APOTHECARY WEIGHT**
1 kilogram = 1000 grams	1 scruple (Ə) = 20 grains (gr)
1 gram = 1000 milligrams	60 grains = 1 dram (ʒ)
1 milligram = 1000 micrograms	8 drams = 1 ounce (ʒ)
1 microgram = 0.001 milligram	1 ounce = 480 grains
1 milligram = 0.001 gram	12 ounces = 1 pound
1 gram = 0.001 kilogram	
	AVOIRDUPOIS WEIGHT
VOLUME	1 ounce (oz) = 437.5 grains
1 deciliter = 100 milliliters	1 pound (lb) = 16 ounces
1 liter = 1000 milliliters	
1 milliliter = 0.001 liter	**APOTHECARY VOLUME**
1 deciliter = 0.1 liter	60 minims (♏) = 1 fluidram (flʒ)
	8 fluidrams = 1 fluid ounce (flʒ)
LENGTH	1 fluid ounce = 480 minims
1 centimeter = 10 millimeters	16 fluid ounces = 1 pint (pt)
1 decimeter = 10 centimeters	
1 meter = 10 decimeters	**LENGTH**
1 kilometer = 1000 meters	12 inches = 1 foot
1 millimeter = 0.1 centimeter	36 inches = 1 yard
1 centimeter = 0.1 decimeter	3 feet = 1 yard
1 decimeter = 0.1 meter	5280 feet = 1 mile
1 meter = 0.001 kilometer	1760 yards = 1 mile

Continued.

Metric and common system equivalents

MILLIGRAMS	GRAMS	GRAINS		
			1 gram	= 15.4 grains
			1 grain	= 64.8 milligrams
.1	.0001	1/600	1 ounce (℥)	= 31.1 grams
.2	.0002	1/300	1 ounce (oz)	= 28.3 grams
.3	.0003	1/200	1 pound (lb)	= 453.6 grams
.4	.0004	1/150	1 kilogram (kg)	= 2.2 pounds
.5	.0005	1/120	1 milliliter (ml)	= 16.23 minims
.6	.0006	1/100	1 minim (♏)	= 0.06 ml
1.0	.001	1/60	1 fluid ounce (fl℥)	= 29.5 ml
2.0	.002	1/30	1 pint	= 473 ml
10	.01	1/6	1 meter	= 39.3 inches
15	.015	1/4	1 kilometer	= .6 mile
30	.03	1/2	1 mile	= 1.6 mile
45	.045	3/4	1 inch	= 2.54 cm
60 (65)	.06	1	1 foot	= 30 cm
300 (330)	.3	5	1 yard	= .9 meter
600 (650)	.6	10		
1000	1.0	15		
2000	2.0	30		
3000	3.0	45		

Approximate household measurements

1 teaspoonful		5 ml
1 dessertspoonful		10 ml
1 tablespoonful	½ fl oz	15 ml
1 jigger	1½ fl oz	45 ml
1 wineglassful	2 fl oz	60 ml
1 teacupful	4 fl oz	120 ml
1 glassful (tumblerful)	8 fl oz	240 ml

Temperature conversion table

F	C	F	C	F	C
95.0	35.0	98.4	36.9	101.8	38.7
.2	35.1	.6	37.0	102.0	38.8
.4	35.2	.8	37.1	.2	38.9
.6	35.3	99.0	37.2	.4	39.1
.8	35.4	.2	37.3	.6	39.2
96.0	35.5	.4	37.4	.8	39.3
.2	35.6	.6	37.5	103.0	39.4
.4	35.7	.8	37.6	.2	39.5
.6	35.9	100.0	37.7	.4	39.6
.8	36.0	.2	37.8	.6	39.7
97.0	36.1	.4	37.9	.8	39.8
.2	36.2	.6	38.1	104.0	40.0
.4	36.3	.8	38.2	.2	40.1
.6	36.4	101.0	38.3	.4	40.2
.8	36.5	.2	38.4	.6	40.3
98.0	36.6	.4	38.5	.8	40.4
.2	36.7	.6	38.6	105.0	40.5

$C° = 5/9 \, (F° - 32°); \ F° = 9/5 \, C° + 32°$

Continued.

Weight conversion table

lb	kg	lb	kg	lb	kg
5	2.3	105	47.7	210	95.5
10	4.5	110	50	220	100
15	6.8	115	52.3	230	104.5
20	9.1	120	54.5	240	109
25	11.4	125	56.8	250	113.6
30	13.6	130	59	260	118.2
35	15.9	135	61.4	270	122.7
40	18.1	140	63.6	280	127.2
45	20.4	145	66	290	131.8
50	22.7	150	68.1	300	136.4
55	25	155	70.5	310	140.9
60	27.3	160	72.7	320	145.5
65	29.5	165	75	330	150
70	31.8	170	77.3	340	154.5
75	34.1	175	79.5	350	159
80	36.4	180	81.8	360	163.6
85	38.6	185	84.1	370	168.2
90	40.9	190	86.4	380	172.7
95	43.2	195	88.6	390	177.2
100	45.4	200	90.9	400	181.8

1 lb = 0.454 kg; 1 kg = 2.2 lb

Formulas for the calculation of infants' and children's dosages

Children's dosages

Bastedo's rule:

Child's approximate dose $= \dfrac{\text{age in years} + 3}{30} \times \text{adult dose}$

Clark's rule:

Child's approximate dose $= \dfrac{\text{weight of child (in pounds)}}{150} \times \text{adult dose}$

Cowling's rule:

Child's approximate dose $= \dfrac{\text{age (in years on next birthday)}}{24} \times \text{adult dose}$

Dilling's rule:

Child's approximate dose $= \dfrac{\text{age (in years)}}{20} \times \text{adult dose}$

Young's rule:

Child's approximate dose $= \dfrac{\text{age of child (in years)}}{\text{age} + 12} \times \text{adult dose}$

Infants' dosages (younger than 1 year of age)

Fried's rule:

Infant dose $= \dfrac{\text{age (in months)}}{150} \times \text{adult dose}$

Pediatric emergency drug dosages*

Drug	Dosage	10 pounds (4.5 kg)	20 pounds (9.1 kg)	30 pounds (13.6 kg)	40 pounds (18.2 kg)	50 pounds (22.7 kg)	60 pounds (27.3 kg)	Reference
Atropine sulfate 0.4 mg/1 ml ampules	0.01 mg/kg/dose IV (maximum, 0.4 mg)	0.045 mg (0.11 ml)	0.09 mg (0.22 ml)	0.14 mg (0.35 ml)	0.18 mg (0.45 ml)	0.23 mg (0.58 ml)	0.27 mg (0.68 ml)	Shirkey Schwerman
Calcium chloride (10%) solution 100 mg/ml-10 ml ampules; contains 270 mg Ca^{++}/10 ml	0.2 ml/kg IV (equivalent to 5 mg Ca^{++}/kg) (maximum, 1 ml/5 kg) Administer at rate of 1 ml/min	22.5 mg (0.90 ml)	45.0 mg (1.82 ml)	68.0 mg (2.70 ml)	91.0 mg (3.64 ml)	113.5 mg (4.54 ml)	136.5 mg (5.46 ml)	Schwerman AHA Nelson
Calcium gluconate 100 mg/ml-10 ml ampules; contains 97 mg Ca^{++}/10 ml	0.52 ml/kg IV (equivalent to 5 mg Ca^{++}/kg) (maximum, 10 ml) Inject at 1 ml/min	22.5 mg (2.34 ml)	45.0 mg (4.68 ml)	68.0 mg (7.02 ml)	91.0 mg (9.36 ml)	97 mg (10.0 ml)	97 mg (10.0 ml)	Schwerman Kempe
Digoxin (Lanoxin) IM, IV 0.5 mg/2 ml ampules	Premature: 0.015 mg/kg STAT, then 0.0075 mg/kg q 12 hr × 2 doses 2 weeks to 2 years: 0.02 mg/kg STAT, then 0.01 mg/kg q 12 hr × 2 doses	0.068 mg/ 0.27 ml then 0.034 mg/ 0.14 ml 0.09 mg/ 0.36 ml then 0.045 mg/ 0.18 ml	0.18 mg/ 0.72 ml then 0.09 mg/ 0.36 ml	0.27 mg/ 1.08 ml then 0.135 mg/ 0.54 ml	0.36 mg/ 1.44 ml then 0.18 mg/ 0.72 ml	0.45 mg/ 1.80 ml then 0.23 mg/ 0.9 ml	0.54 mg/ 2.16 ml then 0.27 mg/ 1.08 ml	Shirkey

Phenytoin (Dilantin) IV 50 mg/ml in a 2 ml syringe	Anticonvulsant dose: 1 to 5 mg/kg/24 hr Single dose or divide into 2 doses Give IV slowly (50 mg/min) NOTE: Values given are for single dose	4.5 mg/ 0.09 ml to 22.5 mg/ 0.45 ml	9.1 mg/ 0.18 ml to 45.0 mg/ 0.9 ml	13.5 mg/ 0.27 ml to 67.5 mg/ 1.35 ml	18.2 mg/ 0.36 ml to 90 mg/ 1.8 ml	22.7 mg/ 0.45 ml to 112.5 mg/ 2.25 ml	27.3 mg/ 0.54 ml to 135 mg/ 2.70 ml	Shirkey Kempe
Epinephrine hydrochloride (1:1000) SC 1 ml ampules	0.01 ml/kg/dose (maximum, 0.5 ml) May repeat at 15-min intervals, 2 to 3 times NOTE: Dose given in ml rather than mg	0.045 ml	0.09 ml	0.14 ml	0.18 ml	0.23 ml	0.27 ml	Shirkey
Epinephrine (1:10,000) IV Add 9.0 ml of normal saline to 1.0 ml ampule of epinephrine 1:1000. Resultant solution is 1:10,000 conc. for IV use	0.1 ml/kg/dose Repeat q 3 to 5 minutes to have persistent effect NOTE: Dose given in ml rather than mg	0.45 ml	0.91 ml	1.36 ml	1.82 ml	2.27 ml	2.73 ml	Shirkey AHA
Isoproterenol hydrochloride (Isuprel hydrochloride) 1.0 mg/5 ml ampules	NOT GIVEN DIRECT IV Add 1.0 mg isoproterenol to 250 ml of D-5-W. This provides a solution containing	NOT RECOMMENDED FOR DIRECT IV INJECTION FOR CHILDREN GIVE BY IV INFUSION						Schwerman Kempe

*Shirkey, H. C., editor: Pediatric therapy, ed. 5, St. Louis, 1975, The C. V. Mosby Co.

Continued.

Drug	Dosage	10 pounds (4.5 kg)	20 pounds (9.1 kg)	30 pounds (13.6 kg)	40 pounds (18.2 kg)	50 pounds (22.7 kg)	60 pounds (27.3 kg)	Reference
Isoproterenol hydrochloride—cont'd	4 mcg per ml of isoproterenol HCl. Attach a Mini-Dripper to the IV set and administer at an initial rate of 5 mcgtts/min.							
Levarterenol bitartrate (Levophed) IV 4 ml ampules containing 0.2% levarterenol bitartrate (equiv. to 0.1% base) 1 ml of solution = 1 mg of base	Place 2 ml of 0.2% solution (as supplied by ampule) in 500 ml D-5-W. Administer at 0.5 ml/min to give 2 mcg (base/min). Titrate with blood pressure. To prevent sloughing and necrosis in areas in which extravasation has taken place, infiltrate *as soon as possible* with 10 to 15 ml of normal saline containing 5 to 10 mg phentolamine (Regitine)	DO NOT GIVE DIRECTLY IV, BUT RATHER BY IV INFUSION						Shirkey
Lidocaine hydrochloride IV 2% solution in ampules (100 mg/5	1 mg/kg (maximum, up to 15 mg, if under 55 pounds) (maximum, up to 25 mg,	4.5 mg 0.23 ml	9.1 mg 0.46 ml	13.6 mg 0.69 ml	15.0 mg 0.75 ml	15.0 mg 0.75 ml	25.0 mg 1.2 ml	Shirkey Schwerman

GIVE DIRECTLY IV

Drug								Reference
Naloxone (Narcan) IM, IV 0.4 mg/ml ampules	0.01 mg/kg initially. May repeat at 2- to 3-minute intervals × 2 or 3 doses. Indicated for treatment of diphenoxylate hydrochloride (Lomotil) poisoning. Also propoxyphene hydrochloride (Darvon) overdosage and narcotic analgesic overdoses. Response is diagnostic for narcotic analgesic use.	0.05 mg 0.12 ml	0.09 mg 0.23 ml	0.14 mg 0.35 ml	0.18 mg 0.45 ml	0.22 mg 0.55 ml	0.28 mg 0.7 ml	Shirkey Rumack
Phenobarbital sodium 130 mg/1 ml (Dosette) (Ready for use)	Anticonvulsant dose 3.5 mg/kg/dose IM IF GIVEN IV: DILUTE WITH NORMAL SALINE AND GIVE SLOWLY	15.8 mg (0.12 ml)	31.6 mg (0.24 ml)	47.4 mg (0.36 ml)	63.2 mg (0.48 ml)	79.0 mg (0.6 ml)	94.8 mg (0.72 ml)	Shirkey
Procainamide hydrochloride (Pronestyl) 100 mg/ml 10 ml vials	2 mg/kg/dose IV (maximum, 100 mg) Diluted and given over a period of 5 minutes, IV, and the dose is repeated	9 mg	18.2 mg	27.2 mg	36.4 mg	45.4 mg	54.6 mg	Shirkey Kempe

Continued.

Drug	Dosage	10 pounds (4.5 kg)	20 pounds (9.1 kg)	30 pounds (13.6 kg)	40 pounds (18.2 kg)	50 pounds (22.7 kg)	60 pounds (27.3 kg)	Reference
Procainamide hydrochloride—cont'd	every 10 to 15 minutes until the arrhythmia is controlled. (maximum total dose is 1.0 g) Administration must be continuously monitored by EKG and frequent blood pressures							
Sodium bicarbonate 50 ml syringe containing 1 mEq/ml	2 mEq/kg/dose IV Dose may be repeated in 8 to 10 minutes, but further doses should depend on blood gases	9.0 mEq (9.0 ml)	18.2 mEq (18.2 ml)	27.2 mEq (27.2 ml)	36.4 mEq (36.4 ml)	45.4 mEq (45.4 ml)	50.0 mEq (50.0 ml)	Schwerman Nelson
Diazepam (Valium) 10 mg/2 ml ampules	0.1 to 0.2 mg/kg/dose Because of varied responses to CNS drugs, initiate therapy with lowest dose NOT FOR USE IN CHILDREN UNDER 6 MONTHS OF AGE DO NOT MIX OR DILUTE WITH OTHER FLUIDS OR DRUGS		0.9 mg/ 0.18 ml to 1.8 mg/ 0.36 ml	.36 mg/ 0.27 ml to 2.72 mg/ 0.54 ml	1.82 mg/ 0.36 ml to 3.64 mg/ 0.72 ml	2.27 mg/ 0.45 ml to 4.54 mg/ 0.9 ml	2.73 mg/ 0.55 ml to 5.46 mg/ 1.09 ml	Shirkey

REFERENCES

American Heart Association: Standards for cardiopulmonary resuscitation (CPR) and cardiac care (ECC), JAMA **227:**837-868, Feb. 18, 1974.

Kempe, C. H., et al.: Current pediatric diagnosis and treatment, ed. 3, Los Altos, Calif., 1974, Lange Medical Publications.

Nelson, W. E., et al., editors: Textbook of pediatrics, ed. 9, Philadelphia, 1969, W. B. Saunders Co.

Rumack, B. H., and Temple, A. R.: Lomotil poisoning, Pediatrics **53:**495, 1974.

Schwerman, E., et al.: The pharmacist as a member of the cardiopulmonary resuscitation team, Drug Intell. Clin. Pharm. **7:**298-308, July, 1973.

Shirkey, H. C., editor: Pediatric therapy, ed. 5, St. Louis, 1975, The C. V. Mosby Co.

Drugs excreted in human milk

Agent	Significance
Alcohol	Moderate amounts have little if any effect
Amantadine (Symmetrel)	May cause urinary retention, vomiting, skin rash
Ampicillin (Penbritin, Polycillin, Amcill, Omnipen)	a*
Aspirin	May cause a bleeding tendency by interfering with the function of the infant's platelets or by decreasing the amount of prothrombin in the blood
Atropine sulfate (ingredient in many prescription and nonprescription products)	Inhibits lactation; may cause atropine intoxication in the infant
Barbiturates	a; high doses may cause sedation; may cause induction of drug metabolizing enzymes
Bromides	Reactions include rash and drowsiness
Calciferol (Vitamin D)	May result in hypercalcemia
Carbenicillin (Pyopen, Geopen)	a
Carisoprodol (Soma)	Concentrated in breast milk; may cause CNS depression and gastric upset
Cascara	Increases gastric motility in infant
Chloral hydrate (Noctec, Somnos)	a
Chloramphenicol (Chloromycetin)	Infant has underdeveloped enzyme system, immature liver and renal function; may not have glycuronide system adequately developed to conjugate chloramphenicol; caution advised
Chlorazepate (Tranxene)	May cause drowsiness
Chlordiazepoxide (Librium)	a
Chlorpromazine (Thorazine)	a; may cause galactorrhea
Codeine	a
Contraceptives (oral)	May inhibit lactation if administered during first postnatal weeks; possible gynecomastia in male infants
Cyanocobalamin (Vitamin B_{12})	a

*a = Not significant in therapeutic doses to affect infant.
Adapted from O'Brien, T. E.: Excretion of drugs in human milk, Am. J. Hosp. Pharm. **31**:846-853, Sept., 1974. Copyright © 1974, American Society of Hospital Pharmacists, Inc. All rights reserved.

Agent	Significance
Cyclophosphamide (Cytoxan)	Nursing should be discontinued
Dextrothyroxine	a
Diazepam (Valium)	Infant reported lethargic and experienced weight loss; may cause hyperbilirubinemia
Diphenhydramine (Benadryl)	a
Ergot (Cafergot)	Symptoms range from vomiting and diarrhea to weak pulse and unstable blood pressure
Erythromycin (Ilosone, E-Mycin, Erythrocin)	Greater concentrations in milk than in plasma
Fluoxymesterone (Halotestin, Ultandren)	Used to suppress lactation
Folic acid	a
Guanethidine (Ismelin sulfate)	a
Heroin	Not enough to prevent withdrawal in addicted infants
Hydrochlorothiazide (Hydro-Diuril, Esidrix)	To be avoided based on manufacturer's recommendation
Indomethacin (Indocin)	a
Iodides	May affect infant's thyroid gland
Iopanoic acid (Telepaque)	a
Isoniazid (INH)	Monitor closely for toxicity
Kanamycin (Kantrex)	Monitor closely for toxicity
Lincomycin (Lincocin)	a
Lithium carbonate (Eskalith, Lithane)	Monitor closely for toxicity
Mefenamic acid (Ponstel)	a
Meperidine (Demerol)	a
Meprobamate (Equanil)	Present in milk at 2 to 4 times maternal plasma level; monitor for toxicity
Mesoridazine (Serentil)	a
Mestranol	see Contraceptives
Methenamine	a
Methocarbamol (Robaxin)	a
Metronidazole (Flagyl)	Apparently not significant in therapeutic doses
Morphine	a
Nalidixic acid (NegGram)	a
Nicotine	No effect with less than 20 cigarettes per day
Norethindrone (Norlutin)	see Contraceptives
Norethynodrel (Enovid)	see Contraceptives
Oxyphenbutazone (Tandearil)	a
Penicillin G	May sensitize infant to penicillin
Phenformin (DBI)	a
Phenobarbital (Luminal)	see Barbiturates
Phytonadione (Vitamin K_1, Aquamephyton)	a
Piperacetazine (Quide)	Unknown
Potassium iodide	May affect infant's thyroid
Primidone (Mysoline)	May cause undue drowsiness

Continued.

Agent	*Significance*
Prochlorperazine (Compazine)	a
Propoxyphene (Darvon)	a
Pyrimethamine (Daraprim)	Unknown
Quinine sulfate	a
Reserpine (Serpasil)	May produce galactorrhea
Salicylates	a
Sulfisoxazole (Gantrisin)	May cause kernicterus; to be avoided during first 2 weeks postpartum
Tetracycline hydrochloride	Theoretically may cause discoloration of teeth
Thiamine	Necessary for normal development
Thiazides (Diuril, Hydro-Diuril)	To be avoided based on manufacturer's recommendation
Thiopental (Pentothal)	a
Thioridazine hydrochloride (Mellaril)	a
Thiouracil	Higher concentrations in milk than serum; may cause goiter or agranulocytosis in nursing infant; to be avoided
Thyroid	a
Tolbutamide (Orinase)	a
Tranylcypromine sulfate (Parnate)	a
Trifluoperazine hydrochloride (Stelazine)	a
Trimeprazine tartrate (Temaril)	a
Warfarin (Coumadin)	Infant should be monitored along with mother

Agents that discolor the feces

Agent	Color
Aluminum hydroxide preparations	Whitish discoloration or speckling
Antibiotics, oral	Greenish gray color caused by undigested material
Barium	Clay, putty
Bismuth compounds	Black
Charcoal	Black
Iron	Black
Lead	Bloody or black caused by presence of lead sulfide
Phenylbutazone (Butazolidin, Azolid)	Black caused by intestinal bleeding
Pyrvinium pamoate (Povan)	Red
Rifampin (Rifadin)	Orange-red
Salicylates	Pink to red to black resulting from internal bleeding
Senna	Yellow, yellow-greenish cast
Warfarin (Coumadin)	Pink to red to black caused by internal bleeding

Adapted from Baran, R. B., and Rowles, B.: Factors affecting coloration of urine and feces, J.A.Ph.A. NS **13:**139-142, 155, Mar., 1973.

Agents that discolor the urine

Agent	Color
Amitriptyline hydrochloride (Elavil)	Blue-green
Azuresin (Diagnex Blue)	Blue or green
Cascara	Red in alkaline urine
Chloroquine (Aralen)	Rust yellow or brown
Deferoxamine mesylate (Desferal)	Red
Furazolidone (Furoxone)	Brown, orange-brown
Indigo blue	Green or blue
Indigo carmine	Green or blue
Indomethacin (Indocin)	Green caused by biliverdinemia
Iron IV	Blackening
Levodopa (Dopar, Larodopa)	Darkening of urine on standing
Methocarbamol (Robaxin)	Brown to black to green on standing
Methyldopa (Aldomet)	Red to black caused by standing in a hypo-chloride solution
Methylene blue	Bluish-green, green
Metronidazole (Flagyl)	Darkened urine
Nitrofurantoin (Furadantin, Macrodantin)	Rust yellow or brownish
Phenacetin	Dark brown to black on standing
Phenazopyridine hydrochloride (Pyridium)	Red or orange
Phenolphthalein	Red in alkaline urine
Phenolsulfonphthalein (PSP)	Red in alkaline urine
Phenothiazines	Pink to red or red-brown
Phensuximide (Milontin)	Pink to red to red-brown
Phenytoin (Dilantin)	Pink or red to red-brown
Primaquine phosphate	Darkening of the urine
Quinacrine hydrochloride (Atabrine)	Yellow
Quinine	Brown to black
Resorcinol	Dark green
Riboflavin (Vitamin B_2)	Yellow
Rifampin (Rifadin, Rimactane)	Bright red-orange
Salicylazosulfapyridine (Azulfidine)	Orange-yellow in alkaline urine
Sulfonamides	Rust yellow or brownish
Triamterene (Dyrenium)	Pale blue fluorescence
Warfarin sodium (Coumadin sodium)	Orange

Adapted from Baran, R. B., and Rowles, B.: Factors affecting coloration of urine and feces, J.A.Ph.A. NS **13:**139-142, 155, Mar., 1973.

Contents of general emergency cart

Quantity	Medication	Concentration	Size
2	Aminophylline	25 mg/ml	10 ml
2	Amyl nitrite perles		0.3 ml
5	Atropine sulfate injection*	0.5 mg/ml	1 ml
2	Calcium chloride 10%	100 mg/ml	10 ml
1	Deslanoside (Cedilanid-D)	0.2 mg/ml	4 ml
1	Dextrose 50% injection*	500 mg/ml	50 ml
1	Dexamethasone injection	4 mg/ml	5 ml
2	Digoxin (Lanoxin)	0.25 mg/ml	2 ml
2	Diphenhydramine hydrochloride (Benadryl)	50 mg/ml	1 ml
4	Dopamine hydrochloride (Intropin)	40 mg/ml	5 ml
6	Epinephrine hydrochloride 1:1000*	1 mg/ml	1 ml
4	Epinephrine hydrochloride 1:10,000* (intracardiac needle)	0.1 mg/ml	10 ml
10	Furosemide (Lasix)	10 mg/ml	10 ml
2	Glucagon injection	1 μ/ml	10 ml
4	Isoproterenol 1:5000 (Isuprel)	0.2 mg/ml	5 ml
4	Levarterenol (Levophed)	2 mg/ml	4 ml
1	Lidocaine hydrochloride 2% (anesthetic)		20 ml
1	Lidocaine hydrochloride (drip infusion)	40 mg/ml	50 ml
3	Lidocaine hydrochloride (bolus infusion)*	20 mg/ml	5 ml
4	Metaraminol bitartrate (Aramine bitartrate)	10 mg/ml	10 ml
3	Naloxone (Narcan)	0.4 mg/ml	1 ml
1	Normal saline		20 ml
2	Phentolamine (Regitine)	5 mg/ml	1 ml
4	Physostigmine salicylate (Antilirium)	0.5 mg/ml	2 ml
4	Phenytoin (Dilantin)*	50 mg/ml	5 ml
1	Procainamide hydrochloride (Pronestyl)	100 mg/ml	10 ml
4	Propranolol (Inderal)	1 mg/ml	1 ml
1	Quinidine gluconate	80 mg/ml	10 ml
4	Sodium bicarbonate*	44 meq/50 ml	50 ml
2	Sterile water for injection		30 ml

	IV solutions		
1	Dextrose 5% in 0.2% sodium chloride		1000 ml
4	Dextrose 5% in water		1000 ml
1	Normal saline		500 ml
1	Lactated Ringer's		1000 ml

*Available as a prefilled syringe

Emergency tray contents

Quantity	Medication	Concentration	Size
2	Aminophylline	25 mg/ml	10 ml
4	Atropine sulfate injection*	0.5 mg/ml	1 ml
2	Calcium chloride 10%	100 mg/ml	10 ml
1	Dextrose 50% injection*	500 mg/ml	50 ml
2	Diphenhydramine hydrochloride (Benadryl)*	50 mg/ml	1 ml
4	Dopamine hydrochloride (Intropin)	40 mg/ml	5 ml
4	Epinephrine hydrochloride 1:1000*	1 mg/ml	1 ml
2	Epinephrine hydrochloride 1:10,000* (intracardiac needle)	0.1 mg/ml	10 ml
2	Isoproterenol 1:5000 (Isuprel)	0.2 mg/ml	5 ml
4	Levarterenol (Levophed)	2 mg/ml	4 ml
3	Lidocaine hydrochloride (bolus infusion)*	20 mg/ml	5 ml
2	Metaraminol bitartrate (Aramine bitartrate)	10 mg/ml	10 ml
3	Naloxone (Narcan)	0.4 mg/ml	1 ml
2	Phentolamine (Regitine)	5 mg/ml	1 ml
2	Phenytoin (Dilantin)*	50 mg/ml	5 ml
1	Procainamide hydrochloride (Pronestyl)	100 mg/ml	10 ml
4	Propranolol (Inderal)	1 mg/ml	1 ml
4	Sodium bicarbonate*	44 meq/50 ml	50 ml
1	Sterile water for injection		30 ml

*Available as a prefilled syringe

Nomogram for calculating the body surface area of adults and children

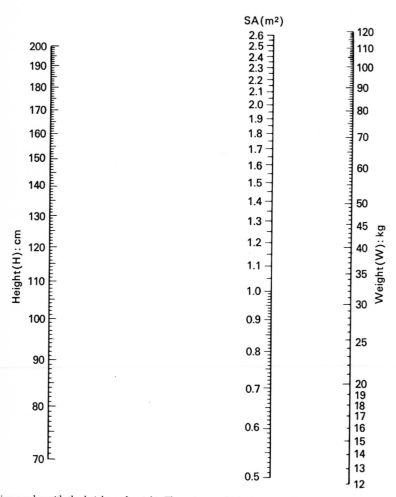

Align a ruler with the height and weight. The point at which the center line is intersected gives the corresponding value for surface area (SA). (From Haycock, G. B.: J. Pediatr. **93**:62-66, July, 1978.)

Continued.

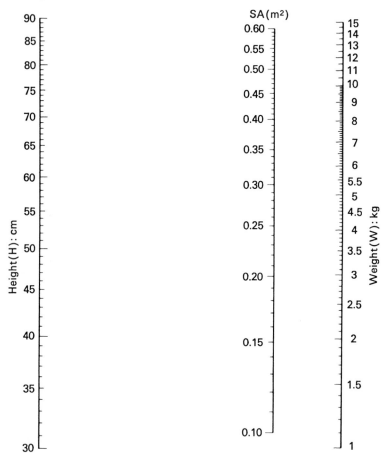

Align a ruler with the height and weight. The point at which the center line is intersected gives the corresponding value for surface area (SA). (From Haycock, G. B.: J. Pediatr. **93:**62-66, July, 1978.)

Bibliography

Aladjem, S., editor: Risks in the practice of modern obstetrics, St. Louis, 1975, The C. V. Mosby Co.

American Academy of Pediatrics: Report of the Committee on Infectious Diseases, ed. 17, Evanston, 1974, American Academy of Pediatrics.

Bergerson, B. S.: Pharmacology in nursing, ed. 14, St. Louis, 1979, The C. V. Mosby Co.

Boedeker, E. C., and Dauber, J. H., editors: Manual of medical therapeutics, ed. 21, Boston, 1974, Little, Brown and Co.

Brunner, L., and Suddarth, D. S.: Lippincott manual of nursing practice, Philadelphia, 1974, J. B. Lippincott Co.

Goodman, L. S., and Gilman, A., editors: The pharmacological basis of therapeutics, ed. 5, New York, 1975, MacMillan Inc.

Goth, A.: Medical pharmacology, ed. 9, St. Louis, 1978, The C. V. Mosby Co.

Govani, L. E., and Hayes, J. E.: Drugs and nursing implications, ed. 3 New York, 1978 Appleton-Century-Crofts.

Greenwald, E. S.: Cancer chemotherapy, ed. 2, Flushing, 1973, Medical Examination Publishing Co., Inc.

Hansten, P. D.: Drug interactions, ed. 3, Philadelphia, 1975, Lea & Febiger.

Hatcher, R. A., et al.: Contraceptive technology, 1978-1979, ed. 9, New York, 1978, Irvington Publishers.

Herfindal, E. T., and Hirschman, J. L., editors: Clinical pharmacy and therapeutics, Baltimore, 1975, The Williams & Wilkins Co.

Johns, M. P.: Pharmacodynamics and patient care, St. Louis, 1974, The C. V. Mosby Co.

Kimble, M. A. and Young, L. Y., editors: Applied therapeutics for clinical pharmacists, Oakland, 1975, Applied Therapeutics, Inc.

Knoben, J. E., et al.: Handbook of clinical drug data, ed. 4, Hamilton, Ill., 1978, Drug Intelligence Publications.

Lichtiger, M., and Moya, F., editors: Introduction to the practice of anesthesia, ed. 2, New York, 1978, Harper & Row, Publishers.

Loebl, S., Spratto, G., and Wit, A.: The nurse's drug handbook, New York, 1977, John Wiley & Sons, Inc.

Lilly Research Laboratories: Diabetes mellitus, ed. 7, Indianapolis, 1973, Lilly Research Laboratories.

Melmon, K. L., and Morrelli, H. F., editors: Clinical pharmacology, basic principles in therapeutics, 2nd ed. New York, 1978, MacMillan Inc.

Metheny, N. M., and Snively, W. D., Jr.: Nurses handbook of fluid balance, ed. 2, Philadelphia, 1974, J. B. Lippincott Co.

Modell, W., editor: Drugs of choice, 1978-1979, St. Louis, 1978, The C. V. Mosby Co.

Physician's desk reference, Oradell, N. J., 1979, Medical Economics Co.

Reilly, M. J., editor: American hospital formulary service, Washington, D.C., 1979, American Society of Hospital Pharmacists, Inc.

Thorn, G. W., et al: Principles of internal medicine, ed. 8, New York, 1977, McGraw-Hill Book Co.

Vickers, M. D., et al.: Drugs in anesthetic practice, ed. 5, Boston, 1978, Butterworth and Co.

Index